ECONOMICS
and
NURSING

**Critical
Professional
Issues**

CYRIL F. CHANG, PhD

Professor of Economics
Department of Economics
The University of Memphis
Memphis, Tennessee

SYLVIA A. PRICE, PhD, RN

Professor (Retired)
College of Nursing
University of Tennessee
Memphis, Tennessee

SUSAN K. PFOUTZ, PhD, RN

Professor
Department of Nursing
Eastern Michigan University
Ypsilanti, Michigan

ECONOMICS
and
NURSING

Critical
Professional
Issues

F A DAVIS COMPANY
PHILADELPHIA

F.A. Davis Company
1915 Arch Street
Philadelphia, PA 19103

Printed in the United States of America

Last digit indicates print number: 10 9 8 7 6 5 4 3 2 1

Acquisitions Editor, Nursing: Joanne P. DaCunha, RN, MSN
Developmental Editor: Suzanne Hall Johnson, RN, MN, CNS
Production Editor: Stephen D. Johnson
Cover Designer: Louis J. Forgione

Library of Congress Cataloging in Publication Data

Chang, Cyril F.
    Economics and nursing : critical professional issues / Cyril F. Chang, Sylvia A. Price,
Susan K. Pfoutz.
        p. ; cm.
    Includes bibliographical references and index.
    ISBN 0-8036-4065-3
    1. Nursing—Economic aspects. 2. Nursing—Supply and demand. 3. Nursing—Effect of managed care on. 4. Managed care plans (Medical care)—Economic aspects. I. Price, Sylvia Anderson. II. Pfoutz, Susan K. III. Title.
    [DNLM 1. Economics, Nursing. 2. Health Services Needs and Demand—economics. 3. Managed Care Programs—economics. 4. Nursing—manpower. WY 77 C456e 2000]
    RT86.7.C47 2000
    338.4'3362173—dc21
                                                                                    00-031474

This book is dedicated to our spouses
Alice, Joe, and Dick
for their understanding, support, and
encouragement
throughout this project

Foreword

Michael Carter

At first glance, one could question the juxtaposition of the concepts of economics and nursing. The commonly held view of nursing is that the field is focused on the care of people. Most of the literature focused on the practice of nursing is concerned with the science base needed for the care of patients. This is understandable, because caring is the central concept of modern nursing. Caring can take many forms, however, and one of those forms is caring about the economics of the services provided.

Today, many clinicians and administrators lack the background in economics to effectively plan and evaluate nursing care and nursing-care delivery. This is curious, in that Florence Nightingale clearly called for nurses to understand this critical component of nursing in her book, Notes on Nursing. She pointed out that nurses have an obligation to attend to the financial matters of their patients and to the financial aspects of the care the patient receives.

The evolution of the modern health-care system in the United States over the past 50 years has meant that nurses have become employees of large, complex organizations. The financing of hospital-based care following the introduction of Medicare and Medicaid in the 1960s led to an even further separation of nursing care from the economics of that care. Hospitals were paid on the basis of their costs plus additional sums for teaching and other purposes. What emerged was that this method of reimbursement by the federal government led to expenditures beyond what the system could afford. Within the hospital, the largest cost was usually nursing. Changes in the payment systems for health care have led to new interests in the economics of care delivery, and nursing is at the nexus of this care delivery.

Today, third-party payers are much less inclined to reimburse on the basis of costs. Rather, these payers have become keen negotiators for the lowest price within an acceptable level of quality. No longer can nurses be passive players within these systems of care delivery; in fact, they must act as leaders in this area. Nursing is the central position for all care delivery within today's complex health-care delivery organizations and nurses must use all available knowledge to advance care.

The health-care system of the United States is quite different from that of any other country in the world. The multiple roles of government at the federal, state, and local levels create strain between government and the private community. Not only does government regulate the provision of care through laws, regulations, and policy, but government is also the largest payer for health-care services. At times, government is also the provider of care, through the Veterans Affairs Health Care System and state health departments. The tensions generated by the conflicting roles of government as regulator, payer, and provider often result in confusion concerning who is in charge, and many decisions are left to the political process. Almost all of the key decisions in health care can best be understood as economic decisions, or at least as having key economic components. Nurses must be well versed in economics if they are to ensure the critical nature of the nursing perspective in the evolution of the health-care system.

Chang, Price, and Pfoutz have cogently and succinctly drawn together the critical economic concepts needed by contemporary nurses. An outstanding group of experts provides key insights into the topics that are covered. Through the various chapters in this book, the reader will gain a strong and highly functional background in economics and in health-care economics in particular. As the authors have pointed out, health care does not always work like other elements of the economy. This means that a broad understanding of economic theory is needed if nurses are to be well prepared. This also means that there are specific theoretical concepts that must be mastered for the nurse to be appropriately educated in the field. Armed with the information provided in this text, nurses will be able to make informed judgments and take actions to ensure the best care for their patients or to operate complex organizations for the care of patients.

This book will provide clinicians, administrators, students, and faculty with the background needed to further develop their expertise in the area of the economics of health care. The broad perspective taken here will arm the reader well to understand and cope with the dynamic changes in the economics of care that characterize the continuing evolution of our health-care industry.

Michael A. Carter, DNSc, RN, FAAN
Professor and Dean
College of Nursing
University of Tennessee
Memphis, Tennessee

Preface

Changes in the way health care is delivered, rapid advances in science and technology, and the influence of consumerism on health care have significantly influenced professional nursing practice. To compete effectively in the job market, nurses must understand the economic and financial realities affecting the health-care delivery system. This knowledge, including a familiarity with changing demands for health-care services, cost-containment measures, and quality-management efforts that promote high-quality client-centered nursing care, enables practicing nurses to collaborate with others in designing and delivering effective health-care services.

Economics focuses on how consumers, business firms, government entities, and other organizations make choices in an environment of scarce resources. An understanding of economic principles is essential to nurses so that they can play a vital role in providing evidence-based services and compete effectively in the health-care marketplace.

As the largest group of direct health-care providers, nurses are critical participants in delivery activities to achieve appropriate resource utilization, cost containment, and high-quality care that the general public can afford. Nurse executives and advanced practice nurses are responsible and accountable for clinical nursing practice, education, and research in a variety of health-care settings. They must have a working knowledge of the theoretical and practical applications of economics. Nurse clinicians also need to apply useful and relevant economic concepts to their decision making regarding patient care for both individuals and groups. In the 21st century it is essential that both nurse executives and practitioners understand the theoretical and practical applications of economics and incorporate these concepts in their practice.

Nurses are examining and analyzing economic factors such as cost, efficiency, and productivity so that the outcome of their work will not only be effective but also cost effective. An effective service or procedure is one that does more good than harm to the individuals to whom it is offered. A cost-effective service or procedure is one that produces the same medical outcome as any other service or procedure but does so at a lower cost.

Economics and Nursing: Critical Professional Issues is a scholarly, comprehensive analysis of economic realities and issues relevant to nursing and health care. It is designed for graduate nursing students, registered nurses in BSN completion programs, and upper-division undergraduate students in nursing. It is also a relevant reference for practicing nurses at all levels in a variety of health-care settings.

It is our intent to offer a nursing economics book that is a valuable resource for nurse executives at all levels and for nurse clinicians, researchers, and educators.

The economic concepts presented in this book are grouped into four major sections:

- **PART I: INTRODUCTION TO ECONOMICS AND NURSING.** This section focuses on the relevance of economics to nursing. The basic economic concepts of supply and demand, and their application to the markets for nursing services, are examined.

- **PART II: THE NURSING LABOR MARKET.** This section presents a conceptual model emphasizing the economics of labor markets, the application of economic principles to nursing, the economic factors influencing nursing education, and the fluctuations in the supply and demand for nurses that affect salary determination.

- **PART III: THE NURSING SERVICE MARKET.** This section analyzes job opportunities for nurses in the health-care market and discusses emerging roles for nurses and professional nursing practice models. The relationship between the changing labor market and the global environment is also examined.

- **PART IV: CRITICAL PROFESSIONAL AND ECONOMIC ISSUES FACING NURSING.** The final section addresses national economic issues confronting nursing. These issues include managed care, access to health care, the relationship between cost and quality, clinical economic analysis, and information technology.

This book is the result of a partnership of two nursing educators and an economics professor. The content of the book progresses from identification of economic concepts to analysis of their impact on health-care delivery. The rise of global markets for health care and the overlap of nursing and medical roles in general practice are also examined. The World Health Organization's goal of health for all by the year 2010 demands a visionary look at caregivers and more involvement on the part of the consumer. The emphasis of the book is on preventive and self-care activities and their financial implications in a variety of health-care settings.

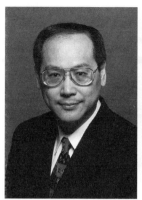

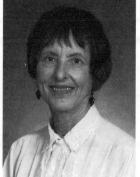

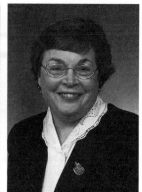

Cyril F. Chang   *Sylvia A. Price*   *Susan K. Pfoutz*

Acknowledgments

Our sincere appreciation to Joanne DaCunha, Nursing Acquisitions Editor, for her support and enthusiasm throughout the project. Special recognition to Suzanne Hall Johnson, Developmental Editor, for her creative contributions, which enhanced both the content and presentation of the book. We also want to acknowledge the following individuals for sharing their clinical experiences that bring economic concepts to life: Marylane Wade Koch, Tom Renkes, Stephanie Myers Schim, Anne Sullivan Smith, and Teresa C. Wehrwein.

Contributors

WILLIAM ROBERT BARTLETT, JR., PHD, RN
Late, Assistant Professor
College of Nursing
Instructor, College of Medicine
Administrator, Memphis Lung Research Program
University of Tennessee
Memphis, Tennessee

KATHY L. BECK, MSN, RN, CPHQ
Chief Nursing Officer
Grenada Lake Medical Center
Grenada, Mississippi

MICHAEL R. BLEICH, PHD, RN, CNAA
Associate Dean for Clinical and Community Affairs
Clinical Associate Professor, Nursing Administration
University of Kansas School of Nursing
Kansas City, Kansas

LORAINE FRANK-LIGHTFOOT, MBA, RN
Director, Nursing and Patient Services
Akron General Medical Center
Akron, Ohio

MARCELLINE HARRIS, PHD, RN
Postdoctoral Fellow, Health Informatics
University of Minnesota/Mayo Foundation
Assistant Professor
Winona State University
Rochester, Minnesota

MARYLANE WADE KOCH, MSN, RN, CNAA, CPHQ
Director of Community Health Outreach
Partnership for Women's & Children's Health
Methodist–LeBonheur–University of Tennessee
Memphis, Tennessee

ROBERT KOCH, DNSc (CANDIDATE), MSN, RN
Assistant Professor
Loewenberg School of Nursing
University of Memphis
Memphis, Tennessee

LILLIAN M. SIMMS, PHD, RN, FAAN
Associate Professor of Nursing Emeritus
University of Michigan
School of Nursing
Ann Arbor, Michigan

REGINA WILLIAMS, PHD, RN, FNS, FAAN
Professor and Department Head
Eastern Michigan University
Department of Nursing
Ypsilanti, Michigan

Consultants

JAN BELCHER, PHD, RN, CS
Assistant Professor
College of Nursing and Health
Wright State University
Dayton, Ohio

ELAINE E. BELETZ, EDD, RN, FAAN
Associate Professor
College of Nursing
Villanova University
Villanova, Pennsylvania

MARY T. BOYLSTON, MSN, RN, CCRN
Assistant Professor
Eastern College
St. David's, Pennsylvania

HARRIET V. COELING, PHD, RN, CS
Associate Professor
College of Nursing
Editor, *Online Journal of Issues in Nursing*
Kent State University
Kent, Ohio

MARY T. DELANEY, PHD, RN
Senior Lecturer
College of Nursing
Wayne State University
Detroit, Michigan

ELAINE A. GRAVELEY, RN, DBA, CNAA
Associate Professor
University of Texas Health Science Center
San Antonio, Texas

MARY ELLEN GROHAR-MURRAY, PHD, RN
Associate Professor of Nursing
School of Nursing
Saint Louis University
St. Louis, Missouri

SUZANNE HALL JOHNSON, MN, RNC, CNS
Director, Hall Johnson Consulting
Editor, *Nurse Author & Editor*
Lakewood, Colorado

MARIAN JOHNSON, PHD, RN
Associate Professor
College of Nursing
University of Iowa
Iowa City, Iowa

SHARON JUDKINS, MS, RN
Faculty
University of Texas at Arlington
Arlington, Texas

VICKI D. LACHMAN, PHD, RN, CS, CNAA
President, V.L. Associates
Philadelphia, Pennsylvania

YOLANDE A. LOCKETT, PHD, RN, CS, PNP
Assistant Professor of Nursing
Rhode Island College
Providence, Rhode Island

MARGARET MCALLISTER, PHD, RN
Coordinator, Nurse Practitioner Programs
University of Massachusetts
Boston, Massachusetts

MARY LYNN MCHUGH, PHD, RNC, ARNP
Associate Professor of Nursing
University of Colorado Health Sciences Center
Denver, Colorado

PATRICIA J. MORIN, PHD, RN
Professor and Chair
Nebraska Wesleyan University
Department of Nursing
Lincoln, Nebraska

JULIE SOCHALSKI, PHD, RN, FAAN
Associate Director
Center for Health Services & Policy Research
Assistant Professor
Health Services Research and Nursing
University of Pennsylvania
Philadelphia, Pennsylvania

JAMES H. SWAN, PHD
Associate Professor
Department of Public Health Sciences
Wichita State University
Wichita, Kansas

LOIS VAN CLEVE, PHD, RN
Professor, Associate Dean
School of Nursing
Loma Linda University
Loma Linda, California

CECILIA VOLDEN, MS, RN
Professor
University of North Dakota
College of Nursing
Grand Forks, North Dakota

MADELINE WAKE, RN, PHD, FAAN
Dean
College of Nursing
Marquette University
Milwaukee, Wisconsin

Contents

xxi

Part I

Introduction to Economics and Nursing

This section introduces the importance of economics to both present and future nurse clinicians as well as nurse leaders. It begins with the concept of *economic perspective*, which emphasizes the necessity of making choices in an environment of scarce resources. Resources can be used at different places for different individuals. Use of health-care resources for one group of people prevents the use of the same resources for others. In a pluralistic society such as that of the United States, where consumers have different wants and preferences, the question of how to allocate scarce resources to best serve the health-care needs of a large number of culturally, racially, and economically diverse people is a daunting challenge facing our health-care system.

Many nurses believe that clinical expertise is their major concern, rather than the financial aspects of care delivery. The first chapter in Part I makes the case that clinical expertise must be applied to the design and delivery of care that results in positive health outcomes at an acceptable price.

The next two chapters present concepts basic to the operation of the health-care system in a predominantly market-driven economy. The concepts of supply and demand describe the activities of providers and consumers that form the basis for price determination of health-care services and products. These concepts, together with the underlying economic principles and specific examples, provide the foundation for an economic understanding of the health-care system.

The final chapter of Part I addresses the complex issues surrounding the question of why health care costs so much. The significance of inflation as a critical health-care issue is discussed, as well as how costs are measured and monitored. The discussion then focuses on the causes of inflation by identifying the key drivers of health-care costs. The recent history of public- and private-sector efforts to contain health-care costs is then reviewed and evaluated. This discussion reinforces the argument that health-care resources are indeed scarce and highlights the consequences of scarcity.

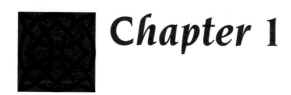

Chapter 1

The Economics of Nursing and Health Care

Sylvia A. Price
Susan K. Pfoutz
Cyril F. Chang

LEARNING OBJECTIVES

- Discuss the value of economics to nursing.
- Define economics and explain how the health economy works.
- Discuss and analyze the scarcity of resources as evidenced by expenditures (hospital, physician, advanced practice nurse, pharmacy, extended-care, and home-care services) and unmet health-care needs of the uninsured and underinsured.
- Give examples of alternative health services and models of care to control costs.
- Describe the impact of values and preferences on the choice of health services.
- Examine the role of consumer information in informed decision making.

 ## WHY SHOULD NURSES LEARN ABOUT ECONOMICS?

Nurses have a long tradition of caring for individuals, families, and groups in a variety of health-care settings. Being able to make a difference in the lives of others is what attracts people to the nursing profession. Regardless of the type of client population or the place of health-care delivery, this caring tradition is central to who nurses are.

An unintended consequence of this caring tradition is that many practicing nurses have not been interested in economic and management issues. Until recently, the cost associated with nursing or health services was not an obvious factor affecting nursing practice. But the health-care milieu has changed. Nurses across a wide range of practice settings are participating in designing nursing services to achieve the best possible care at the lowest cost.

Economics focuses on how consumers, business firms, government entities, and other organizations make choices to overcome the problem of scarcity. The study of economics is essential to nurses so that they can compete effectively in the health-care marketplace. As the largest group of direct health-care providers, nurses are critical participants in delivery activities designed to achieve appropriate resource utilization, cost containment, and high-quality nursing care that the general public can afford. They must be able to conceptualize the economic and financial realities affecting the health-care delivery system. In the 21st century it is essential that both nurse executives and practitioners understand the theoretical and practical applications of economics and incorporate these concepts in their practice arenas.

Nurses are examining and analyzing economic factors such as cost, efficiency, and productivity so that the outcome of their work will be not only effective but also cost effective. An *effective* service or procedure is one that does more good than harm to the individuals to whom it is offered. A *cost-effective* service or procedure, on the other hand, is one that produces the same medical outcome as any other service or procedure but does so at a lower cost.

Cost, efficiency, and productivity are key economic nursing principles today.

In the acute care setting, for example, nurses are witnessing massive changes in how care is delivered. Whatever the reason for hospitalization, patients are being managed in a manner very different from just a few years ago. Before admission, extensive evaluation and diagnostic procedures are performed to shorten the length of stay. Once admitted, the patient's discharge plan is quickly created and put in place to achieve as early a discharge as possible so as to minimize the use of resources and keep the cost of hospitalization within the reimbursable amount. This heightened urgency to "get well and get out" involves in many instances an actual path developed for each patient to reach the discharge point in a given number of days, with specific nursing activities allocated to each day.

Economic knowledge is useful to nurses in other ways. Health-care agencies are all under pressure to provide high-quality, cost-effective, and client-centered care. For example, as recently as the 1980s registered nurses were used for the 24-hour care of patients in a high proportion of hospital settings. Care is now designed to be delivered by an interdisciplinary team using a variety of unlicensed staff who do increasingly more complex patient-care tasks formerly only performed by registered nurses. Nurses are being challenged to prepare their patients and families for posthospitalization care because many patients need continued care to recuperate at home.

Nurses in other settings, such as extended, ambulatory, and home care, see similar trends of doing more with fewer resources. Home-care nurses know that their agencies are being reimbursed less for the care they provide. They also know that reimbursement rules require the use of quality assurance systems to monitor both the amount and the quality of services being reimbursed. Extended-care facilities are struggling to provide care to patients with increasingly more complex conditions with the same or fewer resources. In the public sector, where public health functions are changing and funding for services is limited, there is an ongoing debate about how to deal with the new ambiguities created by the increasingly blurred boundary that used to separate the public and private health-care sectors. Concerns have also been raised about how to avoid duplication of services between the public and private health-care sectors.

In this environment of rapid change, nurses face the challenge of not only doing what is best for their patients but also making the wisest choices for their own career and future. Economic concepts help focus nursing leaders on preparing for the future. As hospitals downsize, units may be closed and nurses laid off. Sometimes, nurses are encouraged to take other positions in the same health-care system or institution. Other times, they are encouraged to go back to school to learn new skills or retool in order to find new jobs in new work settings. It is difficult to predict how to achieve a more stable future. Nurses wonder what positions will remain in demand, what strategies will maximize income, and whether additional education will make them more marketable. Although totally committed to their patients and their practice, nurses are also concerned about their own employment potential and financial security. An understanding of the basic principles of economics and how the health-care economy works can help nurses make better patient-care and career decisions. Figure 1–1 depicts multiple ways in which economic concepts are valuable to nurses.

 ## THE HEALTH ECONOMY

Economics is the science that studies how consumers, business firms, government entities, and other organizations make choices to overcome the problem of scarcity. Scarcity exists because there are not enough resources to satisfy all existing human wants and desires. In the market for ordinary goods and services, consumers purchase the products they desire directly from business firms. However, buyers often do not have sufficient financial resources to buy everything that they want. Similarly, in the health economy most patients and their families do not have the necessary means to obtain all the health services they desire and need. Moreover, the purchasing arrangement in the health economy is more complicated because in addition to the participation of buyers (patients) and sellers (providers), a third party in the form of an insurance company or a government agency is usually involved.

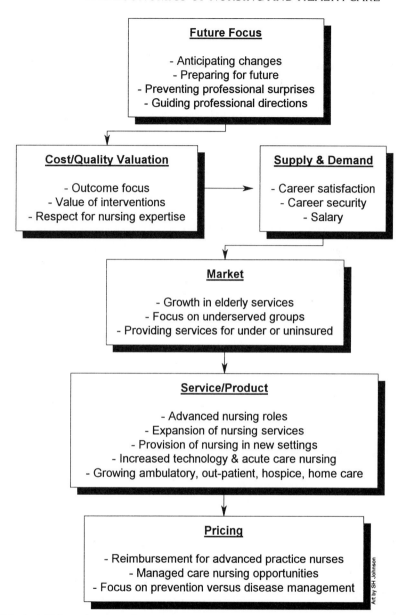

FIG. 1–1. Value of economic concepts to nursing.

Economics *is the science that studies how consumers, business firms, government entities, and other organizations make choices to overcome the problem of scarcity.*

Scarcity *is not having enough resources to satisfy all existing human wants or desires.*

The purchasing arrangement in the health economy is different in another way. Most consumers of health-care services select providers from a list approved by the health plan offered through their employers and do not pay providers directly when service is rendered. A third party pays or reimburses the providers on behalf of the consumers and their employers. In the health economy, the consumers' needs for health services and the breadth and depth of their insurance coverage are the major forces that drive the market for health care.

Health-care providers, like the sellers in a regular market, must deliver the services and products that consumers need at a cost that they and their insurance companies are willing and able to pay. Nurses are a major group of providers who exchange their nursing practice, allegiance, and support of organizational goals for salary, benefits, and other rewards. Nurses must provide these services within the financial constraints of the health-care system that employs them or reimburses for their services.

Health-care providers *include nurses; physicians; occupational, physical, and respiratory therapists; pharmacists; and dentists.*

The health-care system, which comprises individual providers and health-care institutions and facilities such as hospitals, nursing homes, and health maintenance organizations (HMOs), offers a variety of services at a price designed to attract public and private clients. Governments at the local, federal, and state levels also participate in the financing and delivery of health services as insurers who contract for health-care services within the constraints of their annual budgets. Governments also provide services directly: The federal government delivers health services through the Department of Veterans Affairs and military health-care systems, and state and local governments perform a wide range of public health functions.

The health-care system includes institutions and facilities such as hospitals, home-care agencies, extended-care facilities, and health maintenance organizations.

The study of health-care economics analyzes the consequences of limited or scarce resources and the health-care choices that patients, nurses, and other health-care providers make. With an understanding of the economic context of the health-care delivery system, nurses can contribute more effectively to the design and delivery of health services within their organizations. At a larger level, nurses, individually and as a profession, can also actively and fully participate in public debates on health-care issues and in effecting health policy changes.

Although health-care economics is concerned with the distribution of scarce resources in the present, it also projects future trends in the health-care market. Projections of the demographic characteristics of the population, technological advances, and factors affecting costs of services assist health-care providers in planning to meet societal health-care needs. Accurate predictions of health-care needs and economic trends decrease the probability of unexpected demand for services or resources. Nurses who understand economic principles can be active participants in shaping health-care policy and designing futuristic nursing care delivery models.

 ## THE ECONOMIC PERSPECTIVE

An economic framework may seem to be a foreign way to examine health care. How well do these observations explain choices and behavior within health care? A good starting point for an economic examination of the health-care market and its participants is to develop a basic understanding of the economic perspective of health care. Another fundamental concept is that of scarcity in the context of the American health-care system, which is still struggling to satisfy the unmet needs of more than 40 million uninsured individuals. At first glance, it is puzzling that scarcity and inadequate access to health care by a sizable segment of the population can exist in a country with the strongest economy in the world. A review of national health-care expenditure patterns and their historical trends provides a good explanation. But first, what is the economic perspective of health care?

The economic way of looking at the financing and delivery of health services is called the *economic perspective* of health care. According to Victor Fuchs (1998), a noted health economist and a former president of the American Economic Association, the economic perspective is rooted in three fundamental observations about the world:

1. Resources are scarce in relation to the level of consumption that we wish to maintain. For example, individuals must select from a variety of health-care services, many of which are not reimbursed by third-party payers, to serve their needs. Should they invest in preventive services or use the money now for something else or simply save the money away and wait to pay for illness care later? Of all the choices available, which is best suited to a particular individual's constraints of income and other resources?
2. Resources have alternative uses. A choice to expend resources in one area eliminates the use of those same resources for another use. If we wish to build more nursing homes, for example, we must be willing to accept fewer hospitals or less housing, education, or other uses of those same resources.
3. Individuals also want different things or have different preferences. Some people choose alternative treatment modalities such as acupuncture, herbal therapy, or massage therapy rather than traditional health care.

Health care is a multifaceted issue that can be examined from a number of other perspectives, such as those of the sociologist, historian, ethicist, and politician. The value of the economic perspective is not that it is more accurate than the noneconomic perspectives of health care, but that it is able to explain the existence and consequences of scarcity. An economic perspective explains how resources that have alternative uses can be employed by individuals and organizations (who have or represent different values and preferences) to deal with and overcome the problem of scarcity.

SCARCE HEALTH-CARE RESOURCES

Paul Feldstein (1993), a noted health-care economist, described three choices resulting from scarcity of health-care resources—the first component of the economic perspective. These choices are as follows:

1. The amount to be spent on health-care services and the composition of those services
2. The methods for producing those services
3. The method of distribution of health care, which influences the equity of these services to various people within the population

The amount of spending on various health-care services and the composition of these services are annually reported by the Health Care Financing Administration (HCFA) of the U.S. Department of Health and Human Services. A review of the national health-care expenditures and their historical trends provides an overview of the American health-care system and a basic understanding of how health care is financed, produced, and distributed in the United States. It also provides the necessary background for a discussion of the inequity in the distribution of health care and the paradoxical existence of scarcity of health-care resources in the midst of plenty.

NATIONAL HEALTH-CARE EXPENDITURES

How does the United States spend health-care dollars, and what are the trends in those expenditures? Table 1–1 presents detailed data on aggregate national health-care spending and its major components. In 1997, total health-care expenditures in the United States were $1.1 trillion, or $4000 per person (Health Care Financing Administration [HCFA], 1998). This level of total spending represents 13.5 percent of the gross domestic product (GDP).

> **Gross domestic product *is the total market value of all the goods and services produced in a country in a year.***

Where do the funds come from to support such an enormous amount of total spending on health care? In the United States, health-care funding comes from a combination of public and private sources. Part 2 of Table 1–1 shows that in 1997 approximately 53.6 percent of the total national health-care expenditures represents private funding, and the remaining 46.4 percent represents public funding (HCFA, 1998). The private share of health-care funding was much higher in the 1960s and 1970s (HCFA, 1998). The rapid expansion of government programs over the years has reduced the private share from 75.2 percent in 1960 to 53.6 percent in 1997 (HCFA, 1998).

Part 2 of Table 1–1 demonstrates that the rate of increase in spending has declined since the early 1990s as public and private insurers, including Medicare and Medicaid, pursued ways to contain costs, particularly in the public sector. This contrasts with the period from 1970 until 1990, when the increase in health-care spending remained in excess of 10 percent per year (Levit et al., 1996).

Hospital Expenditures

Hospital expenditures are the single largest component of total personal health-care expenditures (PHCEs). In 1997, for example, hospital

TABLE 1–1. NATIONAL HEALTH EXPENDITURES, SELECTED YEARS 1960–1997

	1960	1970	1980	1990	1992	1994	1996	1997
				Part 1: Aggregate and Per Capita Amounts				
					Amount in Billions ($)			
National health expenditures	26.9	73.2	247.3	699.4	836.5	947.7	1,042.5	1,092.4
Private	20.2	45.5	142.5	416.2	483.6	524.9	561.1	585.3
Public	6.6	27.7	104.8	283.2	353.0	422.8	481.4	507.1
Gross domestic product	527	1,036	2,784	5,744	6,244	6,947	7,662	8,111
					Per Capita Amount ($)			
National health expenditures	141	341	1,052	2,690	3,151	3,500	3,781	3,925
Private	106	212	606	1,601	1,821	1,938	2,035	2,103
Public	35	129	446	1,089	1,330	1,561	1,746	1,822

12

Part 2: Percent Distribution and Average Annual Percent Growth

	1960	1970	1980	1990	1992	1994	1996	1997
				Percent Distribution				
National health expenditures	100.0	100.0	100.0	100.0	100.0	100.0	100.0	100.0
Private	75.2	62.2	57.6	59.5	57.8	55.4	53.8	53.6
Public	24.8	37.8	42.4	40.5	42.2	44.6	46.2	46.4
Federal	10.9	24.3	29.1	27.9	30.1	31.8	33.4	33.6
State and local	13.9	13.5	13.3	12.6	12.1	12.8	12.8	12.8
				Percent of Gross Domestic Product				
National health expenditures	5.1	7.1	8.9	12.2	13.4	13.6	13.6	13.5
				Average Annual Percent Growth from Previous Year Shown				
National health expenditures	—	10.6	12.9	10.3	9.1	5.5	4.9	4.8
Private	—	8.5	12.1	10.3	7.7	2.3	4.2	4.3
Public	—	15.3	14.2	10.2	11.0	9.7	5.7	5.3
Gross domestic product	—	7.0	10.4	6.6	5.5	5.9	5.4	5.9

Source: Health Care Financing Administration. (1999). National health expenditures [On-line]. Available: http://www.hcfa.gov/stats/nhe-oact/nhe.htm.

Note: Numbers and percents may not add to totals because of rounding.

13

expenditures were $371.1 billion, or 39.8 percent of PHCEs (see Table 1–2) (HCFA, 1998).

This total amount of hospital expenditures represented a modest 2.9 percent increase from 1996 (see Table 1–3). A slower rate of increase in hospital expenditures reflects a changing use of resources in hospitals. In 1995, federal and non–community hospital inpatient admissions per thousand of the population rose only 0.4 percent for the first time in 10 years. Meanwhile, inpatient days in community hospitals declined by 3 percent (HCFA, 1998; Levit et al., 1996). As a result, overall hospital occupancy fell to less than 60 percent (HCFA, 1998).

Personal health-care expenditures *include all purchased services and products that are associated with individual health care, such as hospital, physician, and dental services; nursing-home care; drugs; and medical supplies. They exclude health-care expenditures for construction, program administration, government health activities, and research.*

Responding to the steady decline in inpatient admissions, hospitals have expanded other services to capture alternative revenue sources such as those offered by an integrated delivery system (IDS) (Duke, 1996). An IDS is a large health-care system that combines hospitals, ambulatory care centers, rural emergency rooms, and home-care agencies under an integrated organization. Duke emphasized that mergers and other contractual agreements between local and national health-care organizations are designed to integrate services, manage competition, and increase cooperation within a managed care environment (Duke, 1996).

Physician Expenditures

Costs for physician services in 1997 were $217.6 billion, which represented 22.5 percent of PHCEs (HCFA, 1998). From 1993 to 1995, the growth of physician expenses was less than the overall growth of health-care spending. In a managed care environment, one way to limit costs is to promote less costly ambulatory or preventive services whenever possible rather than more costly interventions such as hospitalization.

The proportion of Medicare costs devoted to physician services has remained approximately the same. Although the number of Medicare recipients has increased, costs have been contained by the introduction of Medicare Fee Schedules and Volume Performance Standards. Controlling

TABLE 1–2. NATIONAL HEALTH EXPENDITURES: AGGREGATE AMOUNTS BY TYPE OF EXPENDITURE, SELECTED CALENDAR YEARS 1960–1997

Type of Expenditure	1960	1970	1980	1985	1990	1991	1992	1993	1994	1995	1996	1997
					Amount in Billions ($)							
Type of Expenditure												
National health expenditures	26.9	73.2	247.3	428.7	699.4	766.8	836.5	898.5	947.7	993.7	1,042.5	1,092.4
Health services and supplies	25.2	67.9	235.6	412.3	674.8	741.9	809.0	869.5	917.2	963.1	1,010.6	1,057.5
Personal health care	23.6	63.8	217.0	376.4	614.7	679.6	740.7	790.5	834.0	879.3	924.0	969.0
Hospital care	9.3	28.0	102.7	168.3	256.4	282.3	305.3	323.0	335.7	347.2	360.8	371.1
Physician services	5.3	13.6	45.2	83.6	146.3	162.2	175.9	185.9	193.0	201.9	208.5	217.6
Dental services	2.0	4.7	13.3	21.7	31.6	33.3	37.0	39.5	42.4	45.0	47.5	50.6
Other professional services	0.6	1.4	6.4	16.6	34.7	38.3	42.1	46.1	49.6	53.6	57.5	61.9
Home health care	0.1	0.2	2.4	5.6	13.1	16.1	19.6	23.0	26.2	29.1	31.2	32.3
Drugs and other medical nondurables	4.2	8.8	21.6	37.1	59.9	65.6	71.2	76.2	81.6	88.9	98.3	108.9
Prescription drugs	2.7	5.5	12.0	21.2	37.7	42.1	46.6	50.6	55.2	61.1	69.1	78.9

15

TABLE 1–2. (CONTINUED)

	1960	1970	1980	1985	1990	1991	1992	1993	1994	1995	1996	1997
	Amount in Billions ($)											
Vision products and other medical durables	0.6	1.6	3.8	6.7	10.5	11.2	11.9	12.3	12.5	13.1	13.4	13.9
Nursing-home care	0.8	4.2	17.6	30.7	50.9	57.2	62.3	66.4	71.1	75.5	79.4	82.8
Other personal health care	0.7	1.3	4.0	6.1	11.2	13.6	15.4	18.0	21.9	25.1	27.4	29.9
Program administration and net cost of private health insurance	1.2	2.7	11.9	24.3	40.5	40.9	44.9	53.7	55.1	53.3	52.5	50.0
Government public health activities	0.4	1.3	6.7	11.6	19.6	21.4	23.4	25.3	28.2	30.4	34.0	38.5
Research and construction	1.7	5.3	11.6	16.4	24.5	24.9	27.5	29.0	30.5	30.6	32.0	34.9
Research*	0.7	2.0	5.5	7.8	12.2	12.9	14.2	14.5	15.9	16.7	17.2	18.0
Construction	1.0	3.4	6.2	8.5	12.3	12.0	13.4	14.5	14.6	13.9	14.8	16.9

Source: Health Care Financing Administration. (1999) National health expenditures [On-line]. Available: http://www.hcfa.gov/stats/nhe-oact/ nhe.htm.

Note: Numbers may not add to totals because of rounding.

*Research and development expenditures of drug companies and other manufacturers and providers of medical equipment and supplies are excluded from research expenditures, but are included in the expenditure class in which the product falls.

TABLE 1–3. NATIONAL HEALTH EXPENDITURES: AVERAGE ANNUAL PERCENT CHANGE BY TYPE OF EXPENDIGURE, SELECTED CALENDAR YEARS 1960–1997

Type of Expenditure	1960	1970	1980	1985	1990	1991	1992	1993	1994	1995	1996	1997
						Percent						
National health expenditures	—	10.6	12.9	11.6	10.3	9.6	9.1	7.4	5.5	4.9	4.9	4.8
Health services and supplies	—	10.4	13.3	11.8	10.4	9.9	9.1	7.5	5.5	5.0	4.9	4.6
Personal health care	—	10.5	13.0	11.6	10.3	10.6	9.0	6.7	5.5	5.4	5.1	4.9
Hospital care	—	11.7	13.9	10.4	8.8	10.1	8.2	5.8	3.9	3.4	3.9	2.9
Physician services	—	9.9	12.8	13.1	11.8	10.8	8.5	5.7	3.8	4.6	3.3	4.4
Dental services	—	9.1	11.1	10.2	7.8	5.6	11.0	6.8	7.3	6.1	5.6	6.5
Other professional services	—	8.8	16.3	21.2	15.8	10.4	10.0	9.6	7.5	8.1	7.2	7.7
Home health care	—	14.5	26.9	18.9	18.4	22.4	22.3	17.0	14.1	11.0	7.1	3.7
Drugs and other medical nondurables	—	7.6	9.4	11.4	10.1	9.4	8.6	7.1	7.0	9.0	10.6	10.7
Prescription drugs	—	7.4	8.1	11.9	12.2	11.9	10.6	8.7	9.0	10.6	13.2	14.1

TABLE 1–3. (CONTINUED)

Type of Expenditure	1960	1970	1980	1985	1990	1991	1992	1993	1994	1995	1996	1997
						Percent						
Vision products and other medical durables	—	9.6	8.8	12.4	9.2	7.0	6.3	3.4	1.5	4.9	2.3	3.6
Nursing-home care	—	17.4	15.4	11.7	10.7	12.2	9.0	6.7	7.0	6.2	5.2	4.3
Other personal health care	—	6.5	12.0	8.8	12.9	20.7	13.3	17.0	21.8	14.5	9.5	9.0
Program administration and net cost of private health insurance	—	8.9	15.9	15.4	10.8	0.8	9.9	19.5	2.7	−3.2	−1.5	−4.8
Government public health activities	—	13.9	17.5	11.5	11.0	9.2	9.3	8.1	11.3	8.0	11.9	13.1
Research and construction	—	12.2	8.1	7.1	8.4	1.7	10.5	5.3	5.1	0.5	4.3	9.2
Research*	—	10.9	10.8	7.5	9.3	5.8	9.8	2.2	9.6	5.2	2.6	4.7
Construction	—	12.9	6.2	6.7	7.6	−2.4	11.2	8.7	0.5	−4.6	6.3	14.3

Source: Health Care Financing Administration. (1999) National health expenditures [On-line]. Available: http://www.hcfa.gov/stats/nhe-oact/nhe.htm.

Note: Numbers may not add to totals because of rounding.

*Research and development expenditures of drug companies and other manufacturers and providers of medical equipment and supplies are excluded from research expenditures, but are included in the expenditure class in which the product falls.

the cost per procedure has limited the growth in spending for physician services (HCFA, 1996).

Because the way in which physicians are reimbursed has changed, income has declined for specialists and those providers who are procedure dependent (Moser, 1996; Simon & Born, 1996).

Controlling the cost per procedure has reduced spending for physician services.

Pharmacy Expenditures

Another major component of PHCEs is the cost of prescription drugs. In 1997, total spending on prescription drugs was $78.9 billion (HCFA, 1998). Although spending on prescription drugs experienced limited growth in 1993 and 1994, it increased over 10 percent in 1995 (Levit et al., 1996). A large proportion of this increase represents an increase in the number of prescriptions. The proportion of prescription costs paid by third-party payers increased while the cost to consumers decreased.

Another factor in the rising use of prescription drugs is the number of sites where they are available, such as pharmacies, grocery stores, retail stores, and mail order firms. This variety of ways to access prescription drugs increases drug availability and competition for consumers. Advertising by pharmaceutical companies on television and in magazines has also increased, from $256 million in 1994 to $357 million in 1995, which encourages consumers to seek specific name brands (Levit et al, 1996). An opposing trend is the use of a limited drug formulary by managed care organizations. These lists of accepted drugs are usually composed of the generic or less costly brands for the major drug classifications.

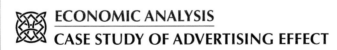

ECONOMIC ANALYSIS
CASE STUDY OF ADVERTISING EFFECT

A woman in her mid-30s suffers from severe spring and summer allergies that she is able to control with antihistamines. When she visits her primary care nurse practitioner for treatment, she requests a prescription for Allegra (fexofenadine hydrochloride). She tells her practitioner that she has read about this medication in *Newsweek* magazine. These ads promise better allergy control with fewer side effects. Allegra costs approximately $63 for a month's supply, compared with $15 for the over-the-counter generic drug. The woman threatens to go to another health-care provider if her request for the medication is not granted.

This case illustrates how pharmaceutical companies can potentially drive increased expenditures for prescription drugs by direct marketing to consumers.

Extended-Care and Home-Care Expenditures

In 1997, $82.5 billion was spent for nursing-home care and $32.3 billion for home care (HCFA, 1998). Medicare and Medicaid financed 57.4 percent of these long term care services, with 42.6 percent paid by the consumer or the consumer's family (HCFA, 1998). Medicare's share of this care has doubled since 1990. The average cost per day of nursing-home care is $127, which reflects an annual cost of $46,000 (HCFA, 1998).

Even with the growth in the percentage of population aged more than 65 years, trends show a declining occupancy in nursing homes, resulting in excess bed capacity, as consumers explore alternative placements such as assisted living and home health care.

Public insurance payers pay the majority (55.3 percent) of home-health-care costs. Consumers pay approximately one-half of the remaining expenses. Home-health-care expenditures have risen dramatically because of expanded coverage, the practice of discharging patients earlier (or "sicker and quicker") from hospitals, the provision of high-technology care in the home, fraud and abuse in billing practices, and the proliferation of home health agencies. However, for the majority of patients home care has been less expensive than hospital care. An estimated three-fifths of hospitals now operate home-care agencies (Meyer, 1997).

Over the past seven years, the percentage of Medicare beneficiaries using home care rose from 5.6 to 10.1 percent, while the average number of visits per patient increased from 33 to 76 and spending dramatically increased (HCFA, 1996; Meyer, 1997). Costs for posthospital services such as skilled nursing and rehabilitation, along with total post–acute care outlays, increased from $8.3 billion to more than $30 billion—about one-sixth of all Medicare expenses (HCFA, 1996; Meyer, 1997).

SCARCITY IN HEALTH CARE: UNMET NEEDS

Can scarcity exist in a country that spends enormous sums of money on health care each year? Yes it can, when human needs exceed what is available to satisfy those needs. Individuals experience unmet health-care needs when they lack health insurance, or their coverage is not sufficient for their needs, or when they lack other financial resources.

The Uninsured

The Bureau of the Census (1998) estimated that 43.4 million individuals, or 16.1 percent of the U.S. population, had no health insurance coverage during the entire year of 1997. Employer insurance represents the major source of health insurance coverage (70.1 percent of the total population). Governmental insurance accounts for 24.8 percent, which includes Medicare (13.2 percent), Medicaid (10.8 percent), and military health care (3.2 percent) (Bureau of the Census, 1998). The percentages of the population groups and subgroups do not add up to the totals because some individuals carry insurance coverage from more than one plan.

Employer insurance *is health insurance coverage provided as an employee benefit.*

The Centers for Disease Control and Prevention published a study in 1997 of access to health care for adults aged 18 to 64 years (Department of Health and Human Services [DHHS], 1997). The data used in this research were from the 1993 Access to Care and Health Insurance surveys of the National Health Interview Survey (NHIS). The sample consisted of 61,287 survey respondents. The results of this study demonstrated that 75 percent of working aged adults had a regular source of medical care, but this percentage declined to 60 percent for those without health insurance. The most frequent reasons given for having no regular source of care were not needing a doctor (49 percent) and lack of insurance or an inability to afford health care (22 percent). More uninsured people (40 percent) reported unmet health-care needs than insured persons (16 percent) (DHHS, 1997).

Several factors influence insurance coverage. Despite the existence of governmental insurance, low-income people are less likely to have insurance. Low-income individuals and their family members include the working poor, those with jobs that do not provide health insurance, those without family coverage, or those who do not meet income criteria for public insurance. Thirty-one percent of the poor have no health insurance, which is double the rate for the nonpoor. Age also influences insurance coverage. Young adults aged 18 to 24 were more likely to lack coverage (28.4 percent), whereas elderly people were least likely to be uninsured (1.1 percent). Poor adults aged 18 to 64 had less insurance coverage than children or the elderly. Race is another factor affecting health coverage. Hispanic persons had the highest proportion of uninsured. Lack of insurance decreases as education increases. Although employers provide insurance coverage for most people, 22.4 percent of part-time employees and 16.4 percent of full-time workers were uninsured. Those of foreign birth were also more likely to be uninsured (33.6 percent) (DHHS, 1997).

Children younger than 19 years are a vulnerable group. Family income level influences their access to health insurance. According to the Census Bureau, the 3-year average from 1994 to 1996 shows that the highest proportion of children below 200 percent of the poverty level live in Washington, D.C. (57.4 percent) and Louisiana (55.6 percent). The state with the lowest percentage of children below 200 percent of the poverty level is New Hampshire (27.8 percent). The state with the highest uninsured population of children under 200 percent of the poverty level is Texas (18.4 percent), and the lowest is Vermont (4.1 percent) (Bureau of the Census, 1999). The number of children without insurance that provides access to primary health care has resulted in policy initiatives that would increase insurance coverage for children.

ECONOMIC ANALYSIS
FAMILY INSURANCE COVERAGE

John and Judy Thomas live in Michigan, and both are self-employed in their home repair and remodeling business. Because they are young and healthy they elected not to purchase health insurance. Judy becomes pregnant. Although the family income does not qualify for traditional Medicaid, their income is within 150 percent of poverty level. Judy, therefore, is eligible for special prenatal Medicaid coverage. The family will then be eligible for children's health insurance at the cost of $5 per month if they are within 200 percent of the poverty level. This situation demonstrates a public policy decision to increase health-care access by providing prenatal and well-child care to families whose parents are working but have no health insurance benefits.

The Underinsured

Another situation that results in unmet needs is insurance that does not provide coverage for prescriptions and services such as home care and long-term care. Limitations in insurance result in consumers making choices among services, delaying obtaining health care, and being unable to implement the prescribed treatment regimen.

Gale and Steffl (1992) describe the coverage for a variety of health-care services in the Medicare program. Tables 1–4 and 1–5 illustrate covered services, uncovered services, deductibles, and copayments for Parts A and B of Medicare. A large gap exists in prescription drug coverage. Medicare covers hospital services completely, but does not cover outpatient prescriptions (with rare exceptions). Many preventive services, such as mammograms, are

TABLE 1–4. MEDICARE BENEFITS 1997: MEDICARE PART A

Benefit	Amount of Service	Medicare Pays	Beneficiary Pays
Hospitalization	First 60 days	All but $760	$760 deductible
Hospitalization	61st to 90th day	All but $190 per day	$190 per day
Hospitalization	91st to 150th day	All but $380 per day	$380 per day
Hospitalization	Beyond 150 days	Nothing	All costs
Skilled nursing facility	First 20 days	100% approved amount;	Nothing
Skilled nursing facility	Additional 80 days	All but $95 per day	$95 per day
Skilled nursing facility	Beyond 100 days	Nothing	All costs
Home health care	Unlimited as long as you meet Medicare requirements	100% approved amount; 80% approved durable medical equipment	Nothing for home health care services; 20% for durable medical equipment
Hospice care	For as long as doctor certifies need	All but limited costs for outpatient drugs and inpatient respite	Limited cost sharing for drugs and inpatient respite
Blood	Unlimited during a benefit period if medically needed	All but first three pints per calendar year	First three pints*

Source: Information adapted from Health Care Financing Administration (1997). Your Medicare handbook 1997: Part A coverage [On-line]. Available: http://www.hcfa.gov/pubforms/mhbkc02.htm.

Note: Most recipients do not have to pay a premium for Part A unless they have less than 40 quarters of Medicare-covered employment.

*To the extent the three pints of blood are paid for or replaced under one part of Medicare, they do not have to be paid for under the other part.

23

TABLE 1–5. MEDICARE BENEFITS 1997: MEDICARE PART B

Benefit	Amount of Service	Medicare Pays	Beneficiary Pays
Medical expenses	Unlimited if medically necessary, except for independent physical and occupational therapists	80% of approved amount after $100 deductible; 50% of approved amount for most outpatient mental health; up to $720 per year each for OTs and PTs	$100 deductible;* 20% of approved amount after deductible; charges above approved amount;† 50% of most mental health; 20% of first $900 for independent OTs and PTs and all after
Clinical laboratory services	Unlimited if medically necessary	Generally 100% of approved amount	Nothing for services
Home health care	Unlimited as long as you meet Medicare requirements	100% of approved amount for services; 80% approved amount for durable medical equipment	Nothing for services, but 20% for durable medical equipment
Outpatient hospital services	Unlimited if medically necessary	Medicare payment to hospital based on hospital costs	20% of whatever the hospital charges after $100 deductible
Blood	Unlimited if medically necessary	80% of approved amount (after $100 deductible and starting with fourth pint)	First three pints plus 20% of approved amount for more pints (after $100 deductible)‡

Source: Information adapted from Health Care Financing Administration (1997). Your Medicare handbook 1997: Part B coverage [On-line]. Available: http://www.hcfa.gov/pubforms/mhbkc02.htm.

Note: 1997 Part B monthly premium is $43.80.

*Part B deductible is paid once per year.

†Federal law limits charges for physican services

‡To the extent the three pints of blood are paid for or replaced under one part of Medicare, they do not have to be paid for under the other part.

OT = occupational therapist; PT = physical therapist.

covered with such limited dollar amounts that high copayments result. Long-term care services, including basic home-health-care or nursing-home services, are also not covered. Although all senior citizens are covered under Medicare, there are many unmet needs. These needs will grow with the aging population.

All people with health insurance have some needs that are not met by insurance. Each policy specifies which services are or are not covered, what amounts will be paid for service, and what copayments and deductibles are required. The uncovered services and out-of-pocket costs result in barriers to service.

ECONOMIC ANALYSIS
UNMET NEEDS

Charles and Julia Douglas are covered by Medicare but do not have any supplemental insurance. Charles has coronary artery disease and arthritis. Julia has Parkinson's disease and congestive heart failure. Their combined medication bill is $400 per month, which is not covered by Medicare. Julia's health-care provider recommends an annual mammogram. Medicare pays only $50 of the $175 cost, so she does not schedule an appointment. This situation demonstrates that having health insurance is not sufficient to meet all health-care needs.

The preceding discussion of unmet health-care needs demonstrates that scarcity exists in the midst of large expenditures on health care. Individuals and families pay for their health care largely through third-party private or public insurers. Each policy or contract defines who is covered, what services are included in the coverage, and what type of payment is available. The options available for payment of health services determine to a large degree one's access to health services.

A NURSING ANSWER TO SCARCITY: ADVANCED PRACTICE NURSING

Advanced practice nurses (APNs) have a significant role in the provision of cost-effective, high-quality client care. Advanced practice nursing comprises the following categories:

- Nurse practitioner (NP)
- Clinical nurse specialist (CNS)
- Certified registered nurse anesthetist (CRNA)
- Certified nurse midwife (CNM)

In 1996, according to the Division of Nursing's most recent survey of registered nurses (Keepnews, 1998), an estimated 71,000 registered nurses were formally prepared as nurse practitioners, 53,799 were prepared as CNSs in advanced clinical practice, and 2,802 were prepared both as NPs and CNSs. There were 6,534 nurse midwives and 30,386 nurse anesthetists. APNs practice in a variety of health-care settings, from primary care clinics and surgical ambulatory care to critical care units in tertiary care referral centers.

Advanced practice nursing can provide increased access to preventive services at an affordable price. APN care is particularly important to populations not previously covered by private insurance (Stanhope, 1995). Several states have requested Medicaid waivers from the Health Care Financing Administration to expand services to geographic areas with limited numbers of health-care providers. Carter (1997) cites TennCare, Tennessee's Medicaid waiver program, as an example of a program that demonstrates that individuals who work without insurance and who cannot purchase insurance because of preexisting conditions can be included in preventive services while still decreasing the overall costs of care. State regulation mandates that nurse practitioners and nurse midwives may participate as primary care case managers. The case manager role is the gatekeeper to the rest of the system.

Advanced practice nursing can increase preventive care.

Brown and Grimes (1995) compared nurse practitioner and certified nurse midwife practice with physician practice by reviewing 210 studies containing data on NP or CNM care. They looked for studies that included the following characteristics:

- An intervention provided by a team composed of an NP or CNM and a physician
- Data derived from patient care provided in the United States and Canada
- Control group patient data derived from physician-managed care
- A measure of outcome in terms of process of care or clinical outcomes
- An experimental, quasi-experimental, or ex post facto research design
- Data that permitted calculation of effect size or determination of direction of effects

Thirty-eight of the 142 NP studies and 15 of the 68 CNM studies met all criteria. Thirty-three outcomes were analyzed from these studies, yielding the following results:

- Greater patient compliance was seen with the treatment recommendations of NPs than of physicians.
- Patient satisfaction and resolution of pathological conditions were greater for patients of NPs.
- CNMs used less analgesia than physicians did in intrapartum care of obstetric patients.
- CNMs achieved neonatal outcomes equivalent to those of physicians.

These studies are limited in their application to practice and do not examine the question of cost effectiveness.

To be acknowledged as a powerful resource for health-care reform, advanced practice nursing must deliver cost-effective care. Research that documents the cost effectiveness of nursing care provided by APNs is limited. One such study described below was conducted by Schaffner and Bohomey (1998), who state that designing treatment plans to limit costs without sacrificing patient care is a pressing concern in the delivery of timely, accessible, appropriate, high-quality patient care.

The cost effectiveness of nutritional support therapies for patients with gastrointestinal impairments was investigated using APNs on the Nutrition Support Team (NST) in the home-care setting. This research was conducted through the University of Rochester. Protocols were established, in collaboration with physicians, for nurses to independently prescribe and intervene in the discharge planning and routine home care of patients. The NST consults on nutritional discharge plans. In the past these plans had frequently consisted of total parenteral nutrition (TPN). Because the goal of the NST is to optimize the use of the gut whenever possible, enteral formulas (ENT) are used when diet is not possible. The costs and patient outcomes of APN consultation and follow-up care for patients referred for TPN were examined.

The annual cost of home TPN was $153,674, which included direct and indirect costs such as $2,119 per year for NST service follow-up. Thus, the cost was $12,802.08 per month, or $426.74 per day. In contrast, ENT had an annual cost of $12,338; thus, the monthly cost of ENT was $1,028.17, with a daily cost of $34.27 (assuming a 30-day month). The cost savings generated in the first quarter of 1996 by patient-appropriate therapy and close monitoring of patient progress, leading to weaning from TPN and ENT use when possible, were $237,440. Subsequent quarterly savings were $236,052, $210,438, and $232,958. These results highlight the ability of APNs to demonstrate their worth to health-care institutions by cost reduction.

In landmark legislation (Public Law PL 105–33), Medicare reimbursement was expanded for nurse practitioners. Nurse practitioners and clinical nurse specialists practicing in any geographic area and clinical setting can be re-imbursed at 85 percent of the physician rates. As of January 1, 1998, Medicare clients, those with mental disorders, and the disabled have had access to the cost-effective, quality health care provided by advanced prac-tice registered nurses in both rural and urban areas and in hospital- and community-based health-care settings. This spending bill included provi-sions to reauthorize the Community Nursing Organization (CNO) demon-stration project. CNOs are pilot managed care programs administered by nurses that offer Medicare benefits to elderly people in noninstitutional settings. These nurse-managed coordinated care programs have been rec-ognized for delivering high-quality, cost-effective patient care since they began in 1994.

> **A *Community Nursing Organization* program is a managed care facility administered by nurses that provides Medicare benefits to elderly people in community-based settings.**

Many current health-care changes result not only from decreased resource use but also from delivery of services in new ways. For example, advanced practice nurses are providing primary care services in community settings at lower costs than physicians' fees for services. Evolving technologies pro-vide an increasing array of services and products from which consumers may choose. This variety of products challenges the abilities of individuals and third-party payers to differentiate what is needed from what is available or desired.

ALTERNATIVE USE OF RESOURCES

The second component of the economic perspective is the notion that re-sources have alternative uses. A direct consequence of scarcity is that when resources are used for one product or service, they are not available for other products and services. Thus when choosing among alternative uses of the same resources, the value of the choice not selected is called an *opportu-nity cost*. Based on this economic concept, the cost of a health service or pro-cedure is best defined as the value of the foregone alternative service or procedure that the same resources could have been used to provide.

> **Opportunity cost *is the value of the alternative resource use that was not selected.***

ECONOMIC ANALYSIS
THE OPPORTUNITY COST CONCEPT IN ACTION

Communities across the United States are concerned about youth violence. In a community of approximately 100,000 citizens, a task force is created to recommend policy to the educational, penal, and family service systems in the area. The school nurse is one member of this task force.

The group meets over a period of time to discuss the philosophy of prevention versus treatment, available community resources of both money and expertise, and alternative ways to address the concern. The following ideas are generated:

- Establishing a kindergarten through high school curriculum that teaches conflict mediation and alternatives to violence
- Creating a coordinated system of youth activities for both grade school and high school students
- Designing a curriculum for parent training to enable parents to work more effectively with children and identify troubling signs
- Hiring additional school counselors so that each student would have at least one adult who could get to know him or her and guide his or her progress
- Building a juvenile facility so that offenders could be incarcerated for longer periods of time when they commit violent offenses
- Hiring additional officers to work more closely with juvenile offenders

This example demonstrates how each problem has many facets. Any community or group has limited resources with which to address a given problem; thus, choices among alternatives are mandatory. Even if the group has a strong preventive focus, members may also want to include means to deal with young people who have committed violent acts. The reality is that there will not be enough resources for all the desired programs. At the point of decision making, one needs to be clear what alternatives are being forgone because of the choices being made and what the value or opportunity cost of those forgone alternatives are.

In general, health-care expenditures can be examined for the alternate use of resources. For example, the United States invests the vast majority of heath-care money into acute care health services. Using alternative re-source analysis, the economist would ask:

- What would be the value of preventive or primary care services produced instead of some critical care services?
- What is the value of nurse practitioner primary care services as an alternative to physician primary care or specialty services?
- What is the value of social or educational resources that could be used to improve health?

Analysis of these questions enables the decision maker to select the most appropriate choice based on the relative cost and outcome of each alternative. Although there are many factors involved in decision making, opportunity cost analysis is an important component of this process.

ECONOMIC ANALYSIS
EXTENDED CARE AND HOME HEALTH CARE

Alternative uses of health-care resources include provision of care in extended-care and home-health-care settings. Population demographics would seem to predict an increase in these types of care. Whereas there were approximately 34.2 million people in the United States over 65 years old in 1995, that number is expected to increase to 52.8 million by the year 2020. Of this population, 11.3 percent are over the age of 85, representing the group most likely to need nursing services provided in extended-care facilities or in a community setting. Contrary to the public image, only 5 percent of elderly people live in extended-care facilities. Ninety-five percent reside in the community. The large percentage of the elderly population over the age of 75 (44 percent) is the group most likely to need supportive nursing services (Social Security Administration, 1996).

Policy makers and health-service professionals trying to meet the needs of this growing population must consider the value of a variety of alternatives, including extended care, home care, and day care for supportive nursing services. Extended care in a nursing home would be the most costly of these choices.

With the cost of health care rising and demographic trends creating pressure, it is likely that health-care expenditures will continue to increase. However, Buerhaus (1998) emphasizes that there is intense pressure on the public sector to control costs because of the budget deficit and the $5 trillion national debt. Because public programs, particularly Medicare and Medicaid, comprise a growing proportion of national health-care expenses (greater than 40 percent), there will be increased pressure to control costs in the public sector.

 ## CONSUMER VALUES AND PREFERENCES

The third component of the economic perspective relates to consumer wants and preferences. People have different values concerning health and the need for health care. Even when individuals seek health-care services, they select among choices such as traditional medicine or alternative therapies. They also select the desired type of health-care provider, for example, a physician or nurse practitioner. These consumer preferences affect the production of health-care products and services. Although individuals differ in their wants and preferences, economic theory assumes that value preferences are stable for individuals.

Value *is the relative importance of health compared with other choices.*

Preferences *refers to the selection of specific health-care services and products among the variety available.*

FACTORS AFFECTING VALUES AND PREFERENCES

What are the factors affecting values and preferences? Shiell, Hawe, and Seymour (1997) argue that basic values for various aspects of life, such as health, are stable, whereas preferences for market services are changeable. The assumption exists that preferences for products and services can be influenced. In health care these preferences include health-care services, types of providers, settings for care, types of treatments, and timing of service (whether for prevention or treatment).

 ### ECONOMIC ANALYSIS
APPLICATION OF PREFERENCES IN MATERNITY SERVICES

As an example of values and preferences, pregnant women choose from a variety of maternity services. Those who prefer specialty care with high technology would likely choose a gynecologist, perhaps at an academic medical center. Those women who prefer a more holistic approach to prenatal care and delivery might choose a nurse midwife who practices at a birthing center. Other women might not seek prenatal care and appear at a care center only at the time of delivery. A variety of factors, including the price and health insurance, also affect the choice of a prenatal care provider; however, preferences affect choice separate from other factors.

CONSUMER INFORMATION

A person's values and preferences are affected by the amount of consumer information he or she possesses. Accurate information is essential for a competitive market to function effectively. Trends affecting participation in health care include promotion of individual responsibility for one's health and lifestyle behaviors, and the expansion of the consumer movement in the United States to include health care.

Enthoven (1993) notes that economists and other proponents of health-care reform have identified informed consumer choice as one element of a better-functioning health-care marketplace. Sangl and Wolf (1996) promote the premise that consumers can be motivated to compare health plans relative to the cost, benefits, and quality-of-care information received and then select the health plans that give the best value. In theory, this process of informed choice would encourage health plans to be responsive to consumers' needs and to compete for enrollees based on both cost and performance. This active participation would then result in greater health-care responsiveness to consumers.

IMPACT OF CONSUMER INFORMATION ON VALUES AND PREFERENCES

Currently there is a time lag in information reaching consumers, which results in less informed consumer decisions. The Health Care Financing Administration is promoting efforts to increase the availability of information that will be useful in health-care decision making. Decisions include choices regarding health care plans, types of provider, setting for care, and types and timing of services. It is a challenge to provide useful information that is appropriate for all individuals because people experience widely varying health states. Comparable data for various health-care service plans are needed. The Agency for Health Care Policy and Research (AHCPR) is collecting survey data from consumers to compile consumer information from the health-care recipient's perspective (McMullan, 1996).

The HCFA is committed to examining consumer needs for information, developing and testing formats for consumer information, and implementing and evaluating key information strategies. Research on consumer use of information assists in the understanding of consumer needs and the implementation of strategies to meet those needs (Hibbard, 1996; Rodwin, 1996).

Nurses are instrumental in the provision of patient education and consumer information. Educational services include provision of the following:

- Preparatory information for procedures and services
- Discharge planning information for self-care
- Support and guidance for individuals, families, and caregivers to prepare for the next phases of health and illness
- Referral information related to community resources
- Advocacy related to obtaining information and services due to consumers
- Information regarding patient rights and responsibilities
- Information regarding advance directives for choice of care when patients are unable to make decisions for themselves

SUMMARY

Although nurses tend to focus on their professional skills to assist clients, knowledge of the economic principles that explain the nature of the health-care market is essential so that they can participate in health-care policy making. All practicing nurses need an understanding of economics, and nurses in leadership and management positions require advanced knowledge to contribute to the health-care systems in which they work. In the 21st century a health-care system that improves the health status of consumers while constraining the use of resources is essential. More nurses than ever before practice in integrated delivery systems composed of insurers, hospitals, physician practices, and other entities that provide health care for a defined population (Shortell, Anderson, Gillies, & Morgan, 1993). Integrated delivery systems and managed care organizations are examples of emerging structures created to provide comprehensive services in a cost-effective environment. These services range from treating a hospital-based illness to emphasizing wellness. Nurses need to understand the forces driving health care that limit health-care expenditures because the scarcity of resources requires choices among competing options.

Consumer preferences as to type of providers, setting for care, and types and timing of services also influence the health-care marketplace. The World Health Organization's goal of health for all by the year 2000 demands a visionary look at the roles of health-care practitioners, such as advanced practice nurses, as well as more active participation by consumers. Nurses need to collaborate with consumers and with other health-care providers to analyze and develop health-care services that incorporate economic principles. Chapters 2 through 4 address the economic principles related to resource allocation and their consequences for nurses.

DISCUSSION QUESTIONS

1. Define economics and health-care economics.
2. Why is it important for nurses to understand the economic principles relative to the cost of nursing care and quality outcomes?
3. What are the three choices that result from scarcity of health-care resources? Give a nursing example that depicts each of these choices.
4. Discuss and analyze two alternative health services and models of care and the impact they have on cost and outcomes for patient care.
5. Give some innovative examples of how nurses could control costs in their practice.
6. What is the impact of values and preferences on the choice of health services?
7. What is the role of nursing in disseminating health information to consumers to enable them to make informed decisions?

 REFERENCES

Brown, S., & Grimes, D. (1995). A meta analysis of nurse practitioners and nurse objectives in primary care. *Nursing Research, 44*(6), 332–339.

Buerhaus, P. I. (1998). Financial challenges and economic implications. In S. Price, M. Koch, & S. Bassett (Eds.), *Managing health care resources: Present and future challenges* (pp. 259–271). St. Louis: Mosby.

Bureau of the Census. (1998, September). Health insurance coverage: 1997 [On-line]. Available: http://www.census. gov/80hhes/hlthins/hlthin97/asc.html.

Bureau of the Census. (1999, June). Low income uninsured children by state [On-line]. Available: http://www.census.gov:80/hhes/hlthins/lowinckid.html.

Carter, M. (1997). The promise of nurse practitioners. *Nursing Administration Quarterly, 21*(4), 19–24.

Department of Health and Human Services. (1997). *Access to health care. Part 2: Working-age adults. Series 10: Data from the National Health Survey.* (DHHS Publication No. 97–1525). Washington, DC: Author.

Duke, K. S. (1996). Hospitals in a changing health care system. *Health Affairs,* 15(2), 49–61.

Enthoven, A. (1993). The history and principles of managed competition. *Health Affairs* Volume 12(Suppl.), 24–48.

Feldstein, P. J. (1993). *Health care economics* (2nd ed.). Albany, NY: Delmar Publishers.

Fuchs, V. (1998). *Who Shall Live?* (Expanded ed.). River Edge, NJ: World Scientific.

Gale, B. J., & Steffl, B. M. (1992). The long-term care dilemma: What nurses need to know about Medicare. *Nursing and Health Care,* 13(1), 34–41.

Health Care Financing Administration. (1996). Overview of the Medicare program. *Health Care Financing Review,* Statistical Supplement.

Health Care Financing Administration. (1998, October). National health expenditures, 1997: Highlights [On-line]. Available: http://www.hcfa.gov/stats/nhe-oact/nhe.htm.

Hibbard, J. (1996, October). *Drawing inferences from quality measures: The $640,000 question.* Paper presented at the conference sponsored by the Henry J. Kaiser Foundation and the Agency for Health Care Policy and Research.

Keepnews, D. (1998). The national sample survey of RNs: What does it tell us? *American Nurse,* 20(3), 10.

Levit, K., Lazenby, H., Braden, B., Cowan, C., McDonnell, P., Sivarajan, L., Stiller, J., Won, D., Donham, A. LongAm, & Stewart, M. (1996). National health care expenditures, 1995. *Health Care Financing Review,* 18(1), 175–214.

McMullan, M. (1996). HCFA's consumer informational commitment. *Health Care Financing Review,* 18(1), 9–14.

Meyer, H. (1997). Home (care) improvement. *Hospital and Health Networks,* 71(8), 40–42.

Moser, J. W. (1996). *Trends and patterns in physician income: Socioeconomic characteristics of medical practice,* 1996. Chicago: American Medical Association.

Rodwin, M. (1996). Consumer protection and managed care: The need for organized consumers. *Health Affairs,* 15(30), 110–123.

Sangl, J. A., & Wolf, L. F. (1996). Role of consumer information in today's health care system. *Health Care Financing Review,* 18(1), 1–8.

Schaffner, R., & Bohomey, J. (1998). Demonstrating APN value in a capitated market. *Nursing Economics,* 16(2), 69–74.

Shiell, A., Hawe, P., & Seymour, J. (1997). Values and preferences are not necessarily the same. *Health Economics,* 6(5), 515–518.

Shortell, S., Anderson, D., Gillies, R., & Morgan, K. (1993). The holographic organization. *Health Forum Journal,* 36(2), 26–29.

Simon, C. J., & Born, P. H. (1996). Physician earnings in a changing managed care environment. *Health Affairs,* 15(3), 124–133.

Social Security Administration, Office of the Actuary. (1996). Unpublished data used in the preparation of the 1996 Trustees' Report. Baltimore: Author.

Stanhope, M. (1995). Primary health care practice: Is nursing part of the solution or the problem? *Family and Community Health,* 18(1), 49–68.

 ## SUGGESTED READING

Betts, V. T. (1996). Nursing's agenda for health care reform: Policy, politics, and power through professional leadership. *Nursing Administration Quarterly,* 20(3), 1–8.

Catalano, J. T. (1996). *Contemporary professional nursing.* Philadelphia: FA Davis.

Feldstein, P. J. (1999). *Health care economics* (5th ed.). Albany, NY: Delmar Publishers.

Fuchs, V. R. (Ed.). (1986). *The health economy.* Cambridge, MA: Harvard University Press.

Mankiw, N. G. (1998). *Principles of economics.* Fort Worth, TX: The Dryden Press.

Phelps, C. E. (1997). *Health economics* (2nd ed.). Reading, MA: Addison-Wesley.

Shi, L., & Singh, D. A. (1998). *Delivering health care in America: A systems approach.* Gaithersburg, MD: Aspen Publishers.

Smith, S. P., & Flarey, D. L. (1999). *Process-centered health care organizations.* Gaithersburg, MD: Aspen Publishers.

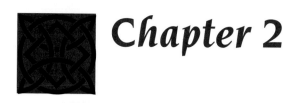

Chapter 2

Market, Demand, and Supply

Cyril F. Chang

LEARNING OBJECTIVES

- Define the concepts of market, demand, and supply.
- Describe how the market system works in a free enterprise economy.
- Explain the relevance and applications of basic economic concepts to nursing and health care.
- Identify the tools and building blocks necessary for the analysis of price determination and its resource allocation functions.
- Discuss the concept of elasticity and its relevance to nursing and health care.

Health care is a major component of the U.S. economy, accounting for about 14 percent of the gross domestic product (GDP). It both affects and is affected by the economic system of the United States—a free enterprise system characterized by the principle that goods and services are bought and sold by individual consumers and business firms in the *market*. An understanding of how a market economy works is a necessary first step for understanding the health economy and the various critical economic issues facing nursing and other health-care professionals.

A market *comprises a group of buyers and sellers who engage in trade.*

A market economy *is an economic system that is based on private ownership of resources and that allocates resources through the interactions of individuals and business firms.*

This chapter begins a two-chapter examination of what a market is and how it functions in a market economy, which is also referred to as a *free enterprise system*. This chapter defines the concepts of market, demand, and supply—the conceptual building blocks that form a market system. A major objective is to explain how these underlying economic principles make market economies work. This chapter also provides the necessary conceptual tools for analyzing how demand and supply work in a market to determine the price of a health-care service or product—the focus of the next chapter.

THE MARKET SYSTEM

THREE FUNDAMENTAL QUESTIONS

An *economic system* is the network of institutions, laws, and rules created by a society to answer three essential economic questions:

1. *What* goods and services shall be produced?
2. *How* shall they be produced?
3. *For whom* shall they be produced? (Baumol & Blinder, 1991)

These three questions are so essential to the proper functioning of an economic system that economists call them the *three fundamental questions*.

THE MARKET SYSTEM'S ANSWERS

The economies of the United States, Japan, and most western European countries are based on a type of economic system called the *market system*. It is a system that relies on market interactions of the competitive forces of supply and demand to coordinate diverse and complex production and consumption decisions by business firms and individual consumers. The three fundamental economic questions can be used to analyze the health-care economy, which is a part of the overall market system.

1. What services are to be provided? Goods and services in a market economy are produced for consumers who express their preferences by choosing those products for which they are willing to pay. For example, as the general population becomes older and more health conscious, food manufacturers introduce low-fat and low-calorie products to meet the changing preferences of consumers. Meanwhile, new businesses, such as home health agencies and wellness and fitness centers, emerge to provide services to the increasingly greater number of health-conscious individuals who are willing and able to pay for these services and products.
2. How will services be provided? Sellers and manufacturers of goods and providers of services must strive to minimize their costs of production and delivery. Otherwise, they cannot compete successfully and earn a sufficient rate of return for their efforts to compensate them for the investment risks that they have undertaken. For example, hospitals in the new, competitive managed care environment increasingly use temporary employment or staffing agencies to meet their nursing workforce needs. Although how much of the staffing needs should be outsourced (i.e., hired from an outside agency) is still being debated, the trend of out-

sourcing many of a hospital's administrative and operational functions reflects an attempt by both nonprofit and for-profit managers to economize and reduce costs.

3. <u>For whom are the services provided?</u> In a market economy, goods and services are produced for those who are able and willing to pay for them. For example, hospital care and physician services in the United States are delivered to those who have insurance coverage. Those who have no insurance or have insufficient insurance coverage must go without the needed services or seek help from charitable organizations or the government.

ECONOMIC ANALYSIS
COSTLY USE OF THE EMERGENCY DEPARTMENT FOR PRIMARY CARE

The "what," "how," and "for whom" economic concepts can be used to analyze the problem of emergency department use for nonurgent primary care by some patients. A mismatch in what is provided (emergency department services) versus what is needed (primary care and transportation to it) causes a problem for poor and uninsured patients and for the health-care system. In the United States, many low-income individuals use a taxi or even an ambulance to go to the emergency department for common colds, headaches, and other primary care problems. Recognizing the expense of this problem in money, resources, and poor patient outcomes, many emergency departments have instituted the triage nurse role to refer patients to an emergency department–based advanced practice nurse for nonurgent care.

TYPES OF MARKETS

Business transactions in a market system, including those involving health-care production and delivery, occur in a place called the *market*. A market comprises groups of buyers and sellers who, motivated by their own self-interests, come together to engage in mutually beneficial activities of buying and selling.

Markets are typically grouped according to the type of goods or services that are bought and sold. Some markets are for *consumer goods*, which are goods intended for the final consumption by households and individuals. For example, neighborhood drugstores comprise the local over-the-counter and prescription retail drugs market. Similarly, offices and clinics where physicians and advanced practice nurses practice are part of the local market for primary care services.

Consumers' demands for health-care services create demand for the resources that are needed to provide these health-care services. These resources are bought and sold in markets for the *inputs of production*. Some of these input markets involve the buying and selling of medical equipment and supplies. Others provide the services (that is, hours of work) of people who have the necessary skills and expertise to work together as a team to supply health-care services for patients and consumers. Examples of these markets include the labor markets for physicians, dentists, registered nurses, physical therapists, and other health-care professionals.

Still other markets are for buying and selling *capital goods*, which are goods used for producing consumption goods or other capital goods. Examples include x-ray and magnetic resonance imaging (MRI) machines used by hospitals and outpatient surgical centers for diagnostic screening of patients. These machines are not immediately used by patients; rather, they are operated by health-care institutions such as hospitals and doctors' offices to provide services for patients who have the financial means to pay for them.

DEMAND AND SUPPLY IN MARKETS

Demand and supply refers to the buying and selling activities of consumers and providers and how they interact with one another in the marketplace. Buyers as a group determine the demand for a service or a product by buying from the providers at a mutually agreeable price. Meanwhile, sellers or providers as a group determine the supply by making the service or product available. The interaction of supply and demand determines the market price and the amounts of the service or product delivered from providers to buyers.

> **Demand and supply *are the buying and selling activities of consumers and sellers who interact with one another in the marketplace.***

 ## DEMAND

Demand refers to the quantity of a service or a product that consumers are willing and able to buy at each of the possible prices. The factors that influence and determine demand can be identified conveniently through an example of the demand for a common over-the-counter product such as vitamin C tablets. Drugstores' advertising, buyers' income, and consumers' health concerns are examples of factors that can affect demand. But whether an individual will buy one brand of the product rather than another brand, or a large bottle containing two hundred 500-milligram tablets rather than a smaller one containing 50 tablets of the same strength, is very much influenced by the price of the product. We therefore will focus first on the influence of price on demand and then proceed to analyze the influences of other factors. We will assume, for simplicity, that all vitamin C tablets sold in local drugstores have the same strength, are packaged in the same 100-tablet bottles, and are homogenous in quality.

> **Demand *is the amount of a service or a product that consumers are willing and able to purchase at specified prices.***

PRICE AS A DETERMINANT OF DEMAND

Table 2–1 illustrates the relationship between the price of a bottle of vitamin C tablets and the total quantity demanded in a local market. At the relatively expensive price of $5 per bottle, consumers buy only 40,000 bottles per month. But when the price is lowered to $4 per bottle, buyers increase their purchases, taking home about 60,000 bottles per month. When stores run sales and drop the price to the rock-bottom level of $3 per bottle, customers rush to the stores and buy as many as 80,000 bottles per month.

The figures in Table 2–1 make up a market *demand schedule*, that is, a table or list that reveals the relationship between the price of a product and the quantity demanded by all of the buyers in a market, holding constant all other factors that can also influence demand. *Quantity demanded* refers to the amount of service or product that all consumers in a market are prepared to buy at a given price.

TABLE 2–1. THE MARKET DEMAND SCHEDULE FOR VITAMIN C TABLETS

Price per Bottle ($)	Quantity Demanded per Month (1000s)
5.00	40
4.50	50
4.00	60
3.50	70
3.00	80

A demand schedule *is a table or list that shows the relationship between the price of a product and the quantity demanded by all of the buyers in a market, holding constant all other factors that can also influence demand.*

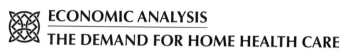

ECONOMIC ANALYSIS
THE DEMAND FOR HOME HEALTH CARE

Medicare recently expanded insurance coverage for home health care. The main purpose of this policy change was to reduce the length of hospital stays and the use of more expensive inpatient care so that scarce resources could be more appropriately distributed. This expansion of insurance coverage reduced the costs of home health care to elderly patients and their families. As a result, the demand for this service increased, opening up new job and career opportunities to many nursing professionals.

Figure 2–1 graphically depicts the demand schedule presented in Table 2–1. In economics, the price of the product is traditionally graphed on the vertical axis and the quantity demanded on the horizontal axis. The downward sloping curve (it has been drawn as a line for simplicity here) that relates the price of vitamin C tablets and the quantity demanded is called the *market demand curve*. The curve is sloped downward to the right to reflect

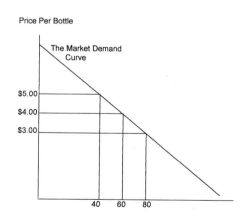

FIG. 2–1. The market demand for vitamin C.

the inverse relationship between the quantity demanded and the price of the product.

NONPRICE DETERMINANTS OF DEMAND

Price is frequently the most important factor in determining whether buyers of a consumer product will actually buy it and how much they will buy. However, price is not the most important factor affecting a patient's decision to see a physician or an advanced practice nurse, or to check into a hospital. Many nonprice factors influence the demand for a service or product, whether it is a regular consumer good or a critical medical service.

What, then, are these nonprice factors that also play an important role in influencing demand for a product? Three variables are major nonprice determinants of demand: consumer income, tastes and preferences, and prices of related goods (Pauly, 1982).

Income

What happens to demand when consumer income increases? For most goods and services, an increase in income increases demand. That is, consumers buy more at the same prices than before the increase in income. Continuing the vitamin C example, the demand curve relationship for this situation is illustrated in Figure 2–2. An increase in consumer income has resulted in a rightward shift of the demand curve (an increase in demand) from D_1 to D_2. At the price of P_1 (and at each of the other possible prices),

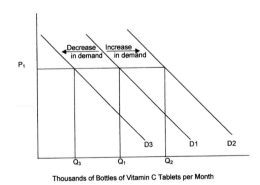

FIG. 2–2. Shifts in market demand curves.

the quantity demanded has increased. Conversely, a decline in consumer income shifts the demand curve to the left (a decrease in demand) from D_1 to D_3.

ECONOMIC ANALYSIS
INCOME AND THE DEMAND FOR HEALTH CARE

The demand for health care also increases and decreases as income fluctuates. When a country becomes more affluent or when tax rates are lowered (which raises household disposable income), the demand for health care in that country will most likely rise. This is especially true in the United States, where increases in income are frequently associated with a steady job that offers insurance coverage, which, in turn, increases the demand for health care. Conversely, people who lose their jobs also lose insurance coverage, causing the demand for health care to decrease.

In economics, the goods and services for which demand increases when consumers earn more money are called *normal goods* (examples in health care are cosmetic surgeries and many alternative and preventive therapies, such as massage therapy and exercise equipment and facilities). An increase in income does not increase the demand for all health-care services, however. Some services, such as those provided at public clinics offered by county health departments or supported by charitable organizations, have higher-priced substitutes. The demand for these services falls when income rises because patients can now afford a higher-priced substitute, such as going to a private clinic for primary care services. These goods and services are called *inferior goods.*

Normal goods *are those services or products that consumers buy more of as their income rises.*

Inferior goods *are those services or products that consumers buy less of as their income rises.*

Tastes or Preferences

Consumer demand is sensitive to buyers' tastes and preferences. For example, the demand for vitamin C tablets is clearly affected by consumers' health concerns and their general understanding of the health effects of nutrition tablets. Frequently, favorable press coverage of the health effects of an over-the-counter drug can push sales to record high levels. Conversely, negative news stories about the newly discovered harmful effects of a drug can seriously reduce its demand and sales. The significance of consumer tastes and preferences is evidenced by the increased attention paid to marketing and public relations by health-care providers and pharmaceutical companies.

Consumer tastes and preferences also present critical challenges to the nursing profession's quest for new roles and professionalism. For example, advanced practice nurses (APNs) face resistance from consumers because of a long-standing preference for services that could in the past be provided only by physicians.

 ## ECONOMIC ANALYSIS
DEMAND AND PRODUCT IMAGE

Most TV commercials use thin models to promote food products. This reflects the belief that the image of a thin model can deflect concerns about perceived adverse effects of food products on buyers' health. Similarly, media promotion of many preventive measures for early detection of a variety of lethal diseases, such as prostate cancer for men and breast cancer for women, minimizes the pain image of the recommended procedure. The fear of pain and side effects in connection with a preventive procedure may cause many people who could potentially benefit from it to stay away.

Prices of Related Goods

The demand for a service or product is also influenced by the prices of related goods. In our ongoing example, suppose the market offers two brands of vitamin C tablets that have no noticeable differences in quality. If the price of brand A increases, consumers will buy less of that brand and more of brand B. In this instance, an increase in the price of one brand results in an increase in the demand for the other (a shift of the demand curve for the substitute brand to the right, from D_1 to D_2 in Figure 2–2).

In this example, the two brands of vitamin C are called *substitutes*. Other examples of substitutes include disposable syringes and reusable syringes, and home health services and semiskilled nursing-home care.

A substitute *is a service or product that can be used to take the place of another service or product.*

Now suppose that the price of home care increases and, as a result, the demand for home-care services decreases. When this happens, the demand for home-care equipment will in all likelihood decrease as well. When an increase in the price of one service causes a decrease in the demand for another (that is, shifting the demand for the related product to the left, from D_1 to D_3 in Figure 2–2), the two goods or services are called *complements*. Additional examples include MRI machines and the complement of skilled radiology technicians who are needed to operate the equipment, and vaccines for the immunization of childhood diseases and the complement of syringes for injecting the vaccines.

A complement *is a service or product that is used together with another service or product.*

ECONOMIC ANALYSIS
ADVANCED PRACTICE NURSES AND PHYSICIANS IN THE EMERGENCY DEPARTMENT

Many types of advanced practice nurses, such as clinical nurse specialists, certified nurse midwives, and certified registered nurse anesthetists, can appropriately perform many of the tasks in a hospital emergency department. If the costs of physician services continue to go up and competition in the health-care market intensifies further, hospital administrators may increasingly find it necessary to substitute advanced nurse practitioners for physicians in their emergency departments.

DETERMINANTS OF DEMAND: A SUMMARY

The discussion to this point has defined the concept of demand and identified two types of factors that influence demand: price and nonprice determinants, the latter of which includes income, tastes and preferences, and prices of related products. This dichotomy of the factors that influence demand into price and nonprice determinants is useful in distinguishing between two important types of changes involving demand, as summarized in Table 2–2:

1. A change in the quantity demanded. When the price of a service increases, the quantity demanded falls, and vice versa. These changes are expressed as movements along a given demand curve. The demand

TABLE 2–2. THE DETERMINANTS OF DEMAND

Variables That Affect the Quantity Demanded	A Change in This Variable Will Cause
Price	A movement along a given demand curve
Income	A shift of the demand curve
Tastes and preferences	A shift of the demand curve
Prices of related goods	A shift of the demand curve

curve therefore shows what happens to the quantity demanded when the price increases or decreases, holding all other factors constant.

2. <u>A change in demand.</u> A change in demand occurs when one of the non-price determinants changes. This is expressed as a shift in the demand curve to the right (an increase in demand) or to the left (a decrease in demand).

A change in the quantity demanded *is a change along a given demand curve in response to a change in the market price.*

A change in demand *is a shift of the demand curve in response to a change in one of the nonprice determinants of demand.*

ECONOMIC ANALYSIS
INCREASING THE EMPLOYMENT OF REGISTERED NURSES

Federal policy makers and nursing leaders have for years tried to increase the employment of registered nurses (RNs). There are two ways to achieve this goal. One way is to increase the demand for RNs. This can be accomplished by increasing the demand for health care through federal and state mandates for insurance coverage for the previously uninsured. An increase in the demand for health care will increase the demand for health-care workers, including RNs. Increases in the demand for RNs (shifts of the demand curve for RNs) not only increase their employment but also their salaries (the price of their services).

Another way to increase the employment of RNs is to make RNs less expensive to hire by, for example, making work rule or wage concessions or by increasing admissions to nursing schools and thereby adding more nurses to the workforce. With RNs costing employers less and becoming more attractive financially (a movement along a demand curve for RNs), more RNs will be hired. Clearly, from the nursing perspective, the first approach is preferable to the second, although both policies can have the same effect of increasing the number of RNs hired.

 ## ELASTICITY OF DEMAND

The demand for a service or product is affected by the product's price and a host of other factors, such as income, tastes and preferences, and the prices of related goods. For example, consumers will buy a smaller quantity of a product if its price increases. But by how much will the quantity demanded fall? The responsiveness of demand to a change in the price of a product is referred to as the *price elasticity of demand*. The formula for measuring the price elasticity is as follows:

$$\text{Price elasticity of demand} = \frac{\text{Percentage change in quantity demanded}}{\text{Percentage change in price}}$$

The responsiveness of demand to a change in the price of a product is referred to as the **price elasticity of demand.**

The formula suggests that the price elasticity of demand is a ratio based on a comparison of two percentage changes. The cause of the change is a change in the price of a product, and the result is a change in the quantity demanded. Since an increase in price always causes a decrease in the quantity demanded, the price elasticity of demand is negative.

When interpreting the price elasticity of demand, however, the sign of the computed ratio is ignored. The demand is said to be *elastic* if the price elasticity of demand is greater than 1, and *inelastic* if the elasticity is smaller than 1.

Elastic demand *is when demand is sensitive to a change in price.*

Inelastic demand *is when demand is insensitive to a change in price.*

ECONOMIC ANALYSIS
THE PRICE ELASTICITIES OF DEMAND FOR HEALTH CARE

Health economists have conducted many empirical studies to estimate the price elasticities of demand for health care and its various components. For example, the demand for primary care services has been determined to be price inelastic, with estimates ranging from −0.1 to −0.8 (Santerre & Neun, 2000). This means that for a 10 percent increase in the price of health care, there will be a relatively small reduction in the demand for health care, in the range of about 1 to 8 percent. The demand for hospitalization has been estimated to be between −0.1 and −0.2 (Manning et al., 1987), and the price elasticity of demand for physician services has been estimated to be about −0.06 (Stano, 1985).

THE DETERMINANTS OF THE ELASTICITY OF DEMAND

The price elasticity of demand varies from product to product. For example, price plays a much smaller role in determining the demand for health-care services than the demand for most consumer goods, such as vacation trips or movie tickets. In general, price elasticity of demand increases (becomes more elastic) when:

- A greater proportion of the household budget is allocated to the purchase.
- Many good substitutes are available.
- The service is unessential to consumers' physical and psychological well-being.
- There is sufficient amount of time available for decision making.

ECONOMIC ANALYSIS
WHY DO HEALTH-CARE SERVICES DIFFER IN ELASTICITY?

Based on the previously identified four factors that affect elasticity, the demand for many types of health care is price inelastic. For example, a lack of time to seek out treatment options and an absence of good substitutes make the demand for hospital emergency department services extremely inelastic. In comparison, the demands for many elective surgeries and "lifestyle" drugs are price elastic. These services are for treating conditions that are not life threatening, and patients have time to seek out various treatment options. Similarly, the demand of surgical patients for intensive care nurses is inelastic, whereas the demand for nursing-home nurses is more elastic in comparison.

 ## SUPPLY

Supply in economics refers to a price-and-quantity relationship expressed in the form of a schedule or a curve. This relationship shows the various quantities of a service or product that providers are willing and able to make available at various prices.

> **Supply *is the quantity of a service or product that providers are willing to sell at particular prices.***

Table 2–3 illustrates the supply relationship for our ongoing example. At a relatively high price of $5 per bottle, drugstores prepare 80,000 bottles per month for sale because they can expect a good profit margin at such a favorable price. At lower prices, profit margins are smaller and the amounts that drugstores are willing to supply are also lower. At the relatively low price of $3 per bottle, for example, some stores cut back the amounts that they are willing to sell and others stop selling the product altogether. As a result, only 40,000 bottles will be made available in the entire market.

Figure 2–3 graphs the figures given in Table 2–3. The upward sloping curve, called the *supply curve*, relates the various quantities of vitamin C tablets that drugstores are willing to supply at each of the prices that stores

TABLE 2–3. THE MARKET SUPPLY SCHEDULE FOR VITAMIN C TABLETS

Price per Bottle ($)	Quantity Supplied per Month (1000s)
5.00	80
4.50	70
4.00	60
3.50	50
3.00	40

Price Per Bottle

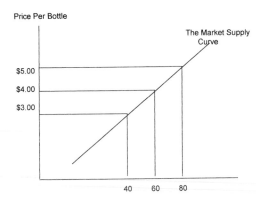

FIG. 2–3. The market supply for vitamin C.

Thousands of Bottles of Vitamin C Tablets per Month

can expect to receive. The curve slopes upward to the right, reflecting a positive relationship between the price and the quantity supplied. At higher prices, sellers expect to realize a larger profit margin and are therefore more eager to supply a greater amount of the product.

The **quantity supplied** *is the total amount of a service or product that sellers in a market are willing to provide at a specific price.*

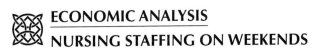

ECONOMIC ANALYSIS
NURSING STAFFING ON WEEKENDS

In many hospitals, nursing administrators find it hard to staff their weekend shifts. However, those that offer full-time pay for two days of 12-hour work usually have no problems finding enough RNs to work on weekends. The number of RNs willing to work at inconvenient and undesirable hours increases as hospitals pay more for each hour of work.

NONPRICE DETERMINANTS OF SUPPLY

Although price is frequently the most influential factor determining the quantity supplied by sellers, several other factors can also influence supply. Most of these factors are related to the cost of production and production

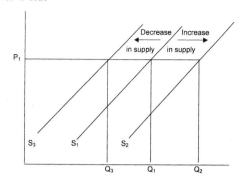

FIG. 2–4. Shifts in market supply curves.

processes, including input prices, technology, changes in related markets, and the length of time needed to alter the capacity of the industry that produces the product.

Prices of Inputs

To produce a health-care product, an assortment of inputs must be used. These include labor, materials, and the services from facilities and equipment. The prices paid for these inputs influence the costs of production and, indirectly, the supply of the final output. For example, if the raw materials used in the production of vitamin C tablets become cheaper, production costs will be reduced and the manufacturer's profit margin will increase. The manufacturer will most likely increase the supply; this situation is represented by a rightward shift in the supply curve from S_1 to S_2, as illustrated in Figure 2–4.

Conversely, if the cost of production increases because of higher input prices, manufacturers will supply less of the product, other things holding constant. This situation is represented by a leftward shift of the supply curve from S_1 to S_3, signifying a decrease in supply.

ECONOMIC ANALYSIS
COST OF NURSING EDUCATION AND THE SUPPLY OF THE NURSING WORKFORCE

The cost of a nursing education and the expenses that nursing students must pay for a nursing degree can significantly influence the supply of the nursing workforce. Since the 1960s, federal and state governments have subsidized nursing education, reducing the cost of a nursing degree. This trend has had a positive impact on the supply of the nursing workforce. But as the federal and state governments cut back their subsidies for nursing education and training, the supply of nursing labor can be expected to decrease.

Technology

The production of health-care products and delivery of health services involves the use of sophisticated medical technologies. The dissemination of these useful technologies reduces costs and increases supply by enabling manufacturers to produce more outputs using the same amount of inputs. However, not all health-care technologies are used for improving the production process and cutting costs. Many are used primarily to increase the sophistication and, presumably, the quality of the service or product. This type of technological advance, which primarily increases the depth and breadth of health care, can actually increase costs and therefore may not increase the supply of health care.

Changes in Related Markets

Most pharmaceutical companies do not manufacture one product only; they produce a host of pharmaceutical product categories called *product lines*. How much of one product, say, vitamin C supplement, that a manufacturer is willing to supply depends in part on the prices of other products that it also produces. For example, if the prices of other products fall and their production becomes less profitable, the company will supply more vitamin C and less of other products.

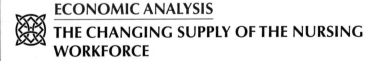

ECONOMIC ANALYSIS
THE CHANGING SUPPLY OF THE NURSING WORKFORCE

The trend of nurses finding employment outside traditional work settings such as hospitals and clinics has had important implications for the supply of the nursing workforce. With new jobs opening up in such nontraditional work settings as pharmaceutical sales, insurance claims processing, and a host of other managerial positions, nurses are increasingly looking for career opportunities outside hospitals and clinics. These employment trends have decreased the supply of the nursing workforce in the traditional work settings where they mainly contribute as providers of patient care.

Changes in the Number of Suppliers

Supply will increase and the supply curve will shift to the right if there is an increase in the number of suppliers or if the existing suppliers expand their capacities. If more colleges and universities set up nursing programs, for example, the supply of the nursing workforce will increase (a rightward shift of the supply curve) when the new schools begin to graduate students. Expanding the class size in existing schools will have the same effect.

DETERMINANTS OF SUPPLY: A SUMMARY

Table 2–4 summarizes the variables that affect supply. A supply schedule or curve reflects the relationship between the quantity of a product that sellers are willing and able to make available during a period of time and its price, holding constant other factors that affect supply. When the price of the product increases or decreases, the *quantity supplied* will increase or decrease along a given supply curve. When one of the nonprice determinants of supply changes, there will be a *change in supply*, which involves shifting the supply curve. Two types of changes involving supply are distinguished:

1. A change in the quantity supplied (caused by a change in the price of the product)
2. A change in supply (caused by a change in one of the nonprice determinants of supply).

TABLE 2–4. THE DETERMINANTS OF SUPPLY

Variables That Affect the Quantity Demanded	A Change in This Variable Will Cause
Price	A movement along a given supply curve
Input prices	A shift of the demand curve
Technology	A shift of the demand curve
Prices of related markets	A shift of the demand curve

A change in the quantity supplied *is a change along a given supply curve in response to a change in the market price.*

A change in supply *is a shift of the supply curve in response to a change in one of the nonprice determinants of supply.*

SUMMARY

In this chapter, we have defined the concepts of market, demand, and supply, and applied them to describe how the market system works in a free enterprise economy. The main purpose is to explain the relevance and applications of basic economic concepts to nursing and health care. We have also discussed the concept of elasticity of demand and other tools of economic analysis. These building blocks for the analysis of price determination and its resource allocation functions are the focus of next chapter.

DISCUSSION QUESTIONS

1. Define the concepts of a market and a market system.
2. Why is it important for nurses to understand how the market works?
3. Describe how the market system works using the concepts of demand, supply, and market.
4. What determines the demand for a common consumer good such as a new computer?
5. What determines the demand for the services of registered nurses?
6. Distinguish between the two types of changes involving demand. What is the significance of making this distinction?
7. Define and explain the concept of price elasticity of demand.
8. What determines the supply of a product?
9. Would a change in medical technology lead to a movement along the supply curve of hospital services or a shift in the supply curve? What other factors can cause the hospital supply curve to shift? Can a change in the price of hospital service cause such a shift?

REFERENCES

Baumol, W. J., & Blinder, A. S. (1991). *Economics* (5th ed.). San Diego: Harcourt Brace.

Manning, W. G., Newhouse, J. S., Duan, N., Keeler, E., Leibowitz, A., & Marquis, M. (1987). Health insurance and the demand for medical care: Evidence from a randomized experiment. *American Economic Review, 77*(3), 261–277.

Pauly, M. V. (1982). Economic aspects of consumer use. In R. D. Luke & J. C. Bauer (Eds.), *Issues in health economics* (pp. 113–139). Rockville, MD: Aspen Publishers.

Santerre, R. E., & Neun, S. P. (2000). *Health economics: Theories, insights, and industry studies.* Orlando, FL: The Dryden Press.

Stano, M. (1985). An analysis of the evidence on competition in the physician's services market. *Journal of Health Economics, 4*(3), 197–211.

 # SUGGESTED READINGS

Feldstein, P. J. (1999). *Health care economics* (5th ed.). Albany, NY: Delmar Publishers.

Fuchs, V. R. (1986). *The health economy.* Cambridge, MA: Harvard University Press.

Mankiw, N. G. (1998). *Principles of economics.* Forth Worth, TX: The Dryden Press.

Phelps, C. E. (1997). *Health Economics* (2nd ed.). Reading, MA: Addison-Wesley.

Rapoport, J. R., Robertson, R. L., & Stuart, B. (1982). *Understanding health economics.* Rockville, MD: Aspen Systems Corporation.

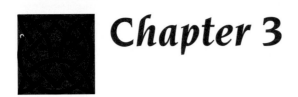

Chapter 3

Market Price
Determination

Cyril F. Chang

LEARNING OBJECTIVES

- Define the concept of market equilibrium.
- Understand how the forces of supply and demand determine the market price.
- Explain what causes the market price to change.
- Provide health-care and nursing examples of the consequences of price changes.
- Discuss the significant role of price in rationing and allocating scarce resources.

The previous chapter used the concepts of the market, demand, and supply to show how a market system worked. This chapter demonstrates how supply and demand interact with each other to set the prices paid by consumers and the quantities of the services or products delivered to them. It then explains what causes the market price to change and how the forces of demand and supply react to stabilize the price. In the process, the powerful and critical role of price in allocating scarce resources in a market is described and discussed.

 ## PRICE DETERMINATION AND MARKET EQUILIBRIUM

THREE KEY PRICING QUESTIONS

The earlier analysis of the market system stated that buyers and sellers, in pursuit of their self-interests, reacted to price changes by adjusting the amounts of a service or product that they were willing and able to buy and sell. The question of how much more or less would be bought and sold was answered by the concept of the price elasticity of demand. Throughout the analysis of a market system, the focus was on the reactions of buyers and sellers to a change in the price of a service or product without asking what had caused the price to change in the first place. This chapter analyzes what causes the market price to change. It begins with an exploration of three central pricing questions:

1. How is the price of a product determined?
2. What causes the price to change?
3. What are the resource-allocation implications of price changes?

PRICE EQUILIBRIUM

Buyers as a group determine the demand for a service or product, and sellers as a group determine the supply. The interaction of demand and supply determines the price and the amount of the service or product delivered from sellers to buyers. Continuing with the example of vitamin C supplements, Figure 3–1 depicts this interaction. The supply curve and the demand curve cross at a point called the market's *equilibrium* (Mankiw, 1998).

The dictionary meaning of the word *equilibrium* is a situation in which the various forces that influence the final outcome of an event are in balance. An *equilibrium price* is therefore one that, once determined, will remain stable. Given the demand for and supply of vitamin C supplements in the ongoing example, the price at which the demand and supply curves cross, at $4 per bottle, is defined as the equilibrium price. The resulting quantity of 60,000 bottles bought and sold per month is referred to as the *equilibrium quantity*. At this price, the amount of a product that sellers are willing and able to sell is exactly equal to the amount that buyers are willing and able to buy. The market hence satisfies both sides.

The **equilibrium price** *is one at which the quantity demanded and the quantity supplied are equal.*

Could the market price be higher or lower than the equilibrium price of $4? In other words, can any price other than the equilibrium one bring the buy-

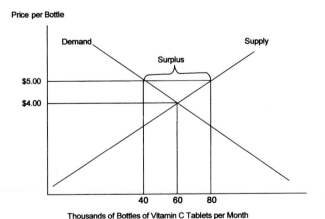

FIG. 3–1. Market surplus.

TABLE 3–1. DEMAND, SUPPLY, AND MARKET EQUILIBRIUM

Price ($)	Quantity Demanded	Quantity Supplied	Surplus (+) or Shortage (−)	Direction of Price Change
5.00	40	80	40	↓
4.50	50	70	20	↓
4.00	60	60	0	Equilibrium
3.50	70	50	−20	↑
3.00	80	40	−40	↑

Note: Quantities are in thousands of bottles.

ers and sellers together so that both sides would be satisfied? The answer is that given the demand and supply curves and the absence of any change in the factors that can influence either the demand or the supply, the only price that can keep the demand and supply in balance is the $4 equilibrium price.

To see this, take a look at any of the nonequilibrium prices. At any of these prices, the amounts demanded and supplied are not equal. This implies a frustrating situation in which either the buyers wish to buy more than the amount that is available or the sellers cannot sell all of what they have prepared to sell. Consequently, dissatisfied buyers and sellers will adjust the amounts that they are willing to buy and sell. These market actions exert pressures on the price to move it toward the equilibrium level. To see this, let us consider the figures in Table 3–1.

Suppose that the market price is initially above the equilibrium price, at $5 per bottle of vitamin C tablets. At this price, the quantity demanded is only 40,000 bottles a month, whereas the quantity supplied is 80,000. The excess quantity of 40,000 bottles supplied per month is called a *surplus*. In Figure 3–1, the surplus is depicted as a gap between the amount supplied (80,000) and the amount demanded (40,000) at the market price of $5.

A surplus *is a market situation in which the quantity supplied exceeds the quantity demanded.*

It does not take long for store owners and sales managers to realize that they must lower their prices to reduce their surplus inventories. The price will continue to fall until it reaches the equilibrium price of $4 at which the quantity demanded is once again equal to the quantity supplied. When this happens, the market equilibrium is said to have been restored.

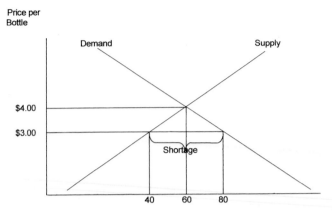

Price per
Bottle

Thousands of Bottles of Vitamin C Tablets per Month

FIG. 3–2. Market shortage.

Suppose now that the initial market price is $3 per bottle, $1 lower than the equilibrium price, as shown in Figure 3–2. The low price will attract extra buyers into drugstores to buy 80,000 bottles a month, whereas the amount that drugstores are willing to make available is only 40,000. The quantity supplied has now fallen short of the quantity demanded, resulting in a shortfall of 40,000 bottles. This imbalance between the quantity demanded and the quantity supplied is called a *shortage*. When this happens, sellers will place additional orders to replenish their inventories and will soon realize that they can earn more profit by charging a higher price. The price of vitamin C tablets begins to rise until the market price reaches the equilibrium level of $4. At this price, the equilibrium is once again restored by the automatic actions of the buyers and sellers who, acting independently of each other, push the market price toward the equilibrium level.

A shortage *is a market situation in which the quantity demanded exceeds the quantity supplied.*

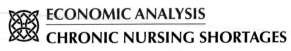

ECONOMIC ANALYSIS
CHRONIC NURSING SHORTAGES

The example of vitamin C supplements suggests that although surpluses and shortages may develop from time to time, permanent market imbalances are not likely. Indeed, this prediction holds true for most consumer products and many of the health-care services that are provided competitively. But the recurring and persistent shortages in the nursing workforce in the United States present a challenge to the economic analysis of the market (Feldstein, 1999).

For a shortage of nursing workforce to exist, the number of nurses needed by employers must exceed the number of nurses willing to work at the going wage rate. The market analysis of demand and supply predicts that employers in such a tight labor market would pay more to attract qualified nurses to work for them. However, this did not happen; nursing wages were stagnant for extended periods of time in the 1960s and 1970s. As a result, workforce shortages of nursing personnel, once developed, lingered for a long time.

Why didn't employers raise wages? Did hospital administrators not understand the concepts of demand and supply? Hospital administrators understood perfectly why it was in their best interest not to raise wage rates to attract nurses. In most cities, hospitals are the largest employers of the nursing workforce. If one hospital raises wages for new hires, it usually cannot avoid raising wages for a large number of existing staff nurses. Thus, the cost of hiring new nurses is far greater than the higher wages needed to attract them. Besides, once a hospital raises its pay scale, other hospitals must follow suit, causing every hospital's labor costs to increase. Thus when the need for a nursing workforce rose after an increase in the demand for hospital care, the reluctance of hospital administrators to raise wages resulted in persistent shortages of nurses (Folland, Goodman, & Stano, 1997).

 ## CHANGES IN THE MARKET PRICE

The analysis has so far focused on the process through which the market equilibrium is determined. In this process, a surplus that results from the market price being above the equilibrium level sends a clear signal to sellers to lower their prices. Lower prices encourage purchases and reduce the surplus. Similarly, a shortage signals to sellers to raise their prices, which, in turn, discourages consumer purchasing and helps to alleviate the shortage. Thus the market has an automatic mechanism to keep the forces of supply and demand in balance and the market price stable via price changes. But what causes the equilibrium price to change? This is an important question because prices of most services and products do fluctuate from time to time. The prices of some products, such as stocks and bonds and most agricultural products, can even change from minute to minute.

SHIFTS IN THE DEMAND AND SUPPLY CURVES

The price of a service or product changes in response to a change in the demand for the product or the supply of it. Chapter 2 described two types of changes involving demand and supply: (1) a change in the quantity demanded (or supplied) and (2) a change in demand (or supply). The former is a movement along a given demand (supply) curve, whereas the latter is a shift of the entire curve. A change in the market price is caused by the second type of change.

A shift in the demand or supply curve is caused by a change in any of the nonprice determinants of demand and supply. Once a market is disturbed by a change in one or more of these determinants, the equilibrium price will change. The following two examples illustrate how the equilibrium market price will change in response to changes from either the demand side or the supply side.

Suppose that a team of researchers from a major research institution has just confirmed the long-suspected benefits of taking vitamin C supplements regularly; that is, the supplements reduce the probability of catching common colds and allow those who have already been afflicted to recover sooner. Shortly after the announcement of this discovery, the demand for vitamin C supplements increases, shifting the demand curve to the right. With consumers increasing their purchases of the product, a temporary shortage ensues and, eventually, the market price moves up to a new equilibrium level.

Suppose next that pharmaceutical companies expand their production capacities by adding manufacturing plants for the production of vitamin C supplements. This expansion of capacity increases the supply. The rightward shift of the supply curve disturbs the market equilibrium, causing the amount supplied to temporarily outstrip the amount demanded. The resulting surplus leads to a serious price cut that eventually lowers the price to a new equilibrium level at which the demand and supply are in balance once again.

WHEN DEMAND AND SUPPLY CHANGE AT THE SAME TIME

Demand and supply can change simultaneously. For example, an increase in demand coupled with a decrease in supply will work together to create a larger shortage than a change in demand or supply could create alone. Conversely, an increase in supply coupled with a decrease in demand will result in a serious oversupply. It is also possible for the forces of supply and demand to work in opposite directions and thus completely or partially cancel out each other's impact on price.

Irrespective of the directions of the changes in supply and demand and the magnitude of these changes, the market price will change and buyers and sellers will respond and adjust. The adjustments they make in terms of how much to buy and sell eliminate the imbalance between supply and demand. These adjustments occur automatically as individual buyers and sellers make buying and selling decisions that are in their own best interests.

 ECONOMIC ANALYSIS
DEMAND AND SUPPLY FOR NURSES

With Americans getting older and hospital patients getting sicker, the demand for nursing services has increased. Meanwhile, nursing schools are admitting fewer students because college-age women are finding job and career opportunities in nonnursing fields. The simultaneous increase in the demand for a nursing workforce and decrease in the supply will create a shortage of nurses. Hospitals and other employers may resort to paying higher wages to attract more nurses or expand the enrollment of hospital-based diploma programs to increase market supply.

 THE RATIONING FUNCTION OF PRICE

Price in the market system functions like a traffic signal at a busy street intersection. Cars and pedestrians in modern cities need traffic signals to regulate their movements. The market price performs a similar function: It directs the flow of goods and services, keeps the market supply and demand in balance, and directs resources to where they are needed the most as indicated by consumers' willingness and ability to pay. This important resource-allocation function is called the *rationing function of price.*

T*he* rationing function of price *refers to the important role played by price in allocating scarce resources in a market economy.*

 ECONOMIC ANALYSIS
A SHORTAGE OF ADVANCED PRACTICE NURSES

Suppose that health maintenance organizations and other cost-conscious health-care delivery organizations have discovered that well-educated advanced practice nurses (APNs) can function cost effectively as providers of certain types of primary care services in the managed care setting. The rightward shift of the demand curve causes the number of APNs demanded to outstrip the number currently available at the prevailing salary level.

How does a freely functioning labor market overcome the problem of a labor shortage? Automatically! Salaries of APNs are likely to rise, increasing the number of these nurses from at least three sources. First, the higher wages will draw some APNs to switch jobs to fill new positions in managed care. Second, some of the increases in the quantity supplied will come from the ranks of inactive APNs who have the training and qualifications but are employed outside the health-care economy or are not employed for a variety of reasons. Third, nursing schools will graduate new APNs in a few years in response to the higher demand.

Meanwhile, higher wages in the short run serve to ration the limited supply of APNs who are currently practicing. The employers who are in desperate need of APNs will pay more for them, while those that cannot afford them or do not feel that they should pay the high salaries will be priced out of the market. The quantity of APNs currently available is then rationed or allocated to those who need them and are willing to pay for them.

SUMMARY

Our discussion has centered on a simple, common household product: vitamin C supplements. But the lessons learned here go far beyond the market for this single and relatively simple product. Price plays an important role that affects the supply and demand of more complicated and far more expensive services and products, such as physician services, nursing care, hospital care, and prescription drugs. Price can even alleviate the problem of nursing shortages or surpluses if the labor market is allowed to function without being overly regulated by the government or influenced by the market power possessed by large employers.

DISCUSSION QUESTIONS

1. Define the concept of market equilibrium and explain why prices have a tendency to move toward equilibrium.

2. Explain how the equilibrium price of a service or product is determined.
3. If prices always tend to equilibrium, what could be reasons for the equilibrium market prices to change?
4. Define the concepts of shortage and surplus. Explain how they can develop and describe how the market system manages to eliminate them.
5. Using the concepts of demand, supply, and market equilibrium, analyze the economic implications of the passage by the U.S. Congress of a universal health insurance legislation. Include in your discussion the impact on the demand for health care, the price of health care, and the future of the nursing profession.
6. Define the rationing function of price.
7. In general, consumers are well served in a market economy where goods and services are allocated by the competitive forces of demand and supply with little interference from the government. Should health care be allocated in a similar manner? Discuss the pros and cons of allocating health care by the private market. (Hint: What would happen to access, cost, and quality of health care?)
8. Should health care be paid by taxpayers so that no one will be denied access to needed health care because of his or her inability to pay? Use the examples of Canada and the United Kingdom to answer this question.

REFERENCES

Feldstein, P. J. (1999). *Health care economics* (5th ed.). Albany, NY: Delmar Publishers.
Folland, S., Goodman, A. C., & Stano, M. (1997). *The economics of health and health care* (2nd ed.). Upper Saddle River, NJ: Prentice Hall.
Mankiw, N. G. (1998). *Principles of economics.* Forth Worth, TX: The Dryden Press.

SUGGESTED READINGS

Cleland, V. S. (1990). *The economics of nursing.* Norwalk, CT: Appleton & Lange.
Fuchs, V. R. (1986). Health care and the United States economic system. In V. R. Fuchs (Ed.), *The health economy* (pp. 11–31). Cambridge, MA: Harvard University Press.
Phelps, C. E. (1997). *Health economics* (2nd ed.). Reading, MA: Addison-Wesley.
Santerre, R. E., & Neun, S. P. (2000). *Health economics: Theories, insights, and industry studies* (Revised ed.). Orlando, FL: The Dryden Press.

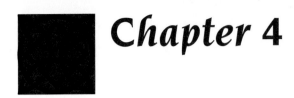

Chapter 4

Why Does Health Care Cost So Much?

Cyril F. Chang

LEARNING OBJECTIVES

- Define inflation and explain why health-care inflation is a critical concern.
- Explore the major trends in inflation and related economic issues.
- Understand how the general price level is measured.
- Discuss why health care is so expensive.
- Discuss why health-care costs are so difficult to control.
- Review the recent history of cost-containment efforts by the government and the private sector.
- Discuss new cost-control strategies such as the prospective payment system and managed care.

 ## WHY IS HEALTH-CARE INFLATION A CONCERN?

The problem of health care inflation has troubled the American health-care system for more than 30 years. Since the implementation of Medicaid and Medicare in the mid-1960s, health-care prices have risen persistently at a rate twice as fast as the general price level. When everyone pays higher prices for health care, insurance and tax rates go up, causing the country as a whole to spend a greater proportion of its national income for health care. This leaves consumers with less to spend on other things that improve the quality of their lives.

Inflation *is an increase in the general price level in an economy.*

Another consequence of high health-care costs is that it exacerbates the critical problem of access to health care. The more costly health care becomes, the heavier a financial burden it places on the nation, making it more difficult to deliver health care to the poor and uninsured. Technologically, American medicine is the envy of the world. But there are 43.4 million uninsured individuals in the United States (Bureau of the Census, 1998), who would probably prefer guaranteed minimum insurance coverage to no health-care coverage at all.

Additional reasons why high health-care costs should be a critical concern were suggested by health economist Victor Fuchs (1993). First, many of the health services utilized by patients do not provide benefits that are commensurate with their costs. These include "defensive medicine," services that provide little or no benefits to patients but are recommended by physicians as protection against possible malpractice lawsuits, as well as many high-cost and low-yield procedures that provide benefits to some patients but on the whole cost more to society than the benefits that they deliver.

Second, the high cost of health care in the United States is partly the result of inefficient use of scarce resources. The American health-care system uses far more resources to produce health-care services than those of Japan, Canada, and most western European countries. The waste and inefficiency are particularly pronounced in three areas: (1) administration, including marketing, insurance claims, and utilization review; (2) excess capacity of facilities, duplication of equipment, and specialized personnel required to operate these facilities and equipment; and (3) fraudulent claims for reimbursements by unscrupulous providers of health-care services and products.

A third reason that Fuchs suggests we should be concerned about health-care inflation is that physicians, hospitals, insurance companies, and pharmaceutical firms in the United States earn high rates of returns to investment. For example, American physicians earn about 35 percent more than their Canadian counterparts (Fuchs, 1993). American pharmaceutical companies consistently earn rates of return higher than the average rates of the manufacturing industry. Lower health-care prices would reduce the abnormally high rates of returns to investment enjoyed by health-care providers in the United States.

This chapter examines why health care is so expensive. It begins with a discussion of how inflation is measured by the federal government and reviews major trends in health-care costs. The root causes of health-care inflation are explored, and past cost-containment policies are reviewed. The chapter ends with a discussion of the reasons for the recent moderation of health-care costs and a prediction of future trends.

 ## MEASURING HEALTH-CARE SECTOR PRICES

WHO MEASURES INFLATION?

Health-care inflation is measured by the Bureau of Labor Statistics (BLS) of the U.S. Department of Labor. This task is performed by the BLS as part of its responsibility to gather and disseminate data on the general price level of the national economy. This is an important governmental function that concerns not only countless numbers of business firms of different sizes but also millions of individual consumers.

The general price level is the average price level of the whole economy.

THE EFFECT OF INFLATION

Figure 4–1 indicates that in 1982 Americans spent an average of $1346 per person for health care (National Center for Health Statistics, 1998). In 1997, the amount measured in current dollars rose to $3925, a 191.6 percent increase in 15 years (Levit et al., 1999). At first glance, this rising trend of health-care spending gives the impression that Americans have vastly increased their use of health-care services. It also implies that in the process, thousands of health-care institutions and organizations, along with the individuals who own them or work in them, have become rich.

Although this is true to some extent, the picture depicted is somewhat exaggerated because of inflation. Although per capita national health-care

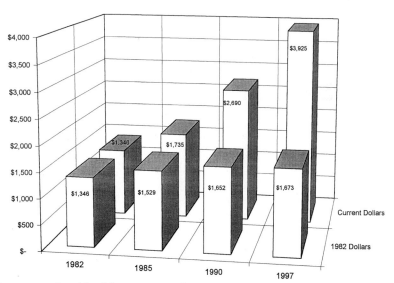

FIG. 4–1. National health-care expenditures in current dollars and 1982 constant dollars. (From National Center for Health Statistics. [1998]. *Health, United States, 1998.* Hyattsville, MD: Public Health Service, p. 344; and Levit, K. R., Cowan, C., Braden, B., Stiller, J., Sensenig, A., & Lazenby, H. (1999). National health expenditures in 1997: More slow growth. *Health Affairs, 17,* 99–110, with permission.)

expenditures rose 191.6 percent from 1982 to 1997, health-care prices increased 2.35 times in the same period (Levit et al., 1999). If health-care prices had not increased, the per capita national health-care expenditures expressed in 1982 dollars would have increased from $1346 to only $1673 ($3925/2.35). This is a much smaller 24.3 percent increase in 15 years. Inflation exaggerates the total amounts of spending because it takes more money to buy the same bundle of services or products when they cost more to consumers.

THE CONSUMER PRICE INDEX

The Bureau of Labor Statistics uses the concept of the *consumer price index* (CPI) to measure the price levels for the economy as a whole and for the major sectors that make up the economy, such as housing, food and clothing, transportation, and health care. For example, the CPI for medical care rose by 128 percent from the base period of 1982–1984 to 1996, whereas the CPI for all goods and services increased by 27 percent (Bureau of Labor Statistics, 1999).

The **consumer price index (CPI)** *is a cost-of-living index that gauges the overall cost (or the price level) of the goods and services bought by a typical household. The federal government reports* **CPI** *estimates for the total economy as well as for major categories of consumer goods such as medical care, food, and energy.*

To calculate the CPI, the BLS collects price data for thousands of goods and services from urban and rural areas across the country. The following example illustrates how the CPI for health care is calculated (Mankiw, 1998). Assume, for simplicity, that patients in a hypothetical health economy utilize two services: hospitalization (in number of inpatient days) and physician or advanced practice nurse services (in number of office visits). The five-step method that the BLS uses to calculate the CPI is as follows (see Table 4–1 for an example):

1. Determine the market basket. The first step in measuring the price index for medical care is to determine which services patients use most often and how much they spend on them. These services are given more weight in the computation of the CPI. The BLS sets these weights by surveying consumers periodically to find out the medical services that consumers typically use. These extensive surveys are conducted once every

decade. This means that the same bundle of goods and services are used as a standard market basket for about 10 years regardless of whether actual spending patterns of consumers have changed within that period. In the example shown in Table 4–1, the typical patient is assumed to visit the physician or advance practice nurse 10 times a year and to stay in the hospital 2 days a year.

TABLE 4–1. CALCULATION OF THE CONSUMER PRICE INDEX AND THE INFLATION RATE FOR THE MEDICAL CARE SECTOR OF THE ECONOMY

Step 1: Survey Utilization Patterns to Determine a Fixed Basket of Medical Services

10 office visits for physician/advanced practice nurse services, and 2 days of hospitalization per year

Step 2: Find the Price of Each Service in Each Year

Year	Price of Office Visits ($)	Price of Hospitalization ($)
1997	50	1000/day
1998	55	1150/day
1999	60	1300/day

Step 3: Compute the Cost of the Basket of Services in Each Year

Year	Cost of Basket
1997	($50 per visit × 10) + ($1000 per day × 2) = $2500
1998	($55 per visit × 10) + ($1150 per day × 2) = $2850
1999	($60 per visit × 10) + ($1300 per day × 2) = $3200

Step 4: Choose One Year as a Base Year (1997) and Compute the Consumer Price Index in Each Year

Year	Consumer Price Index
1997	$(2500/2500) × 100 = 100
1998	$(2850/2500) × 100 = 114
1999	$(3200/2500) × 100 = 128

Step 5: Use the Consumer Price Index to Compute the Inflation Rate from Previous Year

Year	Inflation Rate
1998	(114 − 100)/100 × 100 = 14.0%
1999	(128 − 114)/114 × 100 = 12.3%

The market basket *used in the* CPI *calculation is a hypothetical basket of goods and services that American families typically buy.*

2. Find the prices. The second step is to collect data on the prices of physician visits and hospital days for each time period. Table 4–1 shows the prices paid by patients or their insurance companies for physician or advanced practice nurse visits and hospital care for three different years. Each of the two prices has risen by a different amount from year to year in this example to resemble the patterns of price increases in the actual health-care market.
3. Compute the basket's cost. The next step is to compute the total cost of medical care utilized by the typical patient in each time period. This is done by multiplying the prices at each year by the quantity of services utilized, assuming 10 office visits and 2 hospital days per person per year.
4. Choose a base year and compute the index. The fourth step is to choose a *base year* as the benchmark year against which other years' prices will be compared. In the example in Table 4–1, the year 1997 is chosen as the base year and thus the CPI for that year is set at 100. To calculate the CPI for medical care for 1998, the total amount of medical spending for 1998, $2850, is divided by the base year's total spending of $2500 and multiplied by 100. The CPI for 1998 is thus 114, suggesting that what once cost $100 now costs $114. Similarly, the CPI for 1999 is 128.

Benchmarking *is setting the price level of a particular year as a reference point by which future price levels can be measured.*

5. Compute the inflation rates. The fifth and final step is to use the CPI to calculate the inflation rates. For example, the CPI rose by 14 percent between 1997 and 1998, and 12.3 percent between 1998 and 1999; these percentages are the inflation rates for those periods.

HEALTH-CARE PRICES, 1960–1997

Table 4–2 presents information on the urban CPI, which represents general price levels facing about 80 percent of the noninstitutionalized population in the urban areas of the United States (National Center for Health Statistics, 1998). The price level for the economy as a whole is measured by the data series labeled "CPI for all items." It was 100 for the base period of 1982–1984, and stood at 160.5 in 1997. It is easy to see that the price level has increased by 60.5 percent between 1982–1984 and 1997 (National Cen-

TABLE 4–2. CONSUMER PRICE INDEX FOR ALL ITEMS AND MEDICAL CARE COMPONENTS: UNITED STATES, SELECTED YEARS 1960–1997

Item and Medical Care Component	1960	1965	1970	1975	1980	1985	1989	1990	1993	1994	1995	1996	1997
CPI, all items	29.6	31.5	38.8	53.8	82.4	107.6	124.0	130.7	144.5	148.2	152.4	156.9	160.5
Less medical care	30.2	32.0	39.2	54.3	82.8	107.2	122.4	128.8	141.2	144.7	148.6	152.8	156.3
All medical care	22.3	25.2	34.0	47.5	74.9	113.5	149.3	162.8	201.4	211.0	220.5	228.2	234.6
Medical care services	19.5	22.7	32.3	46.6	74.8	113.2	148.9	162.7	202.9	213.4	224.2	232.4	239.1
Professional medical services	—	—	37.0	50.8	77.9	113.5	146.4	156.1	184.7	192.5	201.0	208.3	215.4
Physicians' services	21.9	25.1	34.5	48.1	76.5	113.3	150.1	160.8	191.3	199.8	208.8	216.4	222.9
Dental services	27.0	30.3	39.2	53.2	78.9	114.2	146.1	155.8	188.1	197.1	206.8	216.5	226.6
Eye care*	—	—	—	—	—	—	112.4	117.3	130.4	133.0	137.0	139.3	141.5
Services by other medical professionals*	—	—	—	—	—	—	114.2	120.2	135.9	141.3	143.9	146.6	151.8
Hospital and related services	—	—	—	—	69.2	116.1	160.5	178.0	231.9	245.6	257.8	269.5	278.4
Hospital rooms	9.3	12.3	23.6	38.3	68.0	115.4	158.1	175.4	226.4	239.2	251.2	261.0	—

75

TABLE 4–2. (CONTINUED)

Item and Medical Care Component	1960	1965	1970	1975	1980	1985	1989	1990	1993	1994	1995	1996	1997
Other inpatient services*	—	—	—	—	—	—	128.9	142.7	185.7	197.1	206.8	216.9	—
Outpatient services*	—	—	—	—	—	—	124.7	138.7	184.3	195.0	204.6	215.1	224.9
Medical care commodities	46.9	45.0	46.5	53.3	75.4	115.2	150.8	163.4	195.0	200.7	204.5	210.4	215.3
Prescription drugs	54.0	47.8	47.4	51.2	72.5	120.1	165.2	181.7	223.0	230.6	235.0	242.9	249.3
Nonprescription drugs and medical supplies*	—	—	—	—	—	—	114.6	120.6	135.5	138.1	140.5	143.1	145.4
Internal and respiratory over-the-counter drugs	—	39.0	42.3	51.8	74.9	112.2	138.8	145.9	163.5	165.9	167.0	170.2	173.1
Nonprescription medical equipment and supplies	—	—	—	—	79.2	109.6	131.1	138.0	155.9	160.0	166.3	169.1	171.5

Source: U.S. Department of Labor, Bureau of Labor Statistics. Consumer price index. Various releases.
Note: 1982–1984 = 100, except where noted.
*Dec. 1986 = 100.
—Data not available.

ter for Health Statistics, 1998). By contrast, the CPI for all medical care increased by 134.6 percent—a rate more than twice as fast as the general price level. When health care is removed from the calculation of the CPI, the resulting measure increased considerably less, by 56.3 percent (National Center for Health Statistics, 1998).

Among the various health-care services, hospital and related services experienced the fastest increase in prices—a 178.4 percent increase from the base period. Prices for physician and dental services also experienced considerable increases: 122.9 percent and 126.6 percent, respectively (National Center for Health Statistics, 1998). Not all health-care prices have risen faster than the general price level. Several categories of services, such as eye care, nonprescription drugs, and medical supplies, experienced slower rates of price increases than the CPI for all items. Note that the services delivered by "other health-care professionals" have in recent years experienced below-average price increases. It is worthy of note that nurses perform many of the services included in this category.

The CPI figures presented in Table 4–2 can be converted into annual percentage changes; these percentage changes are commonly referred to as *inflation rates*. Figure 4–2 presents inflation rates for all items and for medical care, respectively. A careful examination of the average annual percentage

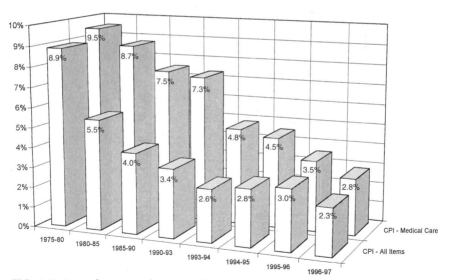

Consumer Price Index (CPI), Annual Percent Change
1982-84=100

FIG. 4–2. Annual percent change in the consumer price index (1982–1984 = 100). (From National Center for Health Statistics. (1998). *Health, United States, 1998.* Hyattsville, MD: Public Health Service, p. 344.)

changes in the CPIs over the entire period from 1975 to 1997 reveals that inflation rates were high from 1975 to 1980, during which time the economy experienced inflation rates of almost 10 percent per year. In recent years, however, prices for both the economy as a whole and the medical care sector have moderated. Today, inflation is less than 3 percent per year for both the overall economy and medical care.

 ## CAUSES OF RISING HEALTH-CARE COSTS

Economists offer two explanations for health-care inflation: the demand-pull theory and the cost-push theory. The *demand-pull theory* hypothesizes that inflation results from too many health-care dollars chasing too few available services. When too much is spent on health care, the demand increases faster than the available supply, causing prices to rise.

> **The demand-pull theory *of inflation hypothesizes that inflation results from too much spending and not enough supply of goods and services.***

The *cost-push theory*, on the other hand, emphasizes four major supply-side factors as the basic driving forces of health-care inflation:

1. The labor-intensive nature of health-care provision and delivery
2. The rising wage rates for health-care workers caused by a persistently strong demand for labor and increased unionization of workers
3. The tendency of the health-care industry to use extremely expensive technology and equipment
4. The fear of malpractice legal actions, which results in the practice of defensive medicine and overuse of resources

> **The cost-push theory *of inflation hypothesizes that inflation results from high and rising costs of doing business.***

The demand-pull and cost-push factors that increase health-care costs, along with the programs and measures that contain costs, are summarized in Figure 4–3.

THE DEMAND-PULL HYPOTHESIS

In the United States, two deep-rooted forces have been responsible for the steady increases in the demand for health care in the last 40 years. The first

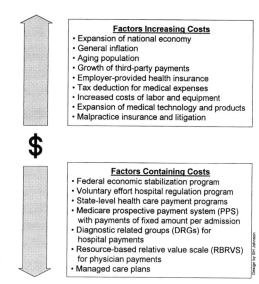

Factors Increasing Costs
- Expansion of national economy
- General inflation
- Aging population
- Growth of third-party payments
- Employer-provided health insurance
- Tax deduction for medical expenses
- Increased costs of labor and equipment
- Expansion of medical technology and products
- Malpractice insurance and litigation

$

Factors Containing Costs
- Federal economic stabilization program
- Voluntary effort hospital regulation program
- State-level health care payment programs
- Medicare prospective payment system (PPS) with payments of fixed amount per admission
- Diagnostic related groups (DRGs) for hospital payments
- Resource-based relative value scale (RBRVS) for physician payments
- Managed care plans

FIG. 4–3. Factors affecting the cost of heath care.

is the gradual rise in living standards, which is supported by the continued long-term expansion of our national economy and the resulting increase in personal incomes. The second is the growth of the population and the accompanying demographic changes, such as the continued aging of the general population. These two factors respond poorly to government programs designed to alleviate the problems caused by these underlying trends.

Rising Income and Aging Population

The living standards of American people have increased steadily since the end of World War II. As income level rises, people desire an increased amount of services that improve the quality of their lives, such as travel, leisure, and, of course, medical care. What were once considered the exclusive privileges of the rich are now deemed necessities for all.

Meanwhile, the population is expanding and getting older. For example, while the general population is projected to grow by 7.1 percent, the "old-old" population (75 and older) will grow 26.2 percent between 1990 and 2000 (Bureau of the Census, 1992). Older persons need more health care. In 1987, people aged 65 and older who had any health-care expenditures spent an average of $4564, compared with $2375 for those aged 45 to 64 and $1250 for those aged 18 to 44 (Prospective Payment Assessment Commission, 1994).

Third-Party Coverage

The American system of health-care financing is referred to as a *third-party payment system* because when services are delivered, patients pay only a relatively small deductible out of their own pockets. Typically, a financial intermediary in the form of a government agency or an insurance company, such as a Blue Cross/Blue Shield Association, pays the bulk of the medical bills based on the costs claimed by the providers. This form of payment arrangement, although providing valuable financial protection for patients, creates several serious side effects with troubling economic consequences.

> **A third-party payment system *is a system of health-care financing whereby providers deliver health care to patients, and a third party or a financial intermediary, usually in the form of an insurance company or a government agency, pays the bill.***

First, cost-based third-party payments eliminate consumers' incentive to economize by shielding them from the financial burden of an unexpected illness. Unless the insurance policy is specially designed to deal with adverse incentive problems, consumers have every reason to demand the best care available even when the potential benefits of treatments cannot justify the costs. Second, until recently, third-party payers routinely paid providers retrospectively on the basis of providers' usual, customary, and reasonable (UCR) charges. This payment method eliminates providers' incentives to behave economically. Worse, it encourages them to overprovide medical care because the more they provide, the more they are reimbursed. Empirical data on third-party payments and health-care inflation provide telling, albeit circumstantial, evidence of this relationship.

> **The UCR charges *are the maximum charges that an insurance company will pay for a given service.***

Over the last four decades, third-party payments as a percentage of total national health-care expenditures grew steadily, from less than 50 percent in 1960 to the present 83 percent (Levit et al., 1999). As third-party involvement increased, out-of-pocket payments by individuals and their families declined and health-care prices spiraled. This link between health-care inflation and third-party payments can be illustrated by an examination of the percentage of third-party coverage of the individual health-care categories.

Table 4–3 shows the proportions of total expenditures covered by third-party payments for several key health-care services from 1980 to 1995. Among the three major health-care items—hospital rooms, physicians' services, and dental services—hospital services have had the highest third-party coverage

TABLE 4–3. PERCENTAGE OF THIRD PARTY COVERAGE

	1980	1985	1990	1995
Hospital rooms	95%	95%	96%	97%
Physicians' services	68	71	82	82
Dental services	34	38	50	53
Other professional services	48	51	59	62
Prescription drugs	19	22	33	40
Eye care	22	26	35	44

Source: Public Health Service, *Health, United States,* various years. Washington, DC: *U.S. Department of Health and Human Services.*

and dental care the lowest. Not surprisingly, there is a close association between the extent of insurance coverage and inflation rates: The more fully health insurance covers the costs of care, the higher the inflation rate.

The more insurance covers health-care costs, the higher the inflation rate.

Favorable Tax Treatment

It has been a workplace tradition since World War II that most Americans obtain their medical insurance coverage through their places of work. In addition, employer-provided health benefits, health insurance premiums, and patients' out-of-pocket medical expenses receive favorable tax treatments under federal income tax laws. These favorable tax treatments encourage the growth of health insurance coverage and, indirectly, the demand for health care. In addition, they discourage substitution of taxable wages or salaries for tax-free insurance benefits. Moreover, they are regressive in that they reduce the tax burden of high-bracket taxpayers more than that of low-bracket taxpayers. These and other favorable tax treatments were originally designed with good intentions to encourage health insurance coverage and provide financial relief to businesses and individuals. However, they have created the unintended side effect of adding pressure on prices by increasing the demand for health insurance coverage and medical services.

THE COST-PUSH HYPOTHESIS

According to the cost-push hypothesis, health-care inflation results from higher prices for the inputs used in the production and delivery of health care. When providers pay higher prices for inputs such as labor and medical equipment, the added costs get passed along to third-party payers. What, then, are the causes of higher input prices?

A major cause is the economy-wide inflation that flared up during most of the 1970s and 1980s. As the general price level rose, hospitals, clinics, and other health-care providers had to pay more for labor, equipment, and supplies to deliver services. Take the cost of hospital care, for instance. A recent study by the congressional Prospective Payment Assessment Commission (1993) suggested that 4.1 percentage points (or 43 percent) of the 9.5 percentage points of the average annual increase in total hospital costs in the period from 1985 to 1991 could be attributed to economy-wide general inflation.

Although general inflation accounts for a substantial portion of health-care inflation, it alone cannot fully explain the persistent high costs of health care, which have consistently outpaced the economy-wide inflation in the last 30 years. The extra inflation in health care is the result of several factors specific to health care.

Technology

Health care is one of the industries that have experienced unprecedented technological changes that few forecasters could have imagined two or three decades ago. Today, in a typical urban community hospital, procedures once considered experimental are performed routinely. Unlike other technology industries, however, technological advances in health care do not reduce costs in general. They do the opposite, in fact.

Medical innovations tend to be inflationary because they are mostly product innovations rather than process innovations, according to health economist Mark Pauly (1978). *Process innovations* are technological advances that enable manufacturers to produce the same products more efficiently and more cheaply. *Product innovations*, on the other hand, are those that improve the product's quality and sophistication. In medicine, the technological progress made in recent years has been mostly the result of product innovations. These innovations are used mostly for improving the breadth and depth of health care and not for reducing costs.

Process innovations *are technological advances that enable providers to deliver the same amount of output more efficiently and cheaply.*

Product innovations *are technological advances that improve the quality and sophistication of a service or product.*

Health-care inflation can be explained as an undesirable consequence of the evolution of medical technology. According to biologist Lewis Thomas (1975), medical technology typically evolves through three stages of development:

1. Nontechnology stage. A period in which technology is primitive, diseases are poorly understood, and patients have little hope.
2. Halfway-technology stage. A period in which better technology adjusts to disease or postpones death at a high cost.
3. High-technology stage. A period in which high technologies, exemplified by immunization, antibiotics for bacterial infections, and nutritional interventions, come from genuine understanding of disease mechanisms. When these technologies become available, they are relatively inexpensive to deliver and are highly effective.

Extending Thomas's observations on the evolution of medical technology, health economist Burton Weisbrod (1991) suggests that "the aggregate effect of technological change in health care costs will depend on the relative degree to which halfway technologies are replacing lower, less costly technologies or are being replaced by new, higher technologies" (p. 534). Unfortunately, few of today's medical technologies fall in the third category of Thomas's classification. Most of the medical technologies that are currently in use are the halfway type, which, though promising in controlling the disease process, deliver half-way results at a very high price.

In nursing, however, opportunities abound to apply technologies that enhance both quality and efficiency, thus controlling costs without sacrificing quality. These include new computer technologies, management information systems for patient care, and new patient management approaches such as nursing case management and total quality management (Zander, 1988).

Malpractice Litigation and Defensive Medicine

In recent years, Americans have turned to the courts in record numbers to redress their health-care grievances. This surge in malpractice litigation has affected health-care delivery and costs in at least three ways (Baily & Cikins, 1984):

1. Malpractice insurance premiums have become increasingly more expensive. In some medical specialties, insurance is unavailable at any price. Court costs, legal fees, and the exorbitant amounts of punitive damages that the courts have often handed down all eventually translate into higher costs for health care.

2. The fear of lawsuits gives rise to the practice of defensive medicine. Providers order tests and procedures that have dubious values to patients in order to protect themselves against possible lawsuits.
3. The threat of litigation and fear of liability slow the progress toward a more efficient and cost-effective system of health-care delivery. Providers and third-party payers may become reluctant to introduce a low-cost style of practice or an alternative delivery system because they may be sued by patients.

How much inflation is caused by malpractice litigation? Physician groups have offered estimates of malpractice costs. For example, the American Medical Association estimated the total costs of unnecessary tests caused by the practice of defensive medicine as $30 billion in 1991 (Eastaugh, 1992). A 1990 Harvard University study provided a lower estimate of $15 billion per year (Eastaugh, 1992). Many economists, although acknowledging the existence of defensive medicine, question whether this practice is caused solely by the fear of malpractice lawsuits. They have suggested the need for more scientific studies, better data collection, and a reduction in the level of emotion and crisis rhetoric that has dominated the current debates on the so-called malpractice crisis.

Interestingly, malpractice claims against nurses have increased in recent years. In one study that examined malpractice claims against nurses filed between 1988 and 1993, nursing negligence was found to have contributed to negative patient outcomes and resulted in a verdict or settlement in 747 cases (Miller-Slade, 1997). In another unusual case, an Arizona hospital's insurance carrier, after settling a case with a patient, sued the insurance carriers of the nurses who allegedly were responsible for the injury resulting in the settlement (Tammelleo, 1997). Today, with hospitals and nursing homes under pressure to cut costs and with nurses, especially advanced practice nurses, taking on additional responsibilities, the chances of nurses getting sued will certainly increase.

 ## COST-CONTAINMENT PROGRAMS

During the last three decades, federal and state governments have attempted a variety of cost-containment programs to restrain the cost of health care. Some of them were carried out through broad-based federal programs that aimed at controlling the general price level of the health-care sector. Others were designed to regulate specific targets, such as the amount of capital investment in the hospital industry or the numbers of medical and nursing school graduates. Still others regulated the prices of specific services, such as physician fees or hospital reimbursement rates. These programs are summarized in this section.

BROAD-BASED COST-CONTROL PROGRAMS

The federal government implemented two broad-based cost-control programs during the inflationary periods of the early and mid-1970s: the Economic Stabilization Program (ESP) and the Voluntary Effort (VE). President Richard Nixon initiated the ESP program in 1971 to combat runaway inflation and stagnant economic growth. During stage I of the program, wages and prices of all goods and services, including health care, were frozen for 90 days. Additional and somewhat less stringent rules and procedures were introduced in the subsequent second, third, and fourth stages. The program formally ended soon after Nixon left the White House in 1974.

The Economic Stabilization Program was the wage and price control program imposed by Richard Nixon in 1971.

After the end of ESP, health-care costs resumed their high rates of acceleration. In response, President Jimmy Carter in late 1977 proposed a program of hospital regulation called the Voluntary Effort, or VE. Hospitals were urged by the federal government to "voluntarily" reduce their rates of cost increases by 2 to 3 percentage points below their previous year's levels. However, the proposal was defeated in Congress in 1979 largely due to the lobbying efforts of the hospital industry. The growth of health spending had also begun to slow, weakening government's justification for the VE program.

The Voluntary Effort was Jimmy Carter's proposal for controlling hospital costs.

The cost-control programs of the Nixon and Carter administrations were mostly ineffective, according to health economists who studied data from that period (Getzen, 1997; Phelps, 1997). Through a combination of mandatory and voluntary cost-control mechanisms, these efforts tended to slow price increases during and immediately after their implementation. But as time went by, with the controls becoming less stringent and providers devising more effective coping strategies, price increases resumed their original long-term growth.

CERTIFICATE OF NEED REGULATION

During the 1970s, when federal broad-based programs were in effect, many states began their own cost-control efforts (Sloan, 1983; Dranove & Cone,

1985). The Certificate of Need (CON) program was widely used by the states to control their hospital costs.

> **T*he* Certificate of Need (CON)** *laws require hospitals to obtain approval from health planning agencies for capital expenditures in excess of a certain threshold amount.*

The CON program aims at regulating hospital expenditures for new beds, equipment purchases, and facility construction. The rationale is that excessive hospital growth is the root cause of hospital inflation because empty beds and underutilized facilities must be maintained. Further, an excess supply of hospital beds presents temptations for hospital administrators and physicians to increase hospital admissions so as to increase occupancy rates for hospitals and income for physicians.

The CON approach to hospital cost control has not been successful, according to many health economists who studied the program (Salkever & Bice, 1979; Feldstein, 1999). It is a conservative approach to cost control that focuses only on hospitals, and it provides no new incentives to change patient or physician behavior.

THE MEDICARE PROSPECTIVE PAYMENT SYSTEM

In October 1983, the federal government changed its method of paying hospitals for treating Medicare patients. Prior to this time, hospitals received cost-based reimbursements from Medicare. That is, hospitals were paid according to their costs irrespective of whether they were high or low compared with other similar hospitals. Because hospitals could shift the costs of treatment to Medicare, they had little incentive to economize. In fact, there existed strong incentives for hospitals to overuse resources because the more they spent, the more they were paid.

In contrast, the prospective payment system (PPS) pays hospitals a fixed, predetermined sum of money for a particular admission. If a hospital can provide the service at a cost below the fixed amount, it pockets the difference. If more resources and money are used than the predetermined amount, the hospital incurs a loss. Under this payment system, hospitals are encouraged to shorten the length of stays and reduce unnecessary resource use to keep costs below the predetermined reimbursement amounts.

> **T*he* prospective payment system (PPS)** *is a hospital payment system that sets payment rates before treatment begins.*

Diagnosis Related Groups

The reimbursement rates under PPS are determined by a patient classification system that relies on Diagnosis Related Groups (DRGs). Medicare patients who need hospitalization are admitted according to their initial diagnosis under 495 DRGs. Each DRG defines a medical condition and its related processes of care. Each DRG is given a flat payment rate based on the national average costs for that DRG. The five leading DRGs based on the number of patients discharged in 1995 are presented in Table 4–4.

Diagnosis Related Groups (DRGs) are the rate-setting categories used by the Medicare PPS to determine payment. Each of the 495 DRGs represents a particular case type. Medicare provides a flat amount of reimbursement for treating patients admitted under a particular DRG.

The DRG rates vary according to several factors. For example, they are modified somewhat for different regions of the country to reflect differences in local wage rates. Rates are also higher for teaching hospitals in recognition that their teaching and training functions necessitate higher costs. Finally, the DRG rates are adjusted annually by Medicare, subject to approval by Congress, to reflect changes in the health-care environment and the resulting increases in national norms of hospital costs.

TABLE 4–4. FIVE LEADING DRGS IN 1995

DRG Code	Description	Average Days of Care	Average Charge per Discharge ($)
005	Extracranial vascular procedures	4.2	13,488
014	Specific cerebrovascular disorders	7.3	10,701
015	Transient ischemic attack and precerebral occlusions	4.3	6,342
024	Seizure and headache, age > 17 with CC	5.7	8,979
075	Major chest procedures	10.9	29,947

Source: Medicare and Medicaid statistical supplement, *Health Care Financing Review,* 1997.

The Prospective Payment System's Effect on Costs

Most hospitals in the United States receive more than half of their revenues from Medicare. How Medicare reimburses hospitals for provision of inpatient and outpatient care has a profound impact on the financial condition and behavior of most hospitals. Moreover, Medicare's influence reaches far beyond the dollars spent directly for care of elderly people and other recipients of Medicare benefits. When Medicare changes its payment system, private health plans usually follow Medicare's lead and implement a similar policy change.

In the first year of PPS (1984), hospitals held their costs down well below the historical growth trend (Prospective Payment Assessment Commission, 1996). The cost per Medicare case rose sharply in the following 6 years, and by the 1990s, hospitals' costs were higher than payments, resulting in negative average margins for hospitals treating Medicare patients. Since the early 1990s, with the economy-wide inflation easing, the overall Medicare costs began to grow more slowly. In 1993, for example, Medicare operating costs per case went up by only 1.2 percent, the smallest increase in the history of the program (Health Care Financing Administration, 1997).

 MANAGED CARE

WHAT IS MANAGED CARE?

Managed care is a health-care system that not only delivers or arranges for the delivery of services but also pays for them. It can therefore be defined as any health-care organization that combines the financing and delivery of health services into one entity. In contrast, the traditional health insurer does not deliver the services itself: It reimburses providers according to the costs of services claimed by the providers (thus the term *fee-for-service* health system).

> **Managed care *is a health-care system that combines the financing and delivery of health services into a single entity.***

When the traditional form of health insurance dominated the health-care industry in the 1960s and 1970s, managed care was seen as an alternative delivery system. But enrollment in managed care grew rapidly in the 1980s and 1990s. Today, according to the statistics presented in Figure 4–4, more than 40 million insured Americans, or 75 percent of the enrolled population

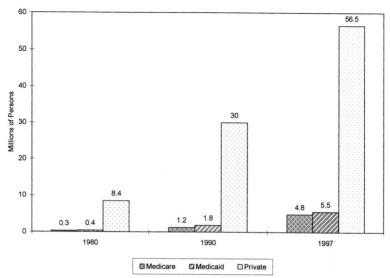

FIG. 4–4. HMO enrollment trends. (National Center for Health Statistics. [1998]. *Health, United States, 1998.* **Hyattsville, MD: Public Health Service, Table 135.)**

in the private sector, are in a managed care health plan of some form, compared with fewer than 50 percent of the insured population in 1990.

The 1990s also saw steady growth of managed care enrollment in the public sector. At present, 32 percent of the Medicaid population and 12 percent of the Medicare population are under managed care (Health Care Financing Administration, 1997). These developments have had remarkable restraining influences on the cost of medical care.

For example, a national study of 11.7 million patients at 3700 acute care hospitals conducted by researchers from the accounting and consulting firm KPMG Peat Marwick concluded that hospital costs vary significantly with the local level of managed care penetration (KPMG Peat Marwick, 1997). Specifically, hospital costs in markets with a high percentage of managed care were approximately 19 percent below those of hospitals in markets with a low percentage of managed care. In addition, hospital stays were 6.32 percent shorter in the former markets than the national average. For years, the medical care CPI grew at a rate twice as fast as the overall CPI for the economy. Since 1990, however, the CPI for all items and the CPI for medical care have been converging. In 1996, the medical care CPI grew 3.5 percent and the CPI for all items less medical care grew 2.9 percent, the narrowest differential since 1991 (Tammelleo, 1997).

ECONOMIC ANALYSIS
IS MANAGED CARE A FRIEND OR FOE?

Many nursing leaders believe that managed care extends many benefits to nursing. For example, managed care has created new professional opportunities, ranging from utilization review to case management. These are satisfying jobs that improve the quality of care by monitoring the appropriateness of the care delivered to managed care patients while economizing on the use of health-care resources.

COST-SAVING MANAGED CARE PRACTICES

Managed care gained popularity in the inflationary periods of the 1980s and early 1990s because it was generally seen as a cost-saving alternative to the traditional fee-for-service delivery system. The following list summarizes practices used by managed care organizations to control resource utilization and health-care costs:

- *Provider networks and selective provider contracting.* Managed care health plans restrict patients' choice of providers. Usually, only those providers who agree to a set of practice rules and standards are invited to participate in a provider network. Some health plans even use providers' practice styles and whether they meet established goals of cost-effective use of resources as criteria for admission into the network. The cost-conscious managed care health plans are also more receptive to nonphysician providers of primary care, such as advanced practice nurses and nurse midwives, than traditional health plans. An increasingly large number of these nonphysician health-care workers now deliver care routinely in the new managed care environment.
- *Payment methods and risk sharing.* An important cost-controlling mechanism used by managed care is an incentive-based reimbursement method that shifts some of the financial risks to providers. For example, many managed care plans use a prospective payment mechanism called *capitation* to pay for services delivered. Instead of paying providers for each service provided, a capitation system pays a lump-sum payment per enrollee per month to providers for all the medically necessary care for an enrolled population. If the providers can keep the enrollees under their care healthy, they pocket the cost savings; if they cannot, they must take a financial loss. Because the amounts of payment are predetermined, the providers share the financial risks with the managed care health plan.

- *Gatekeeping.* Many managed care organizations use primary care physicians or advanced practice nurses as gatekeepers who serve as the patient's primary contact for medical care and referrals to specialists. With gatekeepers directing patients to the most appropriate service setting, managed care health plans reduce unnecessary resource use and the costs of health care.
- *Utilization review.* Utilization review (UR) refers to a variety of managed care practices that rely on rules and incentives to directly affect providers' clinical decisions. Preadmission authorization for the use of hospital inpatient services, case management to monitor the appropriateness of service delivery, and practice guidelines are examples of UR techniques to control unnecessary use of resources. Most managed care organizations use health-care workers with a nursing background to carry out these UR functions.

Utilization review *is a process through which an insurer or health plan reviews the appropriateness of the care delivered by physicians and other providers.*

- *Favorable selection of relatively healthy enrollees.* Because healthier enrollees cost less for a health plan, managed care organizations are known to seek out, or "cherry pick," younger and healthier enrollees and avoid sicker patients. These practices are illegal in most states and are rarely practiced overtly by managed care organizations. However, strong financial incentives exist for managed care organizations to engage in this practice.

SUMMARY

The American health-care system is currently undergoing unprecedented changes that few policy makers could have predicted only a few years ago. Gone are the old-style, cost-based reimbursement mechanisms that routinely allowed providers to shift their costs to insurance companies and other public and private health insurers. In their place, new relationships between providers and third-party payers and among providers themselves have been formed.

Public and private employers have become more aggressive in demanding smaller increases in total health-care spending and the insurance premiums that they pay. They have increasingly encouraged their employees to enroll in a variety of managed care health plans that use incentives to economize the use of scarce health-care resources.

Meanwhile, Medicare and Medicaid, the two largest government-sponsored health insurance programs, began to control aggregate spending by paying hospitals, physicians, and other providers capitated payments for caring for the health-care needs of a given enrolled population. These two government insurance programs have also offered enrollees a variety of incentives to increase managed care enrollment.

As a result of this combination of new public- and private-sector cost-control efforts, health-care prices and national health-care spending have slowed to their lowest levels in the 30 years since the implementation of Medicare and Medicaid in the mid-1960s. Because economy-wide inflation remains low and the health-care system continues to move toward managed care, health-care spending can be expected to remain on its new and slower growth path (Sensenig, Heffler, & Donham, 1997). This has led many forecasters to predict that health-care spending as a percentage of gross domestic product has peaked at 14 percent and will begin to decline.

Although the news from the price front has been encouraging, many difficult issues remain to be resolved. For example, as managed care health plans continue to demand more savings and offer greater incentives to entice providers to economize resources and save money, quality of care and medical outcomes may suffer. This possibility should be carefully monitored to ensure that all Americans, whether young or old, male or female, rich or poor, continue to receive the most cost-effective and high-quality medical care that the health-care system can deliver.

DISCUSSION QUESTIONS

1. Why is health-care inflation a critical concern for all Americans?
2. Define the terms *inflation* and CPI. What are the latest inflation rates for the economy and the various components of health care, such as hospital rooms, physician services, dental care, and prescription drugs? Can you find the Internet home page addresses where inflation and CPI statistics can be downloaded?
3. What are the two economic theories of inflation?

4. Do you agree that medical technology drives the cost of health care? Provide examples of medical technological advances that drive up the cost of health care.

5. Is technology always inflationary? Why is technology inflationary in health care and less so in the rest of the economy?

6. Do you agree with the following statement: "If lawyers were forbidden to sue doctors and hospitals, health-care inflation would be much lower"? Discuss fully.

7. Explain the following statement: "The inflation that we have experienced in health care has more to do with the Internal Revenue Service than with the federal Health Care Financing Administration that administers the Medicaid and Medicare programs."

8. Explain the term *managed care* and contrast it with the traditional form of health insurance that pays providers on a fee-for-service basis.

9. What are the cost-saving techniques used by managed care health plans to economize the use of resources?

10. What has been the major accomplishment of managed care in the last 10 years, and what are the major challenges that it faces today?

 REFERENCES

Baily, M. A ., & Cikins, W. I. (Eds). (1984). *The effects of litigation on health care costs.* Washington, DC: The Brookings Institution.

Bureau of the Census. (1992). *Statistical abstract of the U. S., 1991* (111th ed.). Washington, DC: U.S. Department of Commerce.

Bureau of the Census. (1998). *Current population reports: Health insurance coverage, 1997* (Publication No. P60–202). Washington, DC: U.S. Department of Commerce.

Bureau of Labor Statistics. (1999). Consumer price index [On-line]. Available: http://stats.bls.gov/news.release/cpi.toc.htm.

Dranove, D., & Cone, K. (1985). Do state rate-setting regulations really lower hospital expense? *Journal of Health Economics, 4*(2), 159–165.

Eastaugh, S. R. (1992). *Health economics.* Westport, CT: Auburn House.

Feldstein, P. (1999). *Health economics* (5th ed.). Albany, NY: Delmar Publishers.

Fuchs, V. R. (1993). *The future of health policy.* Cambridge, MA: Harvard University Press.

Getzen, T. E. (1997). *Health economics.* New York: John Wiley & Sons.

Health Care Financing Administration. (1997). Managed care in Medicare and Medicaid: Fact sheet [On-line]. Available: http://www.hcfa.gov/facts/f970128.htm.

KPMG Peat Marwick, LLP. (1997). *The impact of managed care on U.S. markets.* Author. New York.

Levit, K. R., Cowan, C., Braden, B., Stiller, J., Sensenig, A., & Lazenby, H. (1999). National health expenditures in 1997: More slow growth. *Health Affairs, 17*(6), 99–110.

Mankiw, N. G. (1998). *Principles of economics.* Forth Worth, TX: The Dryden Press.

Miller-Slade, D. (1997). Liability theories in nursing negligence cases. *Trial, 33*(5), 52.

National Center for Health Statistics. (1998). *Health, United States, 1998: With socioeconomic status and health chartbook.* Hyattsville, MD: National Center for Health Statistics, 1998.

Pauly, M. (1978). The structure of health insurance and the erosion of competition in the Medicare marketplace. In W. Greenberg (Ed.), *Competition in the health care sector: Past, present, and future* (pp. 270–287). Washington, DC: Federal Trade Commission.

Phelps, C. E. (1997). *Health economics* (2nd ed.). Reading, MA : Addison-Wesley.

Prospective Payment Assessment Commission. (1993). *Medicare and the American health care system* [report to Congress]. Washington, DC: Author.

Prospective Payment Assessment Commission. (1994). *Medicare and the American health care system* [report to Congress]. Washington, DC: Author.

Prospective Payment Assessment Commission. (1996). *Medicare and the American health care system* [report to Congress]. Washington, DC: Author.

Salkever, D. & Bice, T. (1979). *Hospital Certificate-of-Need controls: Impact on investment, costs and use.* Washington, DC: American Enterprise Institute.

Sensenig, A. L., Heffler, S. K., & Donham, C. S. (1997). Hospital, employment, and price indicators for the health care industry: First quarter 1997. *Health Care Financing Review,* 19(1), 207–249.

Sloan, F. A. (1983). Rate regulation as a strategy for hospital cost control: Evidence from the last decade. *Milbank Memorial Fund Quarterly/Health and Society,* 61(2), 196–221.

Tammelleo, A. D. (1997). Hospital's insurer pays $1.4 million and sues nurses' insurer. *Regan Report on Nursing Law,* 38(3), 1.

Thomas, L. (1975). *The Lives of a Cell.* New York: Bantam Books.

Weisbrod, B. A. (1991). The health care quadrilemma: An essay on technological change, insurance, quality of care, and cost containment. *Journal of Economic Literature,* 29(2), 523–552.

Zander, K. (1988). Nursing case management: Strategic management of cost and quality outcomes. *Journal of Nursing Administration,* 18(5), 18–24.

 ## SUGGESTED READING

Fuchs, V. R. (1998). *Who shall live?* River Edge, NJ: World Scientific.

Newhouse, J. P. (1992). Medical care costs: How much welfare loss? *Journal of Economic Perspectives,* 6(3), 3–22.

Schwartz, W. B., & Mendelson, D. N. (1991). Hospital containment in the 1980s. *New England Journal of Medicine,* 324(15), 1037–1042.

Sloan, F. A., Morrisey, M. A., & Valvona, J. (1988). Effects of Medicare prospective payment system on hospital cost containment: An early appraisal. *Milbank Quarterly,* 66(2), 191–219.

Sloan, F. A., & Steinwald, A. B. (1980). Effects of regulation on hospital costs and input use. *Journal of Law and Economics,* 23(1), 81–109.

Part II

The Nursing Labor Market

In addition to being concerned about patient care, nurses should be concerned about their own employment opportunities, compensation, and other career- and job-related issues. To assist nurses in understanding their own labor market, Part II focuses on how market forces affect the supply and demand for nursing services, which are derived from the overall need for health care. An economic model of wage determination is presented to illustrate how the labor market, working through the mechanism of wage adjustment, determines the numbers of nurses at specified wage levels. This wage model is then applied to the fluctuations in the nursing labor market to explain nursing shortages and surpluses.

Nursing education is central to the preparation of clinicians who provide needed bedside services. However, the demand for a nursing workforce has rarely been matched appropriately by the available supply in the past 30 years. These imbalances have led to repeated attempts to examine the supply, demand, and quality of nursing education. For example, the Pew Health Professions Commission has influenced the direction of nursing education at all levels through its involvement in assessing the labor market conditions for

nurses and other health-care professionals. The final chapter
of Part II discusses the labor market for nursing by applying
the economic concepts already presented.

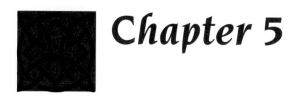

Chapter 5

The Economics of
Labor Markets

Cyril F. Chang
Sylvia A. Price
Susan K. Pfoutz

LEARNING OBJECTIVES

■ Define the concept of a labor market.
■ Introduce the basic economic model of the labor market and the concept of labor market equilibrium.
■ Discuss what determines wages, employment, and labor productivity.
■ Discuss what causes wages and employment to change.
■ Give examples of wage and employment determination in nursing.
■ Discuss the significance of workforce planning.
■ Clarify the complex concepts of labor shortage and surplus.
■ Use the economic model of the labor market to explain the nursing shortage.

According to the Bureau of Labor Statistics, close to 11 million people are employed in the American health-care system, which accounts for nearly 9 percent of the total civilian workforce. Of this total, about 2 million are active nurses of various levels of training and certification. Nurses are the largest group of health-care professionals in the United States.

Over the last 15 years, the nursing profession has experienced faster growth than most other health professions. For example, as shown in Table 5–1, the number of active registered nurses (RNs) increased by 66 percent between 1980 and 1995. In contrast, the number of total active physicians increased by 58 percent during the same period, while that of dentists and pharmacists increased by 34 and 28 percent, respectively.

Nurses are the frontline workers in health care. They traditionally have been employed in hospitals and in doctors' offices. Increasingly, they are finding employment opportunities in a wide variety of alternative clinical and nontraditional practice settings, such as insurance claims administration, case management, managed care gatekeeping, quality assurance, and health-care administration. Irrespective of the work setting, nurses have encountered numerous new challenges in the labor market. These include, but are not limited to, the need for:

• Appropriate cross-training
• Information technology skills

TABLE 5–1. ACTIVE HEALTH PERSONNEL, UNITED STATES, 1980 AND 1995

Occupation	1980	1995	% Change
	Persons in 1000s		
All employed civilians	99,303	124,900	25.8
All active health-care personnel	7,339	11,199	52.6
Physicians	427	673	57.5
Dentists	121	163	34.4
Pharmacists	143	182	27.7
Registered nurses	1,273	2,116	66.2
Associate and diploma	908	1,235	36.0
Baccalaureate	297	673	126.4
Master's and doctorate	67	208	208.3

Source: U.S. Department of Health and Human Services. (1998) *Health, United States.* Washington, DC: Public Health Services. Tables 99 and 103.

- Satisfactory compensations and job security
- Recognition of their professionalism

Nurses, like professionals in other fields, are concerned about their own careers and a wide range of workforce issues, such as compensation, employment opportunities, and professional satisfaction, that can affect their job performance and patient outcomes. Knowledge about these labor market issues is important for understanding how the labor market creates jobs and sets wages. Labor market knowledge is useful in another and more direct way: it helps nurses to make better career choice and job market decisions.

Nursing positions have gone through recurring cycles of ups and downs. During periods of strong demand, many positions open up with few nurses applying for them. But when employers stop hiring, either because of an oversupply of nurses or insufficient demand for health care, many nurses look for few existing vacancies. In most professions, salaries and benefits increase in times of rising labor demand. But in nursing, this does not usually happen, making many nurses wonder whether economics is applicable to health care.

This chapter presents an elementary model of wage determination using the simple concepts of supply, demand, and market equilibrium. Its purpose is to explain the determination of nursing wages and employment and to provide the tools and concepts needed to analyze what causes wage and employment levels to change. These concepts and tools can be used to analyze many economic questions, such as why nursing wages and employment frequently fluctuate with cost-containment efforts and why some specialties of nursing have experienced faster employment growth than other specialties.

 ## AN ECONOMIC MODEL OF THE LABOR MARKET

THE DEMAND FOR LABOR AS A DERIVED DEMAND

The nursing labor market and the market for health care are closely related. The demand for nursing labor is derived from the demand for general health care such as hospital care, nursing-home care, and home health services. As the demand for health services increases, so does the demand for nurses. This close relationship between health care and the nursing workforce will be illustrated using the demand for advanced practice nurses (APNs) as an example, although the economic principles discussed here apply to nurses of all levels of training and certification.

APNs are a group of highly skilled nursing personnel who have earned advanced degrees and received clinical training in a variety of specialties, such as family medicine, pediatrics, anesthesiology, and midwifery. In the current health-care market, the emphasis is on the delivery of primary care and preventive services to reduce the need for costly inpatient services. Health-care employers hire more APNs because they have been shown to be cost effective in delivering primary and preventive services. Thus, as the demand for these health services rises, so does the demand for APNs.

Figure 5–1 illustrates the relationship between the demand for health services and the demand for APNs. Figure 5–1A depicts the determination of the price of primary care delivered by APNs, and Figure 5–1B the determination of the wage level (W) of APNs. The relationship between the two parts of the figure is that changes in the market for primary care (A) create a spillover effect on the labor market for APNs (B). With an increase in the demand for primary care, for example, the demand for APNs increases, resulting in a greater number of APNs hired to satisfy the greater demand for primary care. The demand for APNs or any other type of worker is thus called a *derived demand* because it is usually derived from the demand for the final product or services that a particular type of worker produces. An important implication of this discussion is that health-care workers can benefit from a good understanding of the trends and events in the overall health-care market because what happens there can affect their own job and pay.

A derived demand *is the demand for labor that is derived from the demand for the final product that labor helps to produce.*

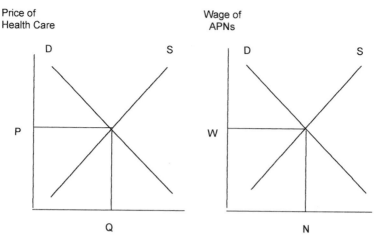

FIG. 5–1. The demand for health care and the demand for advanced practice nurses. *D* = market demand; *N* = number of APNs employed; *P* = market price of health care; *Q* = quantity of health care delivered; *S* = market supply; *W* = market wage. *(A)* The health care market. *(B)* The labor market for APNs.

ECONOMIC ANALYSIS
INSURANCE COVERAGE AND NURSING JOBS

Since the establishment of Medicare and Medicaid, the demand for health care has risen steadily. In 1965, for example, national health-care expenditures were about 5 percent of the gross domestic product (GDP). Today, over 14 percent of the GDP is devoted to the purchase of health-care services. As the demand for health care rose, the demand for nursing personnel increased, resulting in steady increases in the ranks of professional nurses of various training levels and certifications.

AN EMPLOYER'S DECISION TO HIRE

Another useful concept for understanding how the labor market functions is the principle that governs an employer's decision to hire. When employers hire more workers, they create jobs and tend to pay more to achieve the desired size of their workforce. This can be illustrated by how a health-care institution, such as a health maintenance organization (HMO), makes decisions on the number of APNs to hire and the amount of salary to pay. An understanding of this process helps to explain why nurses in some specialties have experienced faster growth in employment and compensation than have nurses in other specialties.

An HMO is a prepaid health plan that takes on the responsibility of satisfying the health-care needs of a group of people, called *enrollees*, in exchange for a prenegotiated monthly premium. Assume that an innovative HMO provides primary care to its enrollees through an APN-led primary care network. When making a decision on the appropriate number of APNs to hire to fully staff the primary care network, an HMO must first know how many patients for whom it is responsible. It must also estimate how much of the various medically necessary services the HMO is obligated to provide and how much care the enrollees are expected to utilize. Once the size of the enrolled population and their health-care needs are known, the number of APNs to hire to deliver the needed primary care service depends on a combination of two additional critical factors:

1. The value to the HMO of an additional APN in terms of the primary care service attributable to that employee
2. The costs of hiring that extra APN

An HMO will hire more APNs as long as the expected contribution of each new hire, in terms of additional patient care provided, exceeds the cost of hiring that person.

How much additional primary care service can one more APN deliver for the HMO? What is the dollar worth of another APN to the employer in terms of the additional output that he or she can produce? The answers depend primarily on the APN's productivity: The more productive the APN is, all other things being equal, the more valuable his or her service is to the organization and the more likely that he or she will be hired. What, then, determines an APN's productivity?

Productivity is the ratio between the amount of input and the quantity of output. Input for health-care services includes health-care workers' time on the job, along with a host of facility, medical supply, and technology factors that make up the work setting. Output includes the numbers and types of services provided and the resulting health-care outcomes. Productivity is said to have increased if more output can be produced with the use of the same number of labor hours.

Harvard economist N. Gregory Mankiw (1998) notes that labor productivity varies with three key economic factors:

1. Physical capital. When workers work with modern equipment and facilities, their productivity increases.
2. Human capital. When workers are more educated, they become more skilled and productive.
3. Technological knowledge. When workers have access to state-of-the-art technologies, they become more productive.

Applying Mankiw's concept of labor productivity to health care, a health-care worker's productivity varies with such personal and work-environment factors as his or her professional training and job skills, the number and types of other health-care workers with whom the employee works, and the medical technologies used in the delivery of health care. Thus, more APNs are likely to be hired if they are productive, highly educated and skilled, work well with complementary workers as a team, and utilize cost-effective technologies.

THE LAW OF DIMINISHING RETURNS

Will an employer hire too many APNs because they are excellent employees considering the costs of hiring them and the quality of their work? No, the labor market has a built-in economic mechanism that prevents this malfunction from happening. As more APNs are hired, assuming the number of other health-care personnel and the size of the facility remain the same, the contribution of the next APN eventually diminishes. This gradual decline in productivity as more of a particular type of health-care worker are hired is called the *law of diminishing returns*. The HMO stops hiring when the next APN costs more than his or her contribution in terms of the market value of the final output contributed.

> **The law of diminishing returns *describes a phenomenon in production whereby adding units of an input (e.g., the service of APNs) to work with fixed amounts of other inputs (e.g., the size of a facility and the number of other types of health-care providers) causes the contribution of the additional input to eventually decline.***

ECONOMIC ANALYSIS
NURSING PRODUCTIVITY IN AMBULATORY CARE

Saint Thomas Hospital recently built an ambulatory cardiac rehabilitation center with state-of-the art cardiac monitoring equipment (physical capital). Sally Jones is a nurse case manager in ambulatory surgery. Jim Smith, a 70-year-old man, requires an angioplasty with a stent. Sally obtains preoperative authorization for the procedure from the managed care organization, schedules preoperative testing, and imparts patient education. On the day of surgery, Bob Jones, a cardiology clinical nurse specialist, greets the patient and family to orient them to the process of care. He monitors the patient before, during, and following the surgical procedure. At discharge, Sally arranges for home health care follow-up because the patient lives alone. This combination of the three factors of physical and human capital and technological expertise enables the delivery of complex health care at decreased cost by eliminating the need for hospitalization.

 ## LABOR MARKET EQUILIBRIUM

Having considered the hiring decision of an individual employer in the previous example, the analysis now shifts to the labor market for nursing as a whole. The central issue here is how wage and employment levels of a particular occupation such as nursing are determined and what role labor demand and supply play in this determination.

THE LABOR DEMAND AND SUPPLY CURVES

Extending the APN example from an individual HMO to the whole managed care industry, we now ask: How many APNs will all HMOs as a group hire? This is a question about the market demand for APNs, in contrast with the demand for APNs by an individual HMO employer.

The labor market demand curve is illustrated in Figure 5–2. This curve (labeled D) slopes downward to the right, indicating that the total number of APNs hired decreases as the market wage level increases. As APNs become more expensive, other things being equal, employers will use other types of personnel who have similar skills as substitutes, thus reducing the number of APNs hired.

Wage

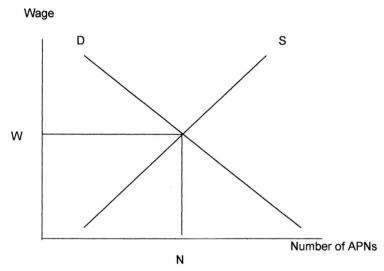

FIG. 5–2. Labor market equilibrium. *D* = market demand for APNs; *N* = equilibrium employment; *S* = market supply of APNs; *W* = equilibrium wage.

The **market demand for labor** *is the relationship between the number of workers that an industry is willing to hire and the possible wage levels.*

The *market supply of labor* is the relationship between the amount of labor services that workers are willing to supply and the possible wage rates. Once again, our illustration focuses on APNs. The market supply curve in Figure 5–2 (labeled S) slopes upward, indicating that at a higher wage rate, a larger number of APNs look for work. Some of the increases in labor services are provided by existing APNs who are willing to work overtime for higher pay, and some by returning APNs who were previously inactive for a variety of reasons and now have reactivated their practice.

The **market supply of labor** *is the relationship between the number of workers willing to work and the possible wage levels.*

In Figure 5–2, the equilibrium wage and employment levels are determined by the interaction of labor market demand (D) and supply (S). The wage that prevails in the market for APNs, called the *equilibrium wage rate*, is labeled W. The resulting quantity of APNs employed, called the *equilibrium level of employment*, is labeled N.

> **The equilibrium wage rate** *is the wage level at the equilibrium point.* **The equilibrium level of employment** *is the total number of employees who have a job at the equilibrium point.*

An important lesson from this market analysis is that the competitive forces of supply and demand have a tendency to drive the labor market to its *equilibrium point*—the point at which the number of APNs willing to work is equal to the number that employers are willing to hire at the prevailing wage rate (W). This intersection point of the demand and supply curves depicts a situation in which the demand and supply are in balance. Because employers have hired the number of APNs that they are willing to hire at the going wage rate and all the APNs willing to work for that wage have been hired, the two sides have little incentive to change.

> **The equilibrium point** *is reached when the number of employees needed (quantity demanded) equals the number available (quantity supplied).*

Once the equilibrium levels of wages and employment are established, can they change? If so, what are the factors that can cause them to change? These questions are discussed in the next section.

SHIFTS IN THE MARKET DEMAND CURVE

Labor markets, like the markets for consumer goods, undergo constant changes. These changes give rise to changes in both how much workers are paid and how many are hired. Now suppose that because patients are being discharged from hospitals sicker and quicker, requiring convalescent or rehabilitation services, the demand for alternative acute care and home health services increases. This results in additional derived demand for RNs who specialize in the treatment of postoperative patients or rehabilitation patients who are recovering at an alternative acute care facility or at home. This increase in the demand for RNs and the resulting impact on wages and employment are illustrated in Figure 5–3, where the demand for RNs has shifted to the right from D_1 to D_2 as a result of an increase in the demand for postoperative and rehabilitative care.

After the demand for RNs has increased from D_1 to D_2, the number of RNs that hospitals and other employers wish to hire (N_3) exceeds the number of RNs who are willing to work (N_1) at the original wage rate of W_1. With the number of RNs demanded outpacing the number supplied, the wage level

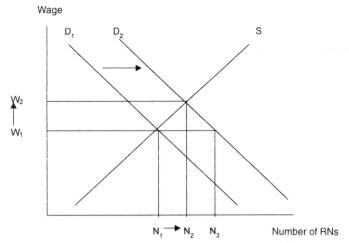

FIG. 5–3. An increase in the demand for registered nurses. D_1 = initial market demand for RNs; D_2 = increased market demand for RNs; N_1 = number of RNs initially employed; N_2 = number of RNs eventually employed after the increase in demand; N_3 = number of RNs demanded by employers at the original wage rate of W_1 immediately after the increase in demand; S = market supply of RNs; W_1 = initial market wage rate; W_2 = market wage rate after the increase in supply.

will rise from W_1 to W_2 and the employment level from N_1 to N_2. This example shows that nurses benefit from greater demand for health-care services and share the prosperity of the entire health-care industry. Workers in other industries, such as steel, automobile, and information technology, understand that their wages and job security are closely tied to the prices paid for the final products of their industry. They have consistently supported measures that increase the demand for the products of their industries. Similarly, nurses have traditionally supported legislation and government programs that expand insurance coverage to the uninsured and underinsured because the added payments for health services increase health-care workers' salaries and job opportunities.

SHIFTS IN THE MARKET SUPPLY CURVE

Although the market demand for labor is subject to change, so is the market supply of labor. The market supply of labor typically changes in response to at least four factors, including immigration, wages in other markets, cost of education, and population changes.

Immigration

The United States has a long history of using foreign-born nurses in times of nursing shortages (Feldstein, 1999). Immigration increases the number of foreign-trained nurses and closes the gap between demand and supply, thus reducing a labor shortage. As time elapses, however, the labor supply curve increases from S_1 to S_2, as depicted in Figure 5–4. When more RNs look for work, the equilibrium wage rate decreases from W_1 to W_2 while more RNs, including many foreign-trained ones, are now employed.

Wage Rates in Other Labor Markets

The supply of RNs is closely linked to wages paid in related labor markets where RNs can find work. For example, many new job opportunities are now opening up in alternative clinical practice settings such as home health care, schools, and occupational health and in nontraditional work settings such as insurance claims processing, gatekeeping in managed care, and pharmaceutical sales. When higher wages are paid in these settings, many RNs leave the traditional workplaces of hospitals and clinics. As a result, the supply of RNs in the traditional labor markets will decrease, as represented by a leftward shift of the supply curve. This will result in a lower employment

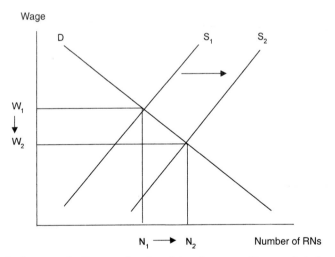

FIG. 5–4. An increase in the supply of registered nurses. *D* = market demand for RNs; *N*₁ = number of RNs initially employed; *N*₂ = number of RNs eventually employed after the increase in supply; *S*₁ = initial market supply of RNs; *S*₂ = increased market supply of RNs; *W*₁ = initial market wage; *W*₂ = the market wage rate after the increase in supply.

level for RNs working in the traditional settings. But those who stay will see their wages rise as demand begins to outstrip the limited supply.

Changes in the Costs of Education and Training

There are strict educational requirements for becoming an RN. The necessary skills and training require both time and money. When the cost of becoming an RN increases, the supply of RNs will decrease (a leftward shift of the market supply curve), raising the wage level but reducing the level of employment. If nursing education and training are subsidized, with nursing students paying only part of the total costs, the supply of RNs will increase (a rightward shift of the market supply curve). This change in policy results in lower wage rates but higher employment. Expansion of nursing school capacity can therefore be a double-edged sword: When more nursing students enter the job market and join the ranks of active nurses after completing their education and training, the added supply, though beneficial to patients, tends to depress wages and benefits.

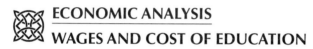

ECONOMIC ANALYSIS
WAGES AND COST OF EDUCATION

Because the cost of collegiate education in nursing continues to rise, there is pressure for an increase in wages for nursing service in hospitals and community agencies. Many clinical ladders (a strategy promoting horizontal advancement of nurses) include wage incentives for graduates holding bachelor of science in nursing (BSN) degrees. This confirms the prediction that higher costs of education reduce labor supply and raise nursing salaries.

Population Changes

The supply of labor can change as a result of population changes. For example, as the number of young people in the age range from 18 to 24 decreases, fewer of them will enter nursing schools. The resulting declines in nursing graduates in a few years will shift the supply of RNs to the left in Figure 5–4. As a result, wage rates will rise but employment will fall. The average age of nurses is rising. In 1997 it was 43.3 years for all nurses and 42.3 years for active nurses (Moses, 1997). There thus may be a shortage of nurses if many retire between the ages of 55 and 65. As they age, nurses tend to work less and to move out of hospital settings (Brewer, 1997).

ECONOMIC ANALYSIS
POPULATION CHANGES

In cities where colleges draw a large percentage of the population, nursing supply can fluctuate based on the college schedule. For example, nurses who are the spouses of students move into the area when school starts and leave when the spouse graduates. This creates a labor shortage of nurses in these areas in the spring of each year and a surplus in the fall.

LABOR MARKET EQUILIBRIUM: A SUMMARY

Several important conclusions regarding nurses' wages and employment emerge from the labor market analysis. They are summarized in the following list to show how the various market forces interact to affect each other.

1. The competitive forces of supply and demand determine the market wage rates for nurses.
2. Nursing wage rates can rise with either an increase in the demand for nursing labor or a decrease in the supply of labor. However, these two changes have opposite effects on nursing employment: The former increases employment whereas the latter decreases it.
3. An increase in the demand for a nursing workforce usually originates from an increase in consumer demand for health care that nurses participate in producing and delivering. These increases cause nursing wages and employment to rise at the same time.
4. A decrease in the supply of the nursing workforce can be accomplished by a tightening up of immigration laws, closing down nursing schools, and increasing the costs of nursing education and training. With fewer nurses available to meet the needs of patients, wages tend to move up. However, a decrease in the supply of labor has the effect of lowering the number of nurses employed.

 WORKFORCE PLANNING

Workforce planning refers to concerted efforts by government agencies and professional organizations to bring the supply of health-care personnel in line with the anticipated demand. This work is important for ensuring an adequate supply of health-care workers. It also has many resource-allocation implications for the health-care system of a country or a state because it costs time and money for educational institutions to redesign their programs and curricula to adjust to an anticipated labor surplus or shortage. No wonder that workforce planning has long played an important role in the U.S. health-care system.

Workforce planning *is a coordinated effort by government and professional organizations to study, plan, and make recommendations to bring the labor supply in line with labor demand.*

Over the years, the federal government has worked closely with the states, their educational institutions, and the various professional organizations to improve the health workforce planning process. A major workforce planning effort by the federal government has been to provide construction subsidies to improve and expand the physical capacity of educational institutions and to provide student loans to make it possible for future health-care workers to acquire the necessary education and training. The success of this effort depends on accurate and reliable estimates of the different types of health-care workers that will be needed at a future point in time. The estimation and planning process begins with a clear understanding of the economic concepts of labor shortage and surplus. Otherwise, the issues of whether the supply of nursing workforce is adequate and, if not, how large a gap exists between the anticipated demand and supply cannot be objectively determined.

LABOR SURPLUSES AND SHORTAGES

A central task of workforce planning for the health-care market is predicting how many of each type of health-care personnel will be needed to maintain the health of a given population. To carry out this task, planners usually consider three key underlying questions to help them define the issues and set the research agenda:

1. How many of each type of health-care professional and other workers are needed to maintain the health of a given population at the present time or at a future point in time?
2. Are there sufficient numbers of professionals and workers to meet the health-care needs given the demand for health care? In other words, will there be a surplus or shortage of health-care personnel?
3. If so, how many more or fewer of what types of professionals and workers will be needed?

These are not easy questions because workforce surpluses and shortages can be defined and measured in at least two different ways: the need-based approach and the economic approach. Much of the confusion about whether a surplus of physicians or a shortage of registered nurses exists results directly from the conceptual differences that underlie these two approaches.

THE NEED-BASED APPROACH

The need-based approach is popular among workforce planners specializing in health-care workforce issues. Sometimes referred to as the *expert determination approach*, the need-based approach is built on the concept of health-care requirements. It begins with assembling a panel of experts to render an informed opinion on the health-care needs of a given population. The experts then estimate the quantities of the various types of health services needed and of the health-care workers required at a particular point in time.

The origin of the need-based approach can be traced to the pioneering work of Roger Lee and Lewis Jones (1933). Interested in the question of current and future physician supply, they provided estimates of the number of physicians required to adequately satisfy the health-care needs of the U.S. population. The following steps for estimating the physician supply summarize the Lee-Jones procedure:

1. Ask a panel of experts to render an opinion on the amount of care needed to keep a given population healthy.
2. Estimate the amount of care each physician is capable of delivering.
3. Estimate the number of physicians needed by dividing the hours of care to be made available and the hours of work that each physician can be reasonably expected to deliver.

The result of this process is a measure called the "physician requirement" that indicates the number of physicians deemed necessary. If the actual number of physicians exceeds the desirable or standard number, there is a surplus. If the reverse is true, there is a shortage.

Based on the estimation of Lee and Jones (1933), the requirement was 134.7 physicians per 100,000 population, or about 165,000 physicians for the United States as a whole in 1933. Over the years, this approach has been used many times to estimate physician shortages and surpluses. For example, in 1995, the third report of the Pew Health Professions Commission (1995) predicted that the United States would soon face a surplus of 100,000 to 150,000 physicians and recommended that medical school spaces be reduced by 20 to 25 percent by the year 2005.

The need-based approach has been extended to the estimation of work-force requirements for many other health-care professionals, such as dentists and nurses. It has been the dominant approach to workforce planning for the last 50 years.

ECONOMIC ANALYSIS
HEALTHY PEOPLE 2000 PROJECT AND WORKFORCE PLANNING

The Healthy People 2000 project represents the health promotion and disease prevention agenda for the United States (National Center for Health Statistics, 1997). This nationwide project has 319 health-related objectives organized into 22 priority areas and has the support of over 350 health-care organizations and 300 state health agencies; it has thus become the de facto mission statement of the American public health system. The Healthy People 2000 goals and objectives have also served as national guideposts that direct the workforce planning efforts of many states and local governments. It is a good example of how a need-based health planning document influences the workforce planning and labor market decisions of many state and local agencies.

THE ECONOMIC APPROACH

Economists take a very different approach to defining workforce shortage and surplus. Instead of asking experts to render an opinion on the adequacy of the numbers of particular types of health personnel, economists rely on the concepts of supply and demand.

The beginning point of the economic approach is the concept of labor market equilibrium. Figure 5–5 depicts this market equilibrium for the labor market for RNs. At the equilibrium wage rate of W_1, the quantity demanded for RNs as indicated by the employment level of N_1 is exactly equal to the quantity supplied. This indicates a situation in which the RNs wishing to work at the going wage rate of W_1 have found jobs in the labor market.

What would happen if the legislature of a state decided to provide subsidized insurance to all the uninsured? Here are the economic approach's predictions:

- The demand for RNs would increase from D_1 to D_2 because more consumers would seek health care now that more people had insurance coverage. A greater demand for health care increases the demand for health-care workers.

- At the going wage of W_1, the number of RNs that employers wish to hire (N_3) would exceed the number of RNs who are willing to work at that wage (N_1) by an amount equal to the difference between N_1 and N_3.
- The resulting gap of excess demand for RNs (from N_1 to N_3) is referred to in economics as a *labor shortage*.

> **An economic shortage of labor** *occurs when employers wish to hire more workers at a particular wage level than there are workers willing to work for that wage.*

An economic shortage therefore is an imbalance between the number of workers willing to work and the number of workers employers are willing to hire at the going wage rate. It occurs when the current wage rate is no longer sufficient to bring the labor market into equilibrium.

In the previous example, the shortage was caused by a sudden increase in the demand for RNs. In the short run, it is very difficult, if not impossible,

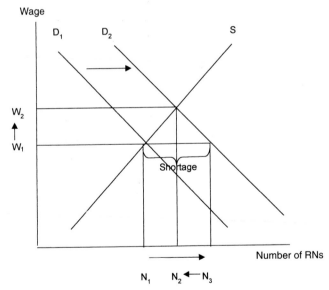

FIG. 5–5. A labor shortage. D_1 = initial market demand for RNs; D_2 = increased market demand for RNs; N_1 = number of RNs initially employed; N_2 = number of RNs finally employed; N_3 = number of RNs that employers would like to hire at the initial wage rate of W_1 immediately after the increase in demand; S = market supply of RNs; W_1 = initial market wage; W_2 = market wage after the increase in demand.

for nursing schools to increase the supply of graduates overnight. This makes it hard for the labor market to provide the additional RNs to meet the rising demand immediately. With employers competing with each other for nurses, wage rates would begin to rise, which would help reduce the size of the labor shortage. With the wage level going from W_1 to W_2, for example, the shortage would shrink and eventually disappear, thereby restoring labor market equilibrium. However, if employers refused to raise wages or raised them too little to close the supply-demand gap, the RN shortage would persist.

A labor shortage can also be caused by a decrease in the supply of RNs. For example, as career opportunities in non-health-care fields open up, nurses leave their profession and find employment in nonnursing fields. When this happens, the supply curve of RNs shifts to the left and a shortage develops at the current wage rate. Irrespective of whether the shortage is caused by an increase in the demand for RNs or a decrease in the supply, it is the result of the prevailing wage rate being too low to bring the quantity supplied in line with the quantity demanded. By examining trends in supply, demand, and wages, professional nurses can position themselves to seize opportunities in growth areas in health care.

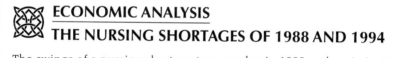

ECONOMIC ANALYSIS
THE NURSING SHORTAGES OF 1988 AND 1994

The swings of a nursing shortage to a surplus in 1988 and again in 1994 were the result of growth in managed care and in the prospective payment mechanisms used by both Medicare and private insurance companies to control hospital costs. In some parts of the country, hospital census dropped below 50 percent as the government and private health plans tightened up hospital reimbursements. This resulted in downsizing of hospitals and a temporary nurse surplus. However, in the long run, as the population ages and new technology fosters more complex treatments, more nurses will be working, although the work settings and training requirements will be different from what they are today.

THE NEED-BASED AND ECONOMIC APPROACHES COMPARED

The need-based and economic approaches to workforce planning are based on very different perspectives. The need-based approach is premised on the concept of medical needs. It largely depends on experts' opinions to determine how large a health-care workforce is required to keep the population healthy. The strength of this approach is that it sets clear national workforce planning goals that are consistent with the overall health objectives for the entire country. It links workforce planning and allocation of human resources to meaningful and measurable health outcomes of the general population.

The major weakness of the need-based approach is that it is a supply-side approach that implicitly assumes that a workforce shortage is a labor supply problem alone. The solutions recommended by the need-based approach therefore tend to be supply-side-oriented, such as reducing nursing school admissions or the number of nursing programs. A workforce surplus or shortage can be caused by unanticipated fluctuations in either supply or demand, however. For example, a sudden expansion of insurance coverage causes the demand for health care and the nursing workforce to rise, whereas a cutback in national health-care spending causes the demand to fall. This suggests that solutions to workforce imbalances can come from either the demand side or the supply side of the labor market. Although supply-side remedies such as adjusting nursing school admissions are helpful and should be taken in times of a nursing surplus, they are not the only solution. Instead, attention should be directed to the demand side—for example, by exploring ways to reverse the decline in demand for health care.

The need-based approach to workforce planning has yet another weakness. Experts' recommendations and the reality in the marketplace can be different. Policies based on expert-perceived needs may lead to too many or too few health-care workers if they are not supported by the actual demand and supply.

The economic approach basically looks on the market as a mechanism for resource allocation. The impersonal market forces of supply and demand determine the wage rates and employment levels. In this system of labor supply and demand, the fluctuation of wage rates serves as a signal to both potential workers and employers to make adjustments that are consistent with their own best interests. Their pursuit of self-interest actually helps to restore market equilibrium.

The strength of the economic approach is that the market is more efficient than the government in allocating scarce resources. The market responds quickly to disturbances and the resulting labor market imbalances. In comparison, the government moves more slowly because of political constraints and bureaucratic burdens.

Another positive feature of the economic approach over the needs-based one is that it not only defines a labor shortage but also suggests alternative solutions. For example, a labor shortage can be eliminated by either an increase in the supply of labor or a decrease in the demand for labor. Either solution can bring the demand and supply back into equilibrium, but the employment consequences of the two proposed solutions are very different: An increase in supply will increase employment, whereas a decrease in demand will reduce employment.

The economic approach suffers from a serious drawback, namely, that markets do not work as competitively and smoothly as assumed. Policy solutions based on the economic approach can take years to accomplish because they involve fundamental changes in the market demand for health care and the supply of the nursing workforce. By the time nursing schools have expanded capacity and graduated new students in an attempt to adjust to a labor shortage that had existed earlier, the demand for health care might have eased, making the expansion of workforce unnecessary.

ECONOMIC ANALYSIS
INFANT MORTALITY AND CERTIFIED NURSE MIDWIVES

Healthy People 2000's objectives on infant mortality provide an excellent comparison of the need-based approach and economic approach. The Healthy People 2000 project has targeted a specific goal of lowering the infant mortality rate to 7 deaths in the first year of life per 1000 live births (National Center for Health Statistics, 1997). To achieve this outcome, several additional objectives for health behavior and prenatal services are identified. This creates a derived demand for nursing services, including certified nurse midwives for delivering prenatal care, community health nurses for health education and follow-up, ambulatory care nurses for monitoring and teaching, and WIC (women, infants, and children) nurses for assessing growth and educating mothers about nutrition.

The economic approach to infant mortality relies on the derived demand for nurses in obstetrical care. The strength of this approach is that it responds to fluctuations in demand for services. It is well documented that infant mortality is most prevalent in minority and lower-income populations. These patients lack resources to enter the health-care market. However, the Healthy People 2000 project has provided a framework for creating programs targeting this population group.

SUMMARY

This chapter introduced the economic concept of the labor market. Understanding how the labor market works will allow nurses to be better prepared to cope with the changing labor market and workforce conditions. The economic knowledge learned can also improve nurses' understanding of the various workforce issues so they can become more informed participants in public policy discussions.

Nurses' salaries and working conditions have improved in the 1980s and 1990s. But the future is full of uncertainty, with both the government and the private sector changing their methods of paying for health care in unpredictable ways. Understanding how the labor market works can affect not only nurses' work and pay but also their professionalism and social status and the future of the profession.

DISCUSSION QUESTIONS

1. Define the concept of derived demand.
2. Define and discuss the concept of labor market equilibrium.
3. Discuss the demand-side factors that can change the equilibrium wage and employment.
4. How can a worker's productivity be improved?
5. Discuss the supply-side factors that can change the equilibrium wage and employment.
6. What are the two different approaches to defining the concept of a labor market shortage? Contrast them and evaluate their strengths and weaknesses.
7. Can a prolonged nursing shortage exist? What are the factors that are preventing the labor market for registered nurses from overcoming the inevitable imbalances between labor demand and supply?
8. Is there a nursing shortage right now in your area? Is there a surplus? What are the labor market signals that indicate to you that such a shortage or surplus exists?
9. What is workforce planning? Discuss and evaluate the contribution of the economic approach and need-based approach to workforce planning.

 ## REFERENCES

Brewer, C. (1997). Through the looking glass: The labor market for registered nurses in the 21st century. *Nursing and Health Care Perspectives*, 18(5), 260–269.

Feldstein, P. (1999). *Health economics* (5th ed.). Albany, NY: Delmar Publishers.

Lee, R., & Jones, L. (1933). *The fundamentals of good medical care*. Chicago: University of Chicago Press.

Mankiw, N. G. (1998). *Principles of economics*. Fort Worth, TX: The Dryden Press.

Moses, E. B. (1997). *Advance notes I and II: From the National Sample Survey of Registered Nurses, March, 1996*. Washington, DC: Division of Nursing, Bureau of Health Professions, Health Resources and Services Administration.

National Center for Health Statistics. (1997). *Healthy People 2000 review*, 1997 (DHHS Publication No. PHS 98–1256). Hyattsville, MD: U.S. Public Health Service.

Pew Health Professions Commission. (1995). *Critical challenges: Revitalizing the health professions for the twenty-first century*. San Francisco: UCSF Center for the Health Professions.

Phelps, C. E. (1997). *Health economics* (2nd ed.). Reading, MA: Addison-Wesley.

 ## SUGGESTED READING

Buerhaus, P. I., & Staiger, D. O. (1996). Managed care and the nurse workforce. *Journal of the American Medical Association, 276*(18), 1487–1493.

Cleland, V. S. (1990). *The economics of nursing*. Norwalk, CT: Appleton & Lange.

Hirsch, B. T., & Schumacher, E. J. (1995). Monopsony power and relative wages in the labor market for nurses. *Journal of Health Economics, 14*(4), 443–476.

Sultz, H. A., & Young, K. M. (1999). *Health care USA*. Gaithersburg, MD: Aspen Publishers.

Yett, D. E. (1975). *An economic analysis of the nurse shortage*. Lexington, MA: DC Heath.

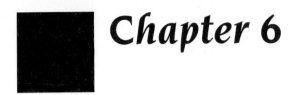

Chapter 6

Application of Economic Principles to Nursing

Susan K. Pfoutz
Sylvia A. Price

LEARNING OBJECTIVES

- Describe and analyze the importance of nurses to cost-effective health care.
- Examine the predicted labor market for nurses.
- Apply economic concepts of supply and demand to nursing.
- Describe the advanced practice opportunities for nursing.
- Describe examples of cost-effective nursing care.

The previous chapters have described the forces affecting the cost of health care. This chapter applies economic principles to nursing and focuses on the role of the nursing profession in influencing those costs. As the largest group of health-care professionals, nurses are integral to the delivery of health care and must be aware of their impact on the cost of client care services and the efficient use of resources. One way to reduce health-care costs is to implement nursing practice models and interventions that use resources efficiently while maintaining or improving the quality of care.

Buerhaus (1998) describes how professional nurses can increase their value to an organization by envisioning themselves as resources in the production of clinical care. From the employer's perspective, the value of nurses increases when nursing demonstrates lower costs in producing care while simultaneously maintaining or improving quality. Organizations reward those who take leadership for eliminating waste and redundancies, abandoning inappropriate activities, and enhancing the quality of care. Using creativity and their unique knowledge of patient needs, nurses can excel in cost-effective care without compromising professional ethics.

Nurses' value increases when nurses provide services that lower cost or increase quality, or both.

Buerhaus predicts that ongoing budget deficits and the increasing proportion of the population using public programs such as Medicare and Medicaid to pay for their health care will result in continuing emphasis on cost containment and price competition for the foreseeable future. As nurses work with the health-care team to provide care that results in desired outcomes while containing resource use, their value is increased and will be recognized.

SUPPLY AND DEMAND CONCEPTS APPLIED TO NURSING

A focus on the cost of health care presents both challenges and opportunities for nursing. Population growth, both in total numbers as well as in the proportion of elderly people, results in continuing demand for preventive and therapeutic health-care services. Services will change, including the use of different types of health-care providers, a wider variety of care settings, and new models of health-care delivery.

Nurses have a long tradition of responding to the health-care needs of society. Evolving nursing roles, particularly in advanced practice nursing, expand ways for nurses to provide care to individuals and families with various health needs across the life span. Nurses have experience in a range of settings, including acute, extended, ambulatory, and community care. After World War II, hospital expansion programs resulted in the majority of nurses practicing in hospital settings for the first time. Lillian Wald pioneered community-based care in the early 1900s. Practicing nurses continue to examine models of care and specific interventions for their potential to improve health-care outcomes while containing costs.

DEMAND FOR NURSING SERVICES

Demand for nurses and nursing care is derived from the broader demand for health care. The current environment, which emphasizes cost containment, is affecting the number of nurses demanded and where those nurses work. Predictions of how those changes will affect the demand for professional nurses vary a great deal.

One widely quoted source used to predict the future of health-care delivery is the Pew Health Professions Commission's series of reports on this subject. The Pew Commission (1995) predicts that by 2005 there will be:

- Health-care systems that integrate financing and service delivery caring for 80 to 90 percent of individuals
- Focus on increased accountability to consumers
- Responsiveness to population needs with broader definitions of health
- Larger focus on prevention
- Focus on effective use of resources
- Greater reliance on evidence of outcomes

Some of the corresponding implications for nursing as a profession and for health-care delivery include the following:

- Closure of up to 50 percent of all hospitals and 60 percent of beds
- Surplus of 200,000 to 300,000 nurses
- Multiple points of entry to the profession, with easier mobility to higher educational levels
- Greater standardization of preparation and job expectations
- Decrease of 10 to 20 percent of associate and diploma schools, with a shift in focus to graduate and nurse practitioner education
- Collaboration between health professionals to identify effective models of practice and interventions that provide evidence of desired outcomes

These predictions suggest that the current supply of nurses is greater than the demand (Pew Health Professions Commission, 1995).

Buerhaus and Staiger (1997) reached different conclusions after examining trends in the nurse labor market. They surveyed a sample of executives from fee-for-service and health maintenance organizations (HMOs). The results predicted a strong nursing labor market for the future. Shifts from institutional to community-based practice are expected to continue. However, these executives doubted that the aging nursing workforce would be able to meet all the needs for care that will emerge. The nursing profession must be ready to respond to changing demands for health care. According to Buerhaus and Staiger (1999), this increased demand is likely to result in a shortage of professional nurses. Participants in the survey questioned whether educational organizations could respond in a timely manner to the rapid changes in health care delivery.

Demand *for nursing care is the need for services, which must be matched with the supply of nurses.*

Using Bureau of the Census Current Population Study data, Buerhaus and Staiger (1999) examined trends in nursing employment and wages from 1983 to 1997. Each month a national representative sample of 100,000 persons were surveyed to examine unemployment, employment, hours worked, and earnings. Such a data set allowed for comparison of various nursing personnel and work trends; however, caution in interpretation is necessary because the definitions of employment changed in 1994. Another concern is that several health-care settings (home health care, free-standing clinics, and HMOs) were grouped in the NEC (not elsewhere classified) category. This grouping of settings precluded specific analyses of each setting. Nursing employment was found to have experienced a reduced growth rate, particularly in the hospital sector. The NEC sector has continued to grow, but at a decreasing rate since the 1994–1997 period. This trend is thought to reflect the cost-containment strategies facing home-health-care agencies (Buerhaus and Staiger, 1999).

Adjusting for inflation, nurses have experienced a flattening of salaries beginning in 1990. There was actually a salary decline in the 1994–1997 period. Although employment in home health care has continued to rise, the rate of growth has slowed as cost-containment efforts continue. (See Chapter 8 for more detail on the economics of nursing salaries.) There was a slight increase in the employment growth for registered nurses (RNs) in 1997, particularly in states with high managed care enrollment (Buerhaus and Staiger, 1999). Whether this increase in nursing employment reflects a temporary correction for skill mix levels or a more stable adjustment is unclear. Although there have been declines in hospital employment, the predicted dramatic declines have not occurred. The trends of slow growth rates for professional nurse employment and salaries are predicted to continue. However, nursing employment opportunities and starting salaries are competitive with other occupations such as elementary and secondary school teachers, and are much higher than those of white-collar professionals such as technical workers and administrative support personnel (Buerhaus and Staiger, 1999).

Nursing salaries are competitive with other similar occupations.

ECONOMIC ANALYSIS
TRANSITION IN NURSING EMPLOYMENT SITES

The Michigan Nurses Association (MNA) recognized the trend in nursing employment of a shift away from the acute care setting. Collaborating with practitioners, educators from Michigan State University and other nursing leaders, the MNA developed a transition program to facilitate the movement of nurses from acute care to community-based settings (Vasquez, 1997). The Department of Labor provided a grant of $248,800 in 1995 to support this project. Over an 18-month period more than 100 nurses participated in the program.

A curriculum was created with a core of information about health-care trends, the role of community settings, and the skills requisite to community practice. Nurses then chose either a home health or an ambulatory care focus. The second portion of the program consisted of skills related to the practice setting. A parallel program was developed for psychiatric nurses to facilitate their transition from psychiatric hospitals to community mental health settings (Vasquez, 1997).

Imagine yourself as a nurse with 10 or more years of experience in acute care nursing. What would encourage you to enroll in such a program? What would you believe that you were gaining and losing?

SUPPLY OF NURSES

Aiken (1995) argues that health-care policy since World War II has focused on increasing the supply of registered nurses rather than examining the need for specific types of nurses. Most of the increase has been absorbed into hospitals, where the ratios of nurses to patients have increased. The research project conducted by Dr. Mildred Montag at Columbia University Teachers College examining the feasibility of associate degree nurses (Montag, 1959) contributed to the blossoming of community college programs, which now prepare 65 percent of the country's nurses each year. Diploma programs currently prepare 7 percent, and baccalaureate nursing programs prepare 25 percent of new nurses (Aiken & Salmon, 1994).

The changing nature of the health-care and economic environments complicates the ability to predict the needs for a nursing workforce. At the present time, the supply of nurses appears to be in excess of the demand (Aiken & Salmon, 1994; Pew Commission, 1995). Historically, the development of new technologies and the fee-for-service reimbursement system contributed to a continuing expansion in the need for health-care and nursing services. Prospective payment systems have led to changes in demand and subsequent declining growth in wages and benefits for nurses, as described earlier. One response to these changes is a slight decline in the percentage of nurses willing to work in these conditions at the prevailing wages. The percentage of nurses working in hospitals is also declining, from 68.1 percent in 1984 to 60 percent in 1996 (Brewer, 1997). Another concern of nurses is that many jobs outside institutional settings pay less.

The supply of nurses is documented in several ways. The National Sample Survey of Registered Nurses in 1996 reported 2.6 million registered nurses, with 82.7 percent being actively employed. This total number of RNs is an increase of 319,000 from 1992 (Moses, 1997). The 1992 survey documented an increased ratio of nurses to population, from 250 nurses per 100,000 population in 1950 to 726 nurses per 100,000 population in 1992 (Moses, 1992). However, there was considerable regional variation. There has been a net increase of 50,000 new nurses in the workforce each year since 1984. Aiken & Salmon (1994, p. 324–7) propose that nurses 1) take a primary role in restructuring the delivery of hospital services, 2) provide primary care services through advanced practice, 3) deliver more primary care services in academic medical centers, 4) care for underserved populations in a variety of settings, and 5) create a new vision for public health population–based practice.

Others dispute the predicted surplus of registered nurses. During the period from 1988 to 1992 when attempts were being made to limit services, particularly hospital days, the employment of nurses increased in every clinical setting (Aiken, 1995; Moses, 1997). In 1996, the Division of Nursing reported that 50 percent of the nursing workforce was over 40 years old (Moses, 1997). This aging of the nursing workforce could alone lead to shortages of nurses early in the 21st century.

The demand for hospital nurses is also interpreted differently by different observers. Currently, two-thirds of the nursing workforce remains employed in hospital settings. Although there has been diminished growth in the number of hospital nurses, by 1994 the number of hospital days had also declined by 55 million compared with 10 years previously. The decline in hospital days has resulted in a shift in the hospital inpatient population to patients who are more severely ill. In response, the ratio of nurses has increased from 50 to 102 per 100 patients (Aiken, 1995). Changes in technology and health-care delivery, an aging population, and more recent labor market data suggest an ongoing demand for hospital nurses that brings the Pew predictions into doubt.

FORECASTING MODEL FOR THE NURSING WORKFORCE

Economics involves predicting the future; thus, it can help predict future nursing workforce changes. Dumpe, Herman, and Young (1998) described a model for forecasting the nursing workforce based on the concepts of supply and demand already described. Building on Prescott's 1991 model, they included variables that improve prediction of the nursing market. The forecasting model is based on two assumptions: The supply and demand forces influencing the market for nurses are similar to those in the market for other goods, and it is possible to forecast the nursing workforce.

The nursing workforce is the predicted number of working nurses required to meet the needs for nursing services.

The supply factors included in the workforce forecasting model are as follows, listed by category:

1. Health-care system: Wages, benefits, and work opportunities
2. Nursing education: The number and types of programs, numbers of graduates, and the amount of funding for nursing education
3. Economic system: Inflation and unemployment in the general economy

4. Demographic features of nurses: Age, gender, race, family constellation, and work satisfaction

The demand factors are as follows:

1. Health-care system: Services provided, technology, kinds of health-care employees, and potential for employee substitution
2. Nursing education: The number and types of programs, which affect the demand for faculty
3. Economic system: Reimbursement for services, and price controls
4. Demographic features of the population: Age, race, geographic distribution, and epidemiology

In addition, five other factors are used in a workforce forecasting model:

1. Contextual factors: The sociocultural values and governmental philosophy that surround health-care needs
2. Aggregate supply of nurses: Total number of nurses available for employment
3. Aggregate demand for nurses: Total number of nurses needed for employment, including all educational levels
4. Market equilibrium: The point at which the supply and demand for nurses meet
5. Nursing workforce: The predicted number of nurses needed to provide desired services

Figure 6–1 illustrates this model. Dumpe, Herman, and Young (1998) believe that incorporation of these factors will result in a more accurate prediction of the need for nurses in the workforce. Although no specific predictions were made, the authors of the model suggest that the educational mix for nurses needs to be raised to meet the demand for baccalaureate and advanced practice nurses.

Workforce forecasting involves predicting the demand for nursing and the supply of nurses at a particular point in the future.

SUMMARY OF NURSING SUPPLY AND DEMAND ISSUES

Although predictions of the demand for nurses vary, trends suggest continued strong employment for nurses. Data demonstrate decreases in the number of hospital days and a slowing of the growth rate for acute care nursing employment. (Chapter 8 describes these economic trends in detail.) The increased level of acute illness has resulted in a higher ratio of

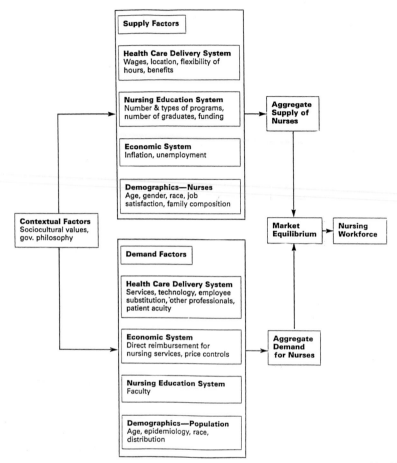

FIG. 6–1. A forecasting model for the nursing workforce. (From Dumpe, M., Herman, J., & Young, S. [1998]. Forecasting the nursing workforce in a dynamic health care market. *Nursing Economics 16*[4], p. 177. Reprinted with permission of the publisher, Janetti Publications, Inc.)

nurses caring for the remaining patients. As health-care systems continue to change, the demand for nurses in acute care practice remains unsure, considering the use of assistive personnel to substitute for nurses, changing practice models, and the expansion of hospital nursing practice with acute care nurse practitioners. It is important to realize that the majority of nurses remain in acute care practice and that the actual decline in the percentage of nurses in acute care settings has been less than predicted. Growth opportunities exist in a variety of positions in community and other settings. A parallel issue is how educational institutions can adapt to supply nurses prepared to meet the existing and emerging practice needs.

Nurses must have the vision to seize opportunities to practice in new ways that meet societal health-care needs. Hesitation to adopt new roles leaves room for others to assume the new opportunities. Timing is crucial for meeting the demands for health care. Subsequent chapters will elaborate on the nursing labor market, the role of nursing education in responding to changing demands for nursing service, and emerging opportunities for nurses in existing and new settings.

Supply timing is important for meeting demand needs when they occur.

 ECONOMIC ANALYSIS
DEMAND FOR OPERATING ROOM ASSISTANTS

There is a demand for assistants to help surgeons in the operating room. Surgeons who have to perform a high number of surgeries in the managed care environment are looking for assistance to increase their productivity. Because operating room nurses may not provide enough assistants from their own ranks or expand their role to meet this need, physicians started training their own technical nonnurse assistants. This is an example of a missed opportunity in which unlicensed technicians provide the labor supply when nursing did not respond rapidly enough.

 ADVANCED PRACTICE OPPORTUNITIES

Some trends in the nursing labor market enable nurses to function as substitutes and complements for other health-care providers. As described in Chapter 2, in economic terms a *substitute* is a service or product that can be used to take the place of another service or product. A *complement* is a service or product that is used with another service or product. For example, a nurse anesthetist and anesthesiologist can substitute for each other in providing many types of surgical anesthesia, whereas a circulating nurse complements either one but is not a substitute for providing anesthesia.

Nurses can provide services that substitute for services by others while providing unique nursing services that complement those of other professionals.

Nurses educated at an advanced level can substitute for physicians in providing certain aspects of medical care. In addition, advanced practice nurses can provide nursing services, such as patient education and other nursing interventions, that complement physician care. One example is nurse midwifery care using certified nurse midwives (CNMs). CNMs can provide well-woman examinations, prenatal care, and delivery for low-risk maternity clients. They may also provide patient education, including childbirth preparation classes and lactation consultation for individuals and groups. These services are part of the traditional nursing role. Some high-risk maternity situations are handled using a system of co-managed care. In this context, a high-risk maternity patient is seen by the obstetrician for prenatal care and medical management of her high-risk condition, while the nurse midwife provides education, support, appropriate coordination of care, and referral services, thus complementing the physician care. Working together, these health-care providers meet more of the maternity client's needs.

Health-care roles are changing as economic factors change, providing opportunities for expanded health-care roles. Health practitioners (HPs) include nonphysician health-care providers, physician assistants (PAs), nurse practitioners (NPs), certified nurse midwives (CNMs), clinical nurse specialists (CNSs), and certified registered nurse anesthetists (CRNAs). These providers require specific educational preparation and certification to practice in their areas of expertise.

Changes in health-care systems provide opportunities for new expanded roles.

From a historical perspective, these additional health practitioners began providing primary care in the mid-1960s. Their numbers reached 22,100 by the end of the 1970s. Substitutability, which refers to a comparable quality of care, has been one criterion for evaluating these practitioners. Reviews of research literature spanning 25 years, such as the ones conducted by the American Nurses Association (1983) and the Office of Technology Assessment (1986), support the observation that the quality of care provided by NHPs is comparable with that provided by physicians.

Research has demonstrated that nonphysician practitioners are acceptable to patients. Given the satisfactory quality of care and patient acceptance, the substitutability of NPs for physicians then depends on such factors as volume of services rendered, costs, and output. For example, McGrath (1990) examined differences in the average salary between physicians and nurse practitioners, including the cost of physician consultation time for NP backup and the cost and time differences for education of physicians versus NPs. In this study one NP was estimated to perform 63 percent of the work of the physician at 38 percent of the cost. In a managed care environment with emphasis on health and prevention, and with emerging models of community-based care, perhaps the discussion should not be about which provider type is best but rather what is the appropriate blend of providers and settings for maximizing cost-effectiveness, access, and improved health in specific populations.

Advanced practice nurses in a managed care organization are both an economic complement and a substitute because their work both increases physician services and provides educational, advocacy, and referral services from nursing. This increases the productivity of the firm and the profits of its owners. Because managed care organizations such as health maintenance organizations operate according to a budget that reflects a specified amount per member per month (capitation), these organizations have an economic incentive to provide health care at the lowest possible cost. In for-profit agencies, any amount of unspent revenues can be retained as profits. In nonprofit agencies, the unspent revenue can be applied to additional services. Similarly, registered nurses who work in the hospital are a complement to physicians. Their work helps to increase the productivity of physicians by providing care to their hospitalized patients while enabling the physicians to maintain their office-based practices. The ability to manage patients in both settings increases physicians' revenues and net income (Walker & Stone, 1996).

ECONOMIC ANALYSIS
ADVANCED PRACTICE NURSES IN THE OPERATING ROOM

The CRNA administers perioperative care to patients who receive anesthesia. The role of the CRNA emphasizes care and comfort measures, distraction techniques and other low-technology interventions, communication, and natural levels of sleep that are consistent with the surgery procedure as well as the immediate administration of anesthesia (Diers, 1992). The CRNA acts as a substitute to the anesthesiologist when administering anesthesia, and functions as a complement when performing the nursing aspects of the role.

 NURSING'S IMPACT ON THE COST OF CARE

Previous chapters as well as the current one have emphasized the importance of limiting the cost of health care. Claire Fagin (1982, 1992), a recognized nursing leader, has promoted the economic value of nursing research and nursing interventions for many years. Her reviews of the literature have highlighted the impact of nursing interventions on patient outcomes and cost in a variety of settings, such as hospitals, nursing homes, community-based care, and home care. Fagin (1992) cautions that it is necessary to examine the populations and interventions to determine whether the delivery of community-based care should be seen as a substitute for other care or as an addition when assessing cost. She emphasizes that many community-based studies demonstrate positive outcomes for the clients and only indirectly address costs. Increasingly, cost is being examined as a relevant outcome for nursing care.

IMPACT OF STRUCTURE AND PROCESS: MAGNET HOSPITALS

The magnet hospital study clearly shows that nursing can be cost-effective and result in quality outcomes (American Academy of Nursing, 1983). This study identified those hospitals throughout the United States that had reputations for being "good places to work" and had been particularly successful in attracting and retaining professional nurses. Forty-one magnet hospitals were identified in the final study. They shared these characteristics:

- 85 percent of all budgeted RN positions were filled on an annual basis.
- The staffs were predominantly composed of professional nurses.
- Well-educated nursing leadership was evident.

Competent, personalized, and cost-effective care was one of the major themes of the study. The conclusion was that a high level of performance by registered nurses is inseparable from high-quality patient care.

High-level nursing care is critical for high-quality patient care.

Kramer (1990) conducted a follow-up interview with 14 chief nurse executives of these magnet hospitals. The most dramatic changes from the earlier study with regard to staff mix were the debureaucratization of the nursing department through flattening of the structure, and the larger percentage of RNs in the work setting. Four of every five employees in the nursing department were registered nurses who were employed in staff positions administering direct care to patients.

In these successful magnet hospitals there was a decrease in the number of nursing administrators. For example, evening and night supervisors were no longer needed because responsible, autonomous staff nurses were functioning more independently. One hospital even eliminated evening and night supervisors altogether, and head nurses were available by beeper for consultation on nursing problems that the staff could not handle. These successful hospitals were redesigning nursing care delivery systems, developing programs and activities to enable or empower staff, strengthening collaborative practice, flattening the organizational structure, and strengthening computerization programs.

Aiken, Smith, and Lake (1994) investigated whether hospitals recognized as good places to practice nursing (magnet hospitals) have lower Medicare patient mortality than hospitals that are similar with regard to a variety of nonnursing organizational characteristics. The researchers believed that nurses had not empirically documented why nursing care is related to patient outcomes. They found that the mortality rate for Medicare patients was lower in 39 of the magnet hospitals than in a sample of 195 nonmagnet hospitals. Mortality rates were 7.7 percent lower (9 fewer deaths per 1000 Medicare discharges) than the matched control hospitals. When adjusting for differences in predicted mortality, the magnet hospitals had a 4.6 percent lower mortality rate.

The nursing skill mix (RNs as a percentage of total nursing personnel) in magnet hospitals is one of their distinguishing characteristics because they have significantly higher ratios of RNs to total nursing personnel and slightly higher nurse to patient ratios. Higher ratios of registered nurses to other nursing personnel have been associated with lower hospital mortality. The data indicate that the lower mortality rates in magnet hospitals are not simply the result of staffing ratios but are related to organizational structures that result in greater professional autonomy for nurses. What nurses do on the units is more important than the number of hands involved in care.

Health-care agencies that facilitate nurses' autonomy to make clinical decisions within their area of clinical expertise and to control their own practice on a routine basis and that foster good relationships between nurses, physicians, and other health-care providers will see positive effects in the quality and outcome of patient care.

EXAMPLES OF COST SAVINGS AND NURSING

Fagin (1992) conducted a review of the literature that demonstrated nursing to be a cost-effective provider of health care. Several research studies have shown the cost-effectiveness of nursing:

- The Office of Technology Assessment (1986) concluded that NPs, PAs, and CNMs provide care that is comparable with physician care. This study also noted that NPs and CNMs are more adept than physicians at providing services that depend on communication with patients or on preventive actions.
- A study on quality of care and health-services utilization was conducted in 30 nursing homes that employed geriatric nurse practitioners and in 30 matched control sites. The sites employing nurse practitioners demonstrated quality improvements such as a reduction in hospital admissions, a reduction in use of restraints, and an increase in the number of patients discharged to home (Kane et al., 1989).
- A study of home nursing care follow-up provided by master's-prepared oncology nurses for a group of patients with progressive lung cancer demonstrated that the patients receiving home care had less symptom distress and social dependency than the group receiving only office care. The total number of hospital days was lower among the specialized home-care group than the control groups (McCorkle et al., 1989).

TECHNIQUES FOR ANALYZING NURSING COSTS

Cost-effectiveness analysis is a specific technique for comparing the costs of achieving similar outcomes. This technique is being used increasingly in nursing and health care, allowing for a standardization of methodology that makes studies more comparable. This technique is presented in Chapter 15.

Cost-effectiveness analysis *compares the costs of achieving similar outcomes.*

A more frequent method of analysis is to examine the cost savings experienced by specific programs or interventions. For example, in a classic study Brooten and associates (1986) examined the outcomes and cost savings of early discharge for infants whose birth weight was less than 1500 grams. This research demonstrated that early discharge resulted in a cost savings of 27 percent in hospital expenditures ($47,520 vs. $64,940) and 22 percent in physician expenditures ($5,933 vs. $7,649). Outcome measures showed no significant difference between the infants in the traditional and short-stay groups.

The recent emphasis on decreased length of hospital stays has led to the use of *clinical pathways* as a mechanism to decrease the cost and length of stays. Clinical pathways outline the activities for each member of the health-care team and the projected resource utilization during the expected inpatient hospital stay. These pathways or guidelines are formulated in conjunction with a specific clinical diagnosis or procedure.

Another tool used in evaluating outcomes is *benchmarking*, which is the process of comparing one facility's selected outcomes with those of another facility that is recognized as an outstanding agency. Benchmarking is identifying what organizations do to achieve better results and then adapting those best practices to improve work processes. Bassett (1998) implies that benchmarking requires individuals to meticulously study work processes in other organizations and apply those processes in their own company. She states that organizations are more open today and are highly recognized for their efforts in benchmarking.

Benchmarking *is identifying and adapting best practices to improve processes of care.*

ECONOMIC ANALYSIS
USE OF BENCHMARKING TO DECREASE THE INCIDENCE OF PRESSURE ULCERS

A nursing home noted that 25 percent of the residents in their facility developed some degree of pressure ulcers within 6 months of admission. The administrators identified this patient discomfort and cost of care as excessive and unacceptable. They therefore contacted nursing-home facilities in the surrounding community that had a reputation for outstanding care in this area. After consulting with personnel from these facilities, the protocols for nursing care in the nursing home were revised. These protocols focused on informally educating personnel and implementing the latest treatment modalities.

After a 6-month period using these protocols, the facility assessed its progress. The pressure ulcer rate had dropped to 15 percent, but was still unacceptable. The protocols were revised and a formal in-service educational program was instituted. Six months later the pressure ulcer rate dropped to less than 5 percent. This situation shows that the use of benchmarks enables staff to examine work processes in similar agencies that are recognized as outstanding organizations and to apply those processes in their own agency.

Lagoe (1998) described issues that are important in the evaluation of clinical pathways or comparison of facilities. These include the following:

- The sample examined must be sufficient for all the groups within the population (i.e., it must be larger than 30).
- The time of year should be adjusted for, because it may affect length of stay and number of admissions.
- The age of the population affects several aspects of recovery and should be taken into consideration.
- The statistical techniques used should include both the arithmetic mean and the median to more accurately represent the variation in outcomes.

Other nursing research examines smaller innovations that achieve positive outcomes while conserving health-care dollars. For example, Wikblad and Anderson (1995) compared the use of conventional absorbent dressing, semiocclusive hydroactive dressings, and occlusive hydrocolloid dressing on wounds after heart surgery. The conventional absorbent dressing was demonstrated to be more effective in wound healing, with fewer skin changes and less redness than the hydroactive dressing. Although traditional dressings need to be changed more frequently, their cost was still less than the other alternatives.

In another example, Richiuso (1998) demonstrated that activated partial thromboplastin time could be accurately tested by using blood from a heparinized arterial line rather than from an invasive venipuncture technique. Using the arterial line, which is already in place, eliminates the need for another invasive procedure and thus saves staff time and equipment cost.

ECONOMIC ANALYSIS
EXAMINING THE OUTCOMES OF A CHANGE TO BAG BATHS

Nurses understand that skin integrity and hygiene are critical elements of nursing care. Daily sponge baths have been routine for patients who are not ambulatory, even though the patient's skin becomes dry and the sanitary nature of the basin used is questionable. One recent innovation is a bag bath, which involves the use of several washclothes saturated with a moisturizing cleansing solution. Although patient-care staff have had difficulty changing from traditional care—the bed bath—the outcomes of this new method suggest that it is preferable. These outcomes include:

- Patient satisfaction
- Less dry skin

- Less potential nosocomial infections
- Less staff time spent in routine care

The procedure is cost effective because it reduces staff time and decreases skin infections.

SUMMARY

Nurses are in a pivotal position for making a difference in the delivery of patient care. To become equal partners in the evolving health-care system, nurses must position themselves as able and willing to assume these responsibilities. To achieve desired outcomes in health care, the nature of service delivery is becoming more interdisciplinary. Because nursing is a focal point in interdisciplinary care, nurses can demonstrate a leadership role in this area. Continuing educational development is required to function in the emerging health-care delivery system.

Concepts of supply and demand are important for understanding how nursing positions are changing to meet the demands for health care in a cost-conscious environment. A variety of predictions were presented in this chapter. There is still no consensus on the predicted needs for nurses. Various factors affecting the supply and demand of nurses were discussed, and a model incorporating relevant factors to predict the nursing workforce was presented.

Research studies have demonstrated that advanced practice nurses can make significant contributions to controlling health-care costs. It is critical that nurses accept responsibility and accountability for providing cost-effective, high-quality, client-centered health care.

Increasingly, nursing research is using a variety of techniques to examine outcomes related to costs, such as cost-effectiveness analysis. Other techniques for examining costs and outcomes include evaluating cost savings and critical pathways

DISCUSSION QUESTIONS

1. What is the role of nursing relative to the provision of cost-effective health care?

2. What is the predicted labor market for nurses? Why is this an important concept?
3. What are the economic concepts of supply and demand for nursing? Why is this relevant?
4. Cite research studies that document cost-effective nursing care.
5. In your practice setting, give examples of what components of practice could be examined for cost effectiveness.
6. Describe how a service in your nursing setting could be compared with a benchmark from another health care agency. What indicators could be used to evaluate clinical and cost outcomes for comparison of agencies?

 REFERENCES

Aiken, L. (1995). Transformation of the nursing workforce. *Nursing Outlook*, 43(5) 201–209.

Aiken, L., & Salmon, M. (1994). Health care workforce priorities: What nursing should know. *Inquiry*, 31(3), 318–329.

Aiken, L., Smith, H. L., Lake, E. T. (1994). Lower Medicare mortality among a set of hospitals known for good nursing care. *Medical Care*, 32(8), 771–787.

American Academy of Nursing. (1983). *Magnet hospitals: Attraction and retention of professional nurses.* Kansas City, MO: Author.

American Nurses Association. (1983). *Nurse practitioners: A review of the literature (1965–1982).* Kansas City, MO: Author

Bassett, S. (1998). Continuous quality improvement (CQI) principles. In S. Price, M. Koch, & S. Bassett, *Health care resource management: Present and future challenges* (pp. 41–63). St. Louis: Mosby.

Brewer, C. (1997). Through the looking glass: The labor market for registered nurses in the 21st century. *Nursing and Health Care Perspectives*, 18(5), 260–269.

Brooten, D., Kumar, S., Butts, P., Finkler, S., Bakewell-Sachs, S., Gibbons, A., & Delivoria-Papadopoulos, A. (1986). A randomized clinical trial of early hospital discharge and home follow-up of very low birthweight infants. *New England Journal of Medicine*, 315(15), 934–939.

Buerhaus, P. (1998). Financial challenges and economic implications. In S. Price, M. Koch, & S. Bassett, *Health care resource management: Present and future challenges* (pp. 59–71). St. Louis: Mosby.

Buerhaus, P., & Staiger, D. (1997). Future of the nurse labor market according to health executives in high managed-care areas of the United States. *Image: Journal of Nursing Scholarship*, 29(4), 313–318.

Buerhaus, P., & Staiger, D. (1999). Trouble in the nurse labor market? Recent trends and future outlook. *Health Affairs*, 19(1), 214–222.

Diers, D. (1992). Nurse-midwives and nurse anesthetist: The cutting edge in specialist practice. In L. Aiken & C. Fagin (Eds.), *Charting nursing's future: Agenda for the 1990s* (pp. 159–180). Philadelphia: Lippincott.

Dumpe, M., Herman J., & Young, S. (1998). Forecasting the nursing workforce in a dynamic health care environment. *Nursing Economics*, 16, 170–179, 188.

Fagin, C. (1982). The economic value of nursing research. *American Journal of Nursing*, 82(12), 1844–1849.

Fagin, C. (1992). Cost-effectiveness of nursing care revisited: 1981–1990. In L. Aiken & C. Fagin (Eds.), *Charting nursing's future: Agenda for the 1990s* (pp. 13–28). Philadelphia: Lippincott.

Kane, R. L., Garrard, J., Skay, C. L., Radosevich, V. M., Buchanon, J. L., McDermott, S. M., Arnold, S. B., & Kepferle, L. (1989). Effects of a geriatric nurse practitioner on process and outcome of nursing care. *American Journal of Public Health*, 79(9), 1271–1277.

Kramer, M. (1990). The magnet hospitals: Excellence revisited. *Journal of Nursing Administration*, 20(9), 35–44.

Lagoe, R. (1998). Basic statistics for clinical pathway evaluation. *Nursing Economics*, 16(3), 125–131.

McCorkle, R., Benoliel, J. Q., Donaldson, G., Georgiaddou, F., Moinpour, C., & Goodell, B. (1989). A randomized clinical trial of home nursing care for lung cancer patients. *Cancer*, 64(6), 1375–1382.

McGrath, S. (1990). The cost-effectiveness of nurse practitioners. *Nurse Practitioner: The Journal of Primary Health Care*, 15(7), 40–42.

Montag, M. L. (1959). Community college education for nursing. New York: McGraw Hill.

Moses, E. B. (1992). *The registered nurse population: Findings from the National Sample Survey of Registered Nurses, March 1992*. Rockville, MD: U.S. Department of Health and Human Services, Health Resources and Services Administration, Bureau of Health Professions.

Moses, E. B. (1997). *Advance notes I and II: From the National Sample Survey of Registered Nurses, March 1996*. Rockville, MD: U.S. Department of Health and Human Services, Health Resources and Services Administration, Bureau of Health Professions.

Office of Technology Assessment. (1986). *Nurse practitioners, physician assistants, and certified nurse-midwives: A policy analysis* (Health Technology Case Study No. 37 OTA-HCS-37). Washington, DC: U.S. Government Printing Office.

Pew Health Professions Commission. (1995). *Critical challenges: Revitalizing the health professions for the twenty-first century*. San Francisco: UCSF Center for the Health Professions.

Prescott, P. N. (1991). Forecasting requirements for health care personnel. *Nursing Economics*, 9(1), 1–24.

Richiuso, N. (1998). Accuracy of aPTT values drawn from heparinized arterial lines in children. *Dimensions of Critical Care Nursing*, 17(1), 14–19.

Vasquez, J. (1997). Michigan program helps acute care nurses transition to other settings. *American Nurse*, 24(3), 1–2.

Walker, P. H., & Stone, P. W. (1996). Exploring cost and quality: Community-based versus traditional hospital delivery systems. *Journal of Health Care Financing*, 23(1), 23–47.

Wikblad, K., & Anderson, B. (1995). A comparison of three wound dressings in patients undergoing heart surgery. *Nursing Research*, 44(4), 312–316.

 SUGGESTED READING

Cherry, B., & Jacob, S. R. (1999). *Contemporary nursing: Issues, trends, and management*. St. Louis: Mosby.

Forkner, D. J. (1996). Clinical pathways: Benefits and liabilities. *Nursing Management*, 27(1), 35–37.

Gardner, K., Allhusen, J., Kamm, J., & Tobin, J. (1997). Determining the cost of care through clinical pathways. *Nursing Economics,* 15(4), 213–217.

Nunnery, R. K. (1997). *Advancing your career: Concepts of professional nursing.* Philadelphia: FA Davis.

Shindul-Rothschild, J., & Duffy, M. (1996). The impact of restructuring and work design on nursing practice and patient care. *Best Practices and Benchmarking in Healthcare,* 1(6), 271–282.

Tappen, R. M. (1995). *Nursing leadership and management: Concepts and practice.* Philadelphia: FA Davis.

Chapter 7

The Economics of Nursing Education

Regina M. Williams
Susan K. Pfoutz

LEARNING OBJECTIVES

■ Analyze the impact of national reports about nursing on nursing education.

■ Analyze the potential impact of the Pew Health Professions Commission on nursing education.

■ Discuss the importance of the assessment movement for identifying and monitoring outcomes of nursing education.

■ Analyze the issues of productivity and faculty workload determination.

■ Examine the impact of for-profit educational corporations on traditional institutions of higher education.

■ Discuss the trends in student enrollment in all nursing programs compared with the recommendations for needs for nurses.

■ Examine issues concerning the preparation of sufficient faculty for the needs of nursing education programs.

■ Discuss strategies to promote educational mobility for nurses.

■ Describe recommended curriculum components for undergraduate and graduate nursing education.

■ Examine mechanisms for supplying nursing education to wider areas using a variety of technologies.

Nursing education provides the mechanism to prepare nurses to assume the variety of positions needed to staff health care delivery systems. This chapter will explore some of the economic aspects (the production, distribution and use) of nursing education throughout the twentieth century. It will examine factors driving costs of nursing education in universities and community colleges. Trends in higher education that affect nursing education will be addressed. It will provide an overview of some of the major studies of nursing reported in this century with a view to the economic realities identified for nursing education at the time they were written and the recommendations made for improving the foundations of nursing education. The current demand for nursing education will be reviewed including the factors that affect the educational preparation of RNs. New product lines exemplified as distance learning and Internet classes will be discussed. Some economic analyses of innovative strategies used to address current educational needs will be presented. These issues will be examined from the perspective of one or more of the key economic principles that apply to nursing education.

The key economic principles:

- Supply and demand
- Assessment of outcome measures
- Productivity and cost containment
- Financing
- Competition among institutions
- Educational advancement and outreach

In 1965 the American Nurses' Association (ANA) stated in a position paper that the "education of those who are licensed to practice nursing should take place in institutions of higher education" (p. 5). No schedule was given for implementation of this goal; however, state nurses' associations were urged to work toward its accomplishment. Reactions to this position were immediate as spokespersons rallied to the defense of the traditional hospital diploma apprentice system of education (ANA, 1983). In 1978 the ANA delegates voted to endorse the baccalaureate degree as the minimum preparation for entry to professional nursing practice. The target date of 1985 was identified as the time by which this change would be achieved (ANA, 1983).

In 1996 the American Association of Colleges of Nursing (AACN) issued a position statement that said in part, "As health care shifts from hospital centered, inpatient care to more primary and preventive care throughout the community, the health system requires registered nurses who can practice across multiple settings. . . . Accordingly, the AACN recognizes the Bachelor of Science degree in nursing as the minimum educational requirement for professional nursing practice" (AACN, 1990a, p. ii, Executive Summary).

The position statements of these two prestigious professional associations notwithstanding, three decades later a majority (approximately 60 percent) of nurses continue to earn their initial nursing credentials in community colleges and hospital schools. This chapter is not intended to address the reasons for the failure of the profession to implement the desired entry level of education. However, this situation has undeniable economic significance for the future of nursing education, its potential students, practitioners in the field, health-care organizations, and society.

 THE ECONOMIC STATUS OF NURSING EDUCATION

Throughout the history of nursing, national reports on the status of nursing practice and education have provided direction for the future development of the profession. The federal government or private foundations funded many of the reports. Each report contributed to the understanding of the current status of nursing education, including its quality and economic base, and offered recommendations for meeting the economic demands of the nation for nursing care. Most of the reports discuss both the demand for nurses by the public and the supply of new registered nurses (RNs) and advanced practice nurses (APNs) that nursing education must produce.

The supply of new nurses must meet the patient-care demand.

HISTORICAL REVIEW OF NURSING STUDIES

The Goldmark Report, published in 1923 and sponsored by the Rockefeller Foundation, examined the proper training of public health nurses. Interviews with nursing educators and surveys of programs resulted in recommendations for a basic nursing curriculum, the improvement of nursing programs, and the education of nurse leaders in universities. In 1926, the report of the Committee on the Grading of Nursing Schools provided recommendations regarding the supply and demand for nurses, job analysis, and the evaluation of nursing programs (Kalisch & Kalisch, 1995).

Nursing for the Future, a report widely referred to as the "Brown Report," was funded by the Russell Sage Foundation and published in 1948. The thrust of this report was the need for the education of nurses to occur in institutions of higher education. In 1952, Mildred Montag undertook an action research project that developed and evaluated the feasibility of conducting nursing programs at community colleges. After 5 years it was concluded that community college programs could prepare direct-care nurses faster and more economically than a 4-year university program. Production of nurses at community colleges would relieve the existing nursing shortage and facilitate the movement of nursing education programs into institutions of higher education (Kelley,1979; Kalisch & Kalisch, 1995).

Associate degree nursing programs can supply the nurses demanded for direct patient care in a shorter time period than a university program while still moving nursing education into institutions of higher education.

In January 1968, the National Commission on Nursing and Nursing Education was founded with the major objective of improving the delivery of health care to the American people through the analysis and improvement of nursing and nursing education. It published a report in 1970 entitled *An Abstract for Action* that recommended that hospital schools of nursing move systematically and with dispatch to effect interinstitutional arrangements with collegiate institutions so that graduates would receive an academic degree from an educational institution upon completion of their course of study (Lysaught, 1970). In 1981 the National Commission on Nursing issued its initial report and preliminary recommendations for nursing practice, nursing education, and the delivery of nursing care within the health-care system. These studies have helped to inform nursing and the public on issues germane to the improvement of the quality of nursing education. They also served to clarify the critical need to have adequately prepared nurses planning and directing the delivery of health care.

The requirement for baccalaureate preparation for professional nurses is based on the need to supply nurses who have a broad range of knowledge and skills to meet the demand from health services for the provision of more complex services.

PEW HEALTH PROFESSIONS COMMISSION

By the end of the 20th century, another commission was formed that would have great impact on nursing education and practice. Unlike the previous studies, which focused on nursing care delivery, the Pew Health Professions Commission took a broader approach by examining the state of health-care delivery within the emerging health-care system and the implications for the preparation of all health-care professionals. This commission generated three reports. Its recommendations focus on the redesign of the health-care workforce, the determination of the right size of the workforce to meet health-care needs, the restructuring of health professional education, and the revision of regulation of health-care professions for accountability and access. The commission predicted that by 2005 vast changes in health-care delivery will affect the 10 million health-care workers and influence the educational programs in which they are prepared as well as the mechanisms by which practice is regulated. Predicted changes included the following (Pew Health Professions Commission, 1995, p. i–iii, Executive Summary):

- Closure of up to 50 percent of all hospitals and up to 60 percent of beds
- Surplus of 100,000 to 200,000 physicians
- Surplus of 200,000 to 300,000 nurses
- Surplus of 40,000 pharmacists
- Consolidation of the 200 health professions into multiskilled professionals
- Increasing demand for public health professionals

Based on these predictions, the commission recommended that all health-care professionals do the following (Pew Health Professions Commission, 1995, p. iii–iv, Executive Summary):

- Enlarge their scientific base of practice to include psycho-social-behavioral sciences and population and health sciences.
- Maintain some areas of discipline training but integrate many areas of professional preparation with other professional groups.
- Prepare for practice in integrated systems.
- Focus on culturally sensitive care by inclusion of diverse students and curricular content.
- Develop varied partnerships to improve education.
- Revise regulation to become more standardized and accountable.

Several recommendations were directed specifically to nursing. Nurses were encouraged to value the multiple points of entry to nursing, to develop single titles for each level of preparation and practice, and to determine how nurses prepared at different educational levels would practice nursing.

It is more cost efficient to prepare the giver of direct patient care at the associate degree level than at the baccalaureate level.

Based on the different levels of nursing education, the Pew Commission recommended that clear distinctions should exist among levels of nursing education and that opportunities for mobility up the nursing career and educational ladder should be facilitated. Finally, there should be greater integration of nursing education and practice. The commission observed that nurses are the professional group best prepared to respond to the changing health-care delivery system. To support this claim the commission cited the following points (Pew Health Professions Commission, 1995, p. 33–35):

- Nurses' education focuses on the delivery of cost-effective care.
- Nurses have a combination of clinical and management skills.
- Nurses focus on the behavioral aspects of health more than do physicians.
- Nurses are effective workers and leaders.

Studies examining and making recommendations regarding the quality and cost of nursing education influence the supply of nurses available to meet the patient-care demands of society.

 ## ECONOMIC TRENDS IN NURSING EDUCATION

Faced with escalating tuition and fees that exceed the consumer price index, anxious consumers are looking for increased value and social relevance for their educational dollars. Responding to a public grown skeptical over the perception that universities cannot control costs, Congress established the National Commission on the Cost of Higher Education. In a report released in 1998 the commission reported this reality of tuition increases: "In the 20 years between 1976 and 1996, the average tuition at public universities increased from $642 to $3,151 and the average at private universities increased from $2,881 to $15,581" (National Commission on the Cost of Higher Education [NCCHE], 1998, p. 5). Tuition at public 2-year colleges, the least expensive of all types of institutions, increased from an average of $245 to $1245 during this period. The commission has likened this rise to the "sticker shock" of buying a new car.

Rapid increase in the cost of a product, such as education, affects satisfaction with and ability to buy the product.

Although consumers have focused on the price they pay for education in terms of tuition, the commission points out that tuition is only one component of the price of attending college. They explain the difference between cost and price as well as the concept of subsidy and tuition discounting as follows (NCCHE, 1998, p. 1–4):

- *Cost* is what the institution spends to provide education and related educational services to students.
- *Price* is what the students and their families are charged and what they pay.
- *Subsidy* is the difference between what it costs the institution to provide education for the student and the tuition and fees charged to students.
- *Tuition discounting* refers to the practice of charging less for tuition than the institution spends to provide education.

Many factors affect the cost of education in addition to the direct costs of providing classes. Financial aid is one consideration. Institutional costs incurred from providing institutional aid to needy students increased about 180 percent in the 10-year period between the 1987–1988 and the 1996–1997 academic years (NCCHE, 1998, p. 20). Costs beyond the production of education and the sources of revenue beyond tuition and fees vary by the type of institution. Table 7–1 illustrates the rise in tuition costs and indicates additional sources of revenue by type of educational institution.

THE ASSESSMENT MOVEMENT

Assessment is germane to all disciplines in the academy and to institutions of higher education as a whole because it is a requirement of all regional accrediting bodies in the United States. Program assessment is viewed as key in the academy's response to criticisms about the outcomes of higher education. The process of assessment includes measures to validate the outcomes of the total curriculum, with emphasis on the general education courses as well as the major field of study. The goals of assessment are to demonstrate and improve the quality of programs, provide accountability, define a unique organizational mission, enhance declining enrollments through recruitment and retention plans, and evaluate innovations (Banta, 1988).

Assessment of program outcomes has been incorporated into the accreditation processes of both the National League for Nursing Accreditation Commission (NLNAC) and the AACN's Commission on Collegiate Nursing Education. Schools must identify their educational outcomes, describe the assessment process, provide analysis of data collected to evaluate those outcomes, and demonstrate the use of that data for program maintenance and revision (Thompson & Bartles, 1999). Because of the importance of accrediting agencies to institutional viability and the importance of assessment in the accreditation process, assessment makes an economic impact on educational institutions.

The goal of assessment is to make inferences about the learning achieved by students as a basis for program maintenance, revision, or termination.

TABLE 7–1. AVERAGE TUITION GROWTH AND ALTERNATIVE FUNDING SOURCES

Type of Nursing Program	Length and Type of Program	Average Tuition in 1976 ($)	Average Tuition in 1996 ($)	Alternative Funding Sources
Diploma	2–3 years, RN	No information	No information	Hospital, health-care organization, endowments, gifts, Medicare funding, fees
Community college	2 years, associate degree	245	1,245	State funding, county taxes, fees
Public university	4 years, BSN 2–4 years, MSN 4–8 years, PhD	642	3,151	State funding, endowments, gifts, grants for research and training, fees, scholarships, loans
Private university	4 years, BSN 2–4 years, MSN 4–8 years, PhD	2,881	15,581	Organizational sponsorship, endowments, gifts, grants for research and training, fees, loans, scholarships

Source: Adapted from National Commission on the Cost of Higher Education (1998, p. 5). *Straight talk about college costs and prices.* Washington, DC: Author.

Educators can agree on the value of such information; however, the creation of an effective assessment program is daunting. The American Association for Higher Education published nine principles for guiding the assessment of student learning in all disciplines, including nursing (Thompson & Bartles, 1999, p. 171–173):

1. The assessment of student learning begins with educational values.
2. Assessment is most effective when it reflects an understanding of learning as multidimensional, integrated, and revealed in performance over time.
3. Assessment works best when the programs it seeks to improve have clear, explicitly stated purposes.
4. Assessment requires attention to outcomes but also and equally to the experiences that lead to those outcomes.
5. Assessment works best when it is ongoing, not episodic.
6. Assessment fosters wider improvements when representatives from across the educational community are involved.
7. Assessment makes a difference when it begins with issues of use and illuminates questions that people really care about.
8. Assessment is most likely to lead to improvement when it is part of a larger set of conditions that promote change.
9. Through assessment, educators meet responsibilities to students and to the public.

The assessment of learning outcomes has an economic impact on institutions both because of the cost of implementing an assessment program for obtaining accreditation and because a negative assessment can discourage potential applicants.

The assessment process is a mechanism of validating the knowledge and skills or value added as a result of the educational process.

PRODUCTIVITY AND COST CONTAINMENT IN NURSING EDUCATION

Cost containment and productivity are key issues not only in nursing service but also in nursing education. The question to be asked is, What is the impact of the cost of nursing education on the university's quest for cost containment? When a university is pressured to try to contain costs, it begins by examining its productivity. Lea Acord, dean of Montana State University, says, "Because nursing is so expensive, we are the first college to be approached [regarding cost containment] in order to save money for the university. Fortunately, our college of nursing has been around for 60 years and has a lot of community support" (personal communication, September 1, 1999). This statement suggests that is is important for nursing units to partner with their community for mutual benefit.

The unit of productivity in education is *credit hour production*, which refers to the number of credits taken per student multiplied by the number of students in a program. Credit hours can be examined by individual class, program, or department. Each faculty member's productivity is determined by the credit hours generated. A faculty that generates few credit hours contributes to the overall per student cost. Nursing programs are vulnerable to comparisons of credit hours produced for several reasons. The foremost reason is the relatively low student to faculty ratio in clinical courses, which make up the bulk of the courses at the upper level. Second, nursing typically offers few support courses in which nonnurses are enrolled. Therefore, it is vulnerable to decreases in nursing enrollments. These two factors increase the unit cost of educating a nursing student as compared with the cost of educating a student in another discipline.

Productivity as measured by credit hours produced by a nursing class or a nursing program is affected by the low ratio of students to faculty in clinical nursing courses.

When one examines only the unit cost of nursing education, the picture is incomplete, and it appears as though a nursing program's impact on the institution's costs is greater than is really the case. To gain a more accurate perspective, one should view the nursing program's contribution to revenue generation. Nursing programs act as magnets in universities, drawing students who take approximately one-half of their total curriculum in general education courses. The productivity generated by the general education courses usually accrues to departments or colleges other than nursing. Some students drawn to the university for nursing decide to forgo this discipline for another, often in the social or natural sciences. The result is increased credit hour production in general education from nursing and nursing-intent students in courses beyond the nursing major. The accompanying economic analysis illustrates the concept of limited credit hour production.

ECONOMIC ANALYSIS
CREDIT HOUR PRODUCTION IN NURSING

A medium-sized nursing program enrolls 80 students per year. One faculty member can teach the classroom component of the course, but the clinical sections are limited to 8 to 10 students per section depending on the clinical facility, the nature of the clinical care, and the regulations of individual state boards of nursing. These regulations require a faculty member for each section, yielding a student to faculty ratio of 8:1 to 10:1. Other courses in the university can enroll from 100 to 300 students in large lecture classes. Even the breakout discussion sections usually enroll at least 30 students, yielding respective student to faculty ratios of 100:1, 300:1, and 30:1. Other health professions use a preceptor model whereby an individual faculty member is not constantly present with a small number of students. Even when the faculty member is on-site, he or she often has less restriction on the number of students for whom he or she is responsible.

Graduate nursing students use a preceptor model for their clinical courses. However, the faculty may still have close clinical responsibilities for students in programs such as those for nurse practitioners. This smaller ratio of students to faculty in generic undergraduate and some graduate programs makes nursing vulnerable to low credit hour production.

Time spent by the faculty on research and administrative tasks also affects productivity. As the demand for more research by the nursing faculty increases, productivity as measured by the generation of credit hours decreases. This trend will continue until nurses begin to generate greater revenue from funding agencies. Research funding that pays for the direct cost of conducting the research as well as for indirect costs will begin to balance the equation because it buys out research faculty time and pays for lower-cost replacement faculty who generate credit hours.

Cost Containment

The vulnerability of nursing programs to limited credit hour production and limited sources of money has led to a variety of cost-containment measures. As state and federal budget cuts have limited the resources for nursing education, institutions and nursing administrators have looked for ways to contain the rising costs of educating nursing students.

Institutions have begun to form partnerships in an effort to become more cost-effective in the use of resources. Such partnerships are expanding as a variety of pressures threaten to deplete resources. Among these are aging campus infrastructures and projected increases in the number of college undergraduates by the year 2005 (National Center for Educational Statistics, 1995). Both these conditions influence university facilities, which have been identified by the National Commission on the Cost of Higher Education (1998) as one of the drivers of cost and price.

Nursing, like other disciplines in the academy, has experienced decreased federal and state funding. This decrease comes at a time when commissions and professional associations interested in changing health care and health-care policy project an increased need for nurses educated at the baccalaureate and higher degree levels. Pursuing joint ventures with other academic institutions and with business and industry as potential sources of funding support has become an increasing aspect of the role of the academic administrator. Michael Carter, dean of the College of Nursing at the University of Tennessee at Memphis, states, "The role of the dean and faculty in assuring a strong and diversified income base has grown as never before" (personal communication, September 29, 1999). Joint initiatives are welcomed by cost-conscious institutions of education that have limited resources. The accompanying economic analysis describes one such partnership.

Partnerships between academic institutions and health-care systems provide value to both institutions and produce nurses with relevant practice knowledge in a more cost-effective way.

ECONOMIC ANALYSIS
PARTNERSHIP BETWEEN EDUCATION AND PRACTICE

This analysis examines the partnership between Henry Ford Health System (HFHS) in Detroit, Michigan, and Oakland University (OU) as described by two staff members of the Center for Academic Nursing: Stephanie Myers Schim, PhD, RN, CNAA, and Teresa C. Wehrwein, PhD, RN, CNAA.

This partnership was designed to be mutually beneficial to both the service agency and the academic institution. The HFHS sought this alliance to ensure an ongoing pool of qualified nurses to support client care and to participate in nursing curriculum design and delivery that would prepare nurses for roles in the evolving health-care system. HFHS employs 3000 registered nurses, many of whom were graduates of the Henry Ford Hospital School of Nursing and Hygiene. The university partner, OU, sought the alliance to enhance learning through clinical placements and faculty practice, to facilitate faculty practice and research objectives, and to recruit urban and minority students. This comprehensive state-assisted institution enrolls approximately 300 undergraduates, 200 RN to bachelor of science in nursing (BSN) completion students, and 120 master of science in nursing (MSN) students.

In December 1996, after 30 months of planning, a contract was signed that created the Center for Academic Nursing (CAN) as the tangible symbol of the alliance. CAN is located within the corporate headquarters of HFHS. The CAN team includes three administrators, three doctorally prepared nurse scholars, two master's-level education specialists, one BSN lab coordinator, and several support staff. The CAN programs reflect a focus on education, practice, and research to mutually benefit the university and health system.

Nurse scholars teach in OU undergraduate courses and consult with faculty on curriculum design. They have collaborated with faculty on new postbaccalaureate internships in critical care and maternal-child nursing. OU faculty members bring a variety of courses to the HFHS main campus to provide educational access for staff nurses. An academic adviser within the CAN office assists students to plan their educational program. The partnership has resulted in a large increase in the number of OU students having clinical placements in HFHS.

CAN staff consult in various clinical areas, including building consensus regarding the philosophy and scope of nursing practice, encouraging a "baby friendly" maternity service, and implementing a skills competency program in ambulatory care. The CAN teams bring academic and service colleagues together and provide resources and support for professional nursing education.

Research has focused on projects relevant to both the health system and the academic partner. One collaborative research project included two faculty members, a nurse scholar, a primary service site, and a community agency representing the Arab community to study "Partnerships for Cultural Competency: Enhancing Health Service Quality and Access with the Arab Community." Other projects include an examination of the perceptions and barriers for African-Americans regarding the use of hospice services and an assessment of activities, priorities, and perceptions of registered nurses working in ambulatory care.

The initial impetus for the academic alliance grew from both professional needs and the expense of maintaining the Henry Ford School of Nursing. Growth in both the severity of patient illness and the diversity of clinical settings created the need for more nurses with higher educational levels; this need could be met by OU using HFHS funding of $1.2 million.

HFHS's economic outcomes include the following:

1. Recruitment and retention of OU students to HFHS
2. Increased number of nurses completing advanced academic preparation

3. Expanded opportunities to maximize RN capacity and scope of practice
4. Increased use of clinical best practices to enhance patient outcomes
5. Opportunities to promote effective interdisciplinary team-based care

From the academic perspective, the outcomes include the following:

1. Recruitment and retention of HFHS employees as students
2. Curriculum enhancement, including business literacy and nursing in a capitated environment with population and care management components
3. Increased use of educational best practices to enhance student outcomes
4. Expanded access to research and clinical practice sites
5. Anticipated development of the nurse practitioner program
6. Seed money for faculty development and research

The health system and university are partners in the preparation and support of professional nurses for the 21st century. By combining resources in this unique alliance, the service, educational, and economic goals of both parties can be creatively met.

FUNDING FOR NURSING EDUCATION

The changing patterns of nurse employment require changes in nursing education to provide nurses who are educationally prepared for emerging positions. The greatest demand is for nurses prepared at the baccalaureate and graduate levels. Currently only 38 percent of nurses are prepared at those levels, and only 25 percent of new graduates have a baccalaureate education. The seventh report to Congress on the Status of Health Personnel in the United States estimated that by the year 2000 the country would have an excess of associate degree nurses and a shortage of nurses educated at the baccalaureate and higher degree levels. A particular shortage exists among nurses in advanced practice (Aiken, 1995). Most students in such programs work while completing these programs on a part-time basis, further slowing the production of advanced practice nurses.

Current federal funding policy for nursing education does not support the nursing profession's desired levels of educational preparation for nurses. Title VIII funding is the main source of money for graduate nursing education. This funding source is appropriated each year and has remained at approximately $60 million. Fifteen percent of the funds for graduate medical education from Medicare goes for nursing and allied health education. The nursing component of these funds has been approximately $174 million, which is reimbursed to hospitals for nursing education. Unfortunately, this money supports hospital school diploma programs, which have decreased to approximately 145 in the entire United States. These programs are not designed to provide the broad-based education required for the professional nurse of today who must practice in a community-based health-care delivery system. Nor do they provide the basis for continuing on to graduate education (Aiken & Salmon, 1994; Aiken, 1995; Aiken, Gwyther & Whelan, 1996). A national policy directing the appropriation of federal funding for nursing education would provide support for meeting projected nursing needs.

The American Association of Colleges of Nursing is engaged in two ongoing advocacy efforts to increase federal funding for nursing education and research. In the first effort, AACN has asked for a 10 percent increase in appropriations for the Nurse Education Act (Title VIII of the Public Health Service Act), for a total of $74.6 million in fiscal year 2000. This money funds doctoral programs that prepare nursing faculty and supports training grants for graduate students (Aiken, Gwyther & Whelan, 1996).

In the second effort, AACN, as a founding member of the Coalition for Nursing Research Funding, is pushing for a markedly increased budget in fiscal year 2000 for the National Institute of Nursing Research (NINR). This funding would support growth in the number of nurse scientists who also function as faculty members. The NINR has the smallest funding of all entities within the National Institutes of Health (Aiken, Gwyther & Whelan, 1996).

Educational funding could be used to achieve the Pew Commission's recommendations to increase the level of nursing education. There is particular need to increase the numbers of baccalaureate and advanced practice nurses in a variety of clinical specialties

Federal funding to support baccalaureate and advanced practice education for nurses maximizes the benefit of public dollars expended for nursing education.

AN ECONOMIC THREAT: FOR-PROFIT HIGHER EDUCATION

A recent trend in higher education is the emergence of for-profit educational institutions that are challenging the traditional university systems. For-profit organizations develop programs, deliver them in a variety of convenient locations, and implement innovative educational delivery mechanisms without what the National Commission on the Cost of Higher Education refers to as the cost and price drivers that plague traditional university systems (NCCHE, 1998). These drivers include financial aid, people (faculty and staff), facilities, technology, regulation, and expectations (for scheduling and support services).

Competition results when a number of suppliers vie for the business of a group of consumers.

The University of Phoenix, a for-profit institution, now claims to be the largest private university in the United States. This claim is supported by an enrollment that surpassed 50,000 in 1998. The franchise for-profit educational organizations target adult students who are over 25 years old and who are working full-time (Stamps, 1998). This student population requires evening classes. Some sources suggest that the University of Phoenix and other for-profit institutions represent a major challenge to traditional higher educational institutions today (Drucker, 1998; Stamps, 1998).

For-profit educational organizations, free of the cost and price drivers of traditional universities, are earning money while universities are struggling financially. It is estimated that the University of Phoenix is responsible for 80 percent of the $283 million profit of its parent corporation. Tuition is not cheap, averaging approximately $6500 per year. The formula for success includes developing a standardized product, marketing that product to a variety of settings, and using adjunct teachers rather than full-time professors (Stamps, 1998).

The desire of RNs to have greater flexibility in their BSN and MSN programs has not escaped the marketing eye of the for-profit institutions. These institutions have achieved program accreditation from the NLNAC. The nursing programs have a schedule of one night per week at a convenient location. Profit is possible in these institutions because they have lower overhead costs, a small number of standardized programs, temporary rented facilities in any location, and part-time teachers who are not eligible for benefits, promotion, or tenure. Although traditional educational institutions criticize this form of learning, for-profit organizations have motivated traditional schools to alter their teaching methods by incorporating distance learning, convenient schedules, and outreach locations for teaching.

The for-profit nursing education business is pushing traditional institutions to adapt their practices to attract students.

NEW PRODUCT LINES IN NURSING EDUCATION: DISTANCE LEARNING

Given the demand for nurses with advanced preparation, competition for students from for-profit education institutions, and evolving technology, educational institutions have become more creative in developing mechanisms to provide education to students in their immediate geographic area as well as in distant ones.

A specific educational strategy to provide health-care professionals with continuing education and additional professional degrees is distance education. When there are no universities in a geographic area, technology becomes an important adjunct for students to reach their educational goals. Mechanisms vary from audiovisual transmission to synchronous interactive television to asynchronous Internet courses.

> *Productivity in nursing education is enhanced by offering courses and programs to students at a distance through the use of distance education technologies.*

A variety of issues affect successful implementation of distance education at an affordable cost. A partnership of local educational facilities, health-care agencies, and the community facilitates program development that meets community needs. Next, the nature of programming must be established: continuing education, credit courses, or clinical courses. Each type of learning requires specific preparation to achieve desired outcomes (Hartshorn, 1998).

> *Consumer choice is provided by distance education products that include flexibility in both the timing and the format of educational technology.*

Student issues include arranging time to become familiar with the technology that they will be expected to use, preparing for the active participation required, and developing a student support network for completion of the program. Although distance education provides faculty with the opportunity to be creative and innovative in their educational pedagogy, teachers must learn to use the technology and to maximize its advantages. Another concern is finding sufficient faculty members who are willing to teach in distance education classes to meet the demand for the services (Hartshorn, 1998).

One cost of distance education is provision of the support services that are required to make distance learning a success. Technical support includes installation and maintenance of the system and assistance during class for system maintenance and problem solving. Support staff at the receiving location are important to facilitate the logistics of course delivery, including books, reading materials, computer access, and library services. For programs of study, students need a liaison to the educational institution to address admissions, registration, progression, and advising issues.

Administrators are faced with balancing the competing goals of meeting the educational needs of communities and providing cost-effective educational programs. Regardless of the format used, distance education programs require costly investment in equipment and support staff as well as an ongoing investment to update the equipment. Many institutions set minimum class sizes in order to cover the costs of the technology.

Faculty and students must understand the intellectual, ethical, and property rights issues associated with distance education. Faculty members spend much time developing creative materials for the programs they teach. It is important for them to understand the copyright and ownership issues involved. In addition, faculty must obtain copyright permission to broadcast visual images, audio information, or audiovisual materials. Similarly, privacy of student and client information is a prime concern when using technologies such as telephone, fax, and audiovisual technologies (Hartshorn, 1998).

The design and implementation of Internet courses raises parallel issues. These courses allow students to access materials at a time convenient to them, frequently called *asynchronous learning*. This method has been used for individual courses and entire on-line programs. Students require individual or publicly accessed computers and an Internet service provider. Tools utilized in such courses include Internet search engines, electronic mail and file transfer, and other conferencing tools and technologies. Courses facilitate interaction by providing a syllabus on-line that links to materials to prepare for class and by providing a conferencing system. All students are then required to participate in the topic of discussion. The system allows for on-line testing and submission of course projects.

Asynchronous learning *occurs when students participate in educational experiences at a location convenient to them at a time of their choosing.*

The accompanying case example demonstrates how a nursing program can extend programs beyond the campus area to facilitate educational mobility by incorporating partnerships with health-care agencies in other communities.

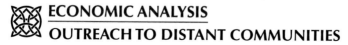

ECONOMIC ANALYSIS
OUTREACH TO DISTANT COMMUNITIES

With enrollments declining in basic baccalaureate programs, Eastern Michigan University chose to enhance enrollments in the RN/BSN

Completion Program. Outreach programs were developed with small to midsized communities that did not have a 4-year university available.

In a local community, a nursing service department negotiated a partnership with the university nursing department to offer the RN/BSN Completion Program to their employees. Agreements were made to offer the classes on one night per week, to locate classes at a site closer to the hospital than the local community college, and to evaluate the experience for continuation. This facility did not want to use distance learning by interactive television for the program, so faculty traveled to the site to hold classes. An information meeting was held to present a model in which the students, the service agency, and the university would come together to meet the challenges inherent in a changed health-care system. Students were asked to commit to the program as a cohort that would enhance retention in the program. The university committed to bringing all nursing courses and sufficient general education courses for program completion to the local site. The agency committed to facilitate schedules and tuition reimbursement. In the initial cohort there were 70 students. Although some original students did not complete the program, additional students joined the program; 63 students completed the program. Following evaluation, the partners agreed to establish a second cohort consisting of 40 students.

Based on this experience, Eastern Michigan University has expanded its outreach to three additional locations for the RN/BSN Completion Program as well as three sites for the MSN program. The MSN program uses interactive television combined with on-site delivery. Plans include incorporation of some Internet courses. The partnerships between service agencies and universities as well as between junior and senior colleges have proved to be cost effective. It is expected that such partnerships will continue to flourish.

 ## DEMAND FOR NURSING EDUCATION

The increased demand for nurses and the problems of supply are discussed in Chapters 5 and 8. The need for health care creates a derived demand for well-educated nurses. This in turn creates a demand for well-educated faculty to teach in nursing education programs.

SUPPLY OF FACULTY FOR NURSING EDUCATION

To prepare a supply of nurses sufficient for health-care demands, there must be a sufficient supply of appropriately educated faculty members. Several factors affect the supply of nursing faculty (AACN, 1998):

- Nursing services in large organizations have begun to hire doctorally prepared nurses as administrators and researchers in their agencies.
- An increase in the number of new programs being developed contributes to the problem that nursing deans have in finding appropriately prepared faculty.
- The annual graduation rate from doctoral programs remains small.
- The time from enrollment to graduation in doctoral programs can be up to 10 years.
- Bureaucratic systems of higher education inhibit organizational change.
- Aging nursing faculty members continue to leave the teaching pool as they retire.

These factors are resulting in a specific shortage of nursing faculty.

In its core guidelines for master's education, the AACN notes that the primary thrust of master's programs is to prepare nurses for clinical practice and that doctoral preparation should be considered the appropriate and desirable credential for a nurse educator. However, of the more than 9000 faculty at AACN-member nursing schools at universities and senior colleges around the country, only slightly more than 50 percent are doctorally prepared. The percentage of master's nursing students pursuing academic careers is in a steep decline, dropping 27.5 percent from 1997 to 1998 alone, according to AACN figures. And with the average age of full-time nursing faculty now 49, a wave of retirements is expected to peak in just 10 years (AACN Bulletin, 1999).

AACN data for 1998 reveal that 411 people graduated from doctoral programs in nursing. Only 43 percent of those graduates had a commitment to becoming a nursing school faculty member. Seventeen percent had accepted nonacademic positions. The master's-level academic track, which is a source of qualified faculty members, is eroding at schools nationwide. This may be a result of focus on practitioner programs. AACN data show that 85 practitioner programs, responding to an AACN survey in 1998, graduated just 348 students, down from 480 in 1997. In 1998, 3.3 percent of master's graduates in nursing were completing of educator tracks, compared with 6.5 percent in 1995 (AACN Bulletin, 1996).

Another challenge for schools of nursing is the discrepancy between the skills and expectations of prospective faculty and the multiple demands of a faculty position. Nursing faculty members are expected to provide excellent teaching, produce contributions to the scholarship of nursing, and participate in service activities related to the educational institution and the professional discipline. Frequently, doctorally prepared nurses do not have skill and experience in teaching. Carole Anderson, nursing dean at the Ohio State University and immediate past president, cites lack of academic experience as a real barrier. Many PhDs, she says, "do not appear to have a 'fundable' program of research defined, or they lack teaching skills." Other candidates "know that research is the name of the game, and that is what they want to do," states Pamela Watson of Thomas Jefferson. "Often they don't want to teach at the baccalaureate level at all—only graduate—and here they only want to teach selected courses; most don't have a clinical specialty." Rita Carty, dean of the College of Nursing and Health Science at George Mason University in Fairfax, Virginia, concurs: "It is becoming increasingly difficulty to have a sufficient resource of doctorally prepared faculty to work at all levels in nursing education, especially clinical supervision of undergraduate students" (AACN Bulletin, 1998).

BUREAUCRACY IN EDUCATIONAL SYSTEMS

Bureaucratic educational systems are another factor affecting the production of nurses with advanced education. The accompanying economic analysis demonstrates how it can take approximately 3 years to create an advanced practice nursing program and an additional 2 years to increase student numbers.

ECONOMIC ANALYSIS
CREATING A NEW NURSE PRACTITIONER PROGRAM

A small public university has an MSN program with a clinical focus on adult health. However, a needs assessment suggests that more students could be recruited if there were a nurse practitioner option. A task force of faculty members is formed to create a post-master's certificate program for adult-health nurse practitioners. This task force reports to the Graduate Curriculum Committee. After 15 months the proposed curriculum is approved by this committee. The proposal is then debated by the entire nursing faculty, the college-level committee, all other colleges, and the university graduate program. During this process, any group can request more information for consideration. When this process is complete the provost must agree to support the proposal in the state-level group of other public universities. This process can take another year, depending on scheduling. During the approval process, the nursing administrator must also seek resources from the university and other sources to fund the program.

When the proposal has been approved, the nursing administrator must then hire sufficient nurse practitioner faculty members and plan for program implementation. Planning could easily take another 6 months. A time frame of 33 months has thus elapsed from program conception until the first cohort of 10 students is admitted.

The nurse administrator believes that such a small program cannot be sustained. She submits another proposal when the first cohort of students is graduated that justifies an increase of the student cohort from 10 to 30 students and two additional faculty based on the need for nurse practitioners, the success of students on their certification exam, and program evaluation. This proposal takes another year to be approved and funded. This lengthy process illustrates the limitations of a bureaucratic organization for responding in a timely fashion to changing demands for nursing education.

MARKETING NURSING EDUCATION

If there are so many opportunities for nurses with baccalaureate and higher degree education, how can the profession use these opportunities for recruitment? The American Nurses' Association and other nursing organizations can employ a variety of marketing strategies to attract students to nursing.

Students should be made aware of the myriad job opportunities for nurses. These opportunities need to be presented in an exciting and appealing manner. Strategies for recruitment should include a variety of media advertising, particularly the Internet. The goal is to counteract existing false nursing images in the media (books, television, and movies) that do not reflect the true work of nurses. Currently, most nursing organizations have Web sites. All media should be designed to be attractive not only to existing nurses but also to potential nurses.

The following key marketing messages could be used to attract new nurses:

- Opportunities to engage in exciting work to help others
- Available jobs in a variety of clinical areas and settings
- Competitive salaries for new graduates
- Science-based, challenging profession
- Geographic diversity of available jobs
- Opportunities for advancement in practice, management, and education or research for those with additional education

To attract registered nurses to return for BSN and graduate education, the strategies would be similar but should focus on the added value of an additional degree and the feasibility of attaining this education while working. Potential students need encouragement to realize that further education is possible.

Some key marketing messages to encourage current nurses to pursue additional education are as follows:

- New job opportunities
- Advancement within a present job location
- Opportunity to learn with other motivated professionals
- Convenient programs, including one evening per week, locations close to students, and distance learning options

PREPARING NURSES WITH THE NEEDED EDUCATION

Supply problems can and do exist in specific nurse markets. There is growing awareness that practicing nurses do not have sufficient educational preparation for their new roles in changing health-care systems (AACN, 1998). Nursing must prepare for the present and future needs in health-care delivery or it will miss opportunities. The respondents to a study by Buerhaus and Staiger (1999) were skeptical about the ability of nursing educators and educational organizations to respond in a timely manner to the rapid changes in health-care delivery.

Supply deficits can exist in total numbers of nurses as well as in specific educational levels.

Aiken argues that health-care policy since World War II has focused on increasing the total supply of registered nurses rather than examining specific needs (Aiken, 1995). The Pew Health Professions Commission recognizes this dilemma of a current oversupply of nurses who are inadequately prepared to meet the challenges of the present and evolving health-care system. It recommends closing 10 to 20 percent of nursing programs, targeting diploma and associate degree community college programs. Along with the closing of programs, the Commission strongly recommends facilitating the educational mobility of nurses seeking to advance their education (Pew Health Professions Commission, 1995). Professional nursing organizations, particularly the National League for Nursing and the American Association of Colleges of Nursing, continually examine the health-care environment and make recommendations for preparing nurses for the future.

A cost-effective means of promoting higher-quality health care is to close up to 20 percent of the nation's associate degree and hospital diploma nursing programs and provide concentrated support for baccalaureate and graduate degree programs.

MOBILITY IN NURSING EDUCATION

To meet the demand for more nurses with baccalaureate and graduate education, mechanisms to promote educational mobility are needed. Because there are multiple educational routes to becoming eligible for licensure to practice nursing, including the diploma, associate degree, baccalaureate degree, and generic master's and doctoral programs, mechanisms are needed to assist nurses to progress to higher levels of nursing education. Enhancing the educational level of practicing nurses who are prepared at less than the baccalaureate degree level is a quick means of developing a larger pool of nurses with a baccalaureate degree.

Educational mobility is a cost-effective process that enables nurses to acquire additional broad-based knowledge and skills.

The goals of educational mobility supported by the AACN (1999a) are to:

- Maintain educational integrity and program quality
- Enhance the professional socialization of students as well as promote the achievement of personal goals
- Focus on attainment of outcomes that reflect a higher level of knowledge, skills, and critical thinking
- Be flexible regarding admission but clear on outcome criteria and standards
- Collaborate among educational institutions for the achievement of optimal transfer of credits

The AACN promotes creative and flexible approaches for achieving the desired educational outcomes rather than the traditional and very rigid requirements that have limited the educational progression of students from vocational nursing, associate degree, and diploma programs. Nursing can no longer afford to squander its human capital by costly repetition of courses by licensed practitioners. The cost to educate an RN with a diploma or an associate degree to the baccalaureate degree level is considerably less than the cost of educating the baccalaureate student because of the relatively high cost of clinical supervision in the latter case. Educating practicing nurses also shortens the time period for supplying more baccalaureate nurses to the health-care system.

With the recognition of the need for more nurses prepared at the baccalaureate and higher degree levels, educators are being urged to eliminate unnecessary educational hurdles and to develop creative mechanisms to foster educational mobility for practicing nurses. Many states are examining creative mechanisms to evaluate prior learning and facilitate the educational mobility and career development of practicing nurses (McClelland et al., 1997). The accompanying economic analysis recounts two different state's initiatives for improving educational mobility.

ECONOMIC ANALYSIS
TWO STATE-LEVEL INITIATIVES TO IMPROVE EDUCATIONAL MOBILITY FOR NURSES

STATE A

Two nursing organizations composed of educators in the state—one of associate degree educators and the other of baccalaureate degree educators—created a task force to develop recommendations for the educational progression of nurses from an associate degree to a baccalaureate degree. The primary goals in this process were to respect prior learning, avoid duplication of previous learning experiences, and maintain desired standards for a baccalaureate-prepared nurse. One strategy to achieve these goals was to hold a forum early in the process that enabled a larger community of nursing educators to participate in this important discussion. The discussion also included strategies for integrating diploma-prepared nurses, who frequently lack credits that can be transferred to an institution of higher education.

The result of the overall process enabled the task force to propose a broad set of criteria to guide baccalaureate programs in accepting and assisting students from associate degree and diploma nursing programs. The five agreed-upon criteria are as follows:

1. The student must hold an active, unencumbered state nursing license.
2. The student must meet the specific admission requirements of the accepting institution (i.e., the institution to which the student is applying for further education).
3. The accepting institution recognizes passing of the National Council Lincensure Examination (NCLEX) as validation of the common core knowledge, attitudes, and skill upon which further nursing education can be built.
4. The sending institution (i.e., the institution from which the student has graduated) and the accepting institution will collaborate concerning curriculum practices to eliminate barriers to educational mobility.

5. To graduate with a degree in nursing, the transfer student will need to satisfy all general education, support, and major core requirements of the accepting institution. In no case should a transfer student be required to duplicate or earn more nursing credits than the generic student.

 ## STATE B:
THE IOWA ARTICULATION STORY

As a result of the Iowa Board of Nursing's Statewide Plan for Nursing in Iowa, an articulation plan was developed that built on the history of articulation between vocational and associate degree nursing programs. The Iowa Board's recommendations included fostering collaboration among educational institutions to facilitate articulation and measuring achieved competencies to minimize repetition in the curriculum.

An Articulation in Nursing Education Committee was composed of representatives from baccalaureate programs, two associate degree programs, diploma programs, and the state-level consultant for Health Occupations Education. The committee's charge was to develop and present a plan to the Iowa Board of Nursing within 2 years. The plan approved was similar to those of Colorado and Maryland but specific to the needs of Iowa. Articulation options included the following:

1. Programs could achieve direct transfer of credits for graduates of Iowa diploma and associate degree nursing programs. Each program would be evaluated using validation criteria, and then at least one-half of the total nursing credits for graduation would be awarded.
2. Students who graduated from an associate degree or diploma program in another state could be awarded at least one-half of their nursing credits by successfully completing standardized examinations.
3. Students from Iowa or any state could receive placement in a baccalaureate program by completing three articulation courses: nursing concepts, scientific concepts, and social science concepts.
4. Students from Iowa or any state could achieve credit for at least one-half of the nursing program by holding those credits in escrow until they had completed three to four credits in the nursing program.

This program was implemented in 1991. All associate degree and diploma schools have been validated for participation. All the baccalaureate programs except one have been validated for participation. A reporting system to the state board of nursing has been created. Three areas provide challenges to the operation of this system: trust, communication, and maintaining NLNAC accreditation. The number of students in the program has increased. Many students choose the option of a direct transfer of credits, but most students by far choose the option to escrow their credits until validated by course work (McClelland et al., 1997).

FACTORS AFFECTING FUTURE NURSING EDUCATION

In addition to supply and demand, competition and the health-care environment, other factors affect nursing education. These include the need for:

- Input from professional organizations regarding curriculum development
- Economic content in nursing education
- Interdisciplinary content in nursing education
- Focus on demographic changes in the population, such as increased diversity of age and ethnicity

PROFESSIONAL ORGANIZATIONS AND CURRICULUM DEVELOPMENT

The dynamic environment of health care requires changes in nursing education. The AACN recommends flexible, innovative curricula based on core nursing values and interdisciplinary collaboration. These curricula should include the following priorities (AACN, 1998a):

- Development of critical thinking and clinical judgment skills
- Recognition of the changing demographics of the population
- Focus on ethnic diversity and skills of cultural competence
- New and expanded roles for nursing
- Provision of care that is high quality, cost effective, and accountable
- Focus on care that is population based
- Increasing focus on primary health care
- Development of system skills of management, health-care policy, economics, quality assessment, financial management, research, and technology

Standardization and quality of nursing education and its graduates are promoted by the identification of essential educational content by professional organizations.

ECONOMIC CONTENT IN EDUCATIONAL PROGRAMS

Health-care trends and the AACN recommendations for curricula highlight the need for content on health-care economics to achieve the goal of "provision of care that is high quality, cost effective and accountable" (AACN, 1995, 1997). This content should include basic economic principles, the working of the health-care market, and mechanisms to achieve cost-effective health care.

Nurses, as the largest group of health-care professionals, need to understand the labor market and how that affects the supply and demand for nurses as well as the wages for the work performed. Knowledge of health-care systems and how they work economically positions nurses to contribute effectively to this system.

INTERDISCIPLINARY HEALTH PROFESSIONAL EDUCATION

Both the AACN and the Pew Health Professions Commission have highlighted the necessity for interdisciplinary health professional education to achieve desired health-care outcomes in a cost-effective manner and to achieve economies in health professional education. Such education also prepares health professionals to work together more effectively.

Traditionally, health professional education has been provided separately within each discipline. Creating models for interdisciplinary education is a challenge for institutions and professions. In an effort to provide direction for this movement, the Institute for Healthcare Improvement initiated the Interdisciplinary Professional Education Collaborative in 1994 (Bellack, 1998). Four universities were selected for a 3-year demonstration project. Each site had to demonstrate commitment to quality improvement, involvement of at least three disciplines (nursing, medicine, and health administration), and commitment of institutional resources to the project. The ultimate goal of each project was to meet the needs of individuals and communities for health care through cost-effective practice. Although each project operated differently, each project identified keys and barriers to success.

The keys to success are as follows (Bellack et al., 1997):

- Clarity of team goals and team dynamics
- Faculty team leaders who are respected within their discipline and institution
- Commitment of high-level organizational leaders

- Campus visibility
- Pilot success

The barriers to success are as follows (Bellack et al., 1997):

- Institutional resistance to change
- Perception that quality improvement is a business rather than an educational issue
- Educational culture and disciplinary traditions
- Hierarchical power structures and imbalances
- Rigidity of curricula, scheduling, and regulations
- Limited institutional commitment
- Lack of faculty experience with interdisciplinary practice and teaching
- Funding and reward structures that reinforce research over practice and interdisciplinary work

This effort supported projects in interdisciplinary health professional education at four sites. The presence of the project allowed learning and progress in interdisciplinary efforts at each site.

DEMOGRAPHIC CHANGES

Population demographics continue to demonstrate more diversity. Institutions of higher education and professional organizations recognize that having a workforce that mirrors the population is one strategy for providing acceptable health care that results in positive health outcomes. The AACN includes race, ethnicity, socioeconomic status, gender, age, religion, sexual orientation, and physical disability in their definition of diversity (AACN, 1998b).

There is both good and bad news about the number of minority nurses in the workforce. Although the total percentage of minority nurses has increased from 6.3 percent in 1977 to 9.7 percent in 1997, this proportion is less than in other health professions (Buerhaus & Averbach, 1999; National League for Nursing [NLN], 1998). Civil rights legislation and affirmative action programs have promoted the entry of minority students to higher education, including nursing programs.

Remaining barriers to recruitment of minority students include inadequate financial assistance, inadequate levels of academic preparation, racism, isolation, alienation, and poor perceptions of nursing by students and parents. Schools can examine their admission requirements, support services, and academic assistance programs as mechanisms to assist all students to be successful (Buerhaus & Averbach, 1999; NLN, 1998).

The accompanying economic analysis describes an initiative to recruit minority students into an interdisciplinary program focused on the preparation of nurse practitioners.

 ECONOMIC ANALYSIS
GREATER DETROIT AREA PARTNERSHIP FOR TRAINING

Anne Sullivan Smith, PhD, RN, with acknowledgment to Joan Urbancic, PhD, RN

The Greater Detroit Area Partnership for Training was initiated in 1995 with funding from the Robert Wood Johnson Foundation. The purpose of the initiative is to develop and implement a regional interdisciplinary educational program to prepare advanced practitioners for clinical practice within underserved areas. The goal is to recruit potential students who live or work in underserved areas, or are minorities, to become community-oriented, culturally competent clinicians committed to the delivery of primary care in medically underserved areas or communities identified as at risk.

Student recruitment is focused on minority students who will practice in underserved areas upon graduation. Faith-based organizations and health-care systems are partners in recommending candidates who are committed to their communities and will return there to practice. The Partnership includes community-based organizations, four universities that offer advanced practice nursing programs, and five health-care systems providing care to the communities of interest.

An initial step was curriculum review to identify similarities and differences among the six program plans. During the planning phase, several work groups were established to develop and implement the joint curriculum. Three courses were identified for priority consideration: Health Promotion Risk Reduction, Health-Care Policy Issues, and Professional Perspectives (a course to foster the transition from student to practitioner). A fourth course was also identified: an enhanced clinical experience with focus on care management, cultural competence, client access to care, and greater satisfaction with care by the medically underserved populations. These course selections were designed to provide opportunities for students to understand their specific contribution to patient care management and to recognize the synergy that arises from interdisciplinary perspectives. The courses that were created incorporated an interdisciplinary paradigm and represented the best content based on input of known faculty experts from the participating programs.

Economies of scale are achieved because faculty rotate responsibility for course teaching, with a section being offered at one neutral site rather than concurrently at all four universities. Opportunities are available for other students to enroll in course offerings. One of the newer graduate programs had not yet developed a Health Promotion Risk Reduction course. Instead of expending the time and talent to build such a course, they are electing to advise their Partnership students to enroll in the course designed for the project. One of the programs elected to offer the Partnership course as that semester's option for all its enrolled advanced practice graduate students.

The enhanced clinical experience has been complemented by cooperative efforts with medical colleagues. A grand rounds presentation is planned for each fall and winter, which includes a lecture on clinical topics of special interest to medically underserved communities and guided on-line interdisciplinary discussion groups. The lectures emphasize cultural congruence relevant to groups in the area. It is anticipated that state-of-the-art care management guidelines will be developed to address the concerns of the populations of interest.

Administration has been designed to minimize barriers to course enrollment and submission of grades across institutions. These decisions have yielded important benefits for the project by eliminating the need to address administrative differences among institutions. These efficiencies have contributed to holding administrative expenses to a minimum. Although it is difficult to measure the benefits of preparing an interdisciplinary group of minority students, students express a continuing commitment to meeting the needs of medically underserved communities, the major goal of the project.

SUMMARY

This chapter presented an overview of nursing and nursing education studies that have influenced the quality and economics of nursing supply and demand throughout the 20th century. It discussed major trends, projections, and recommendations reported by the Pew Health Professions Commission. The economics of higher education was discussed, drawing on the 1998 report of the National Commission on Costs in Higher Education. Issues of productivity and cost containment in nursing education were explored.

The chapter detailed the relationship of nursing productivity and cost containment and suggested that nursing educators must clearly articulate the unit's funding needs to produce an adequate supply of nurses prepared at the appropriate educational levels to meet the needs of society. If institutions of higher education are unable or unwilling to produce sufficient nurses, an industry of for-profit educational programs is building capacity to compete for students. Particularly troubling is the deficit of doctorally prepared nursing faculty members who have requisite clinical and teaching skills. A variety of new educational product lines are being employed to reach students who might not otherwise have access to advanced education.

DISCUSSION QUESTIONS

1. Which of the national reports on the status of nursing practice and education have had the most significant effect on providing direction for the future development of the profession? Explain your position.
2. Analyze the financial pressures for cost containment and productivity in higher education.
3. Compare and contrast the types of program resources required for traditional courses in higher education versus for-profit courses or programs.
4. Educators emphasize that decreasing enrollments do not necessarily mean a declining interest in nursing careers. Do you agree? Defend your answer.
5. What is the feasibility of the Pew Commission recommendation to close up to 20 percent of the nation's associate degree and hospital diploma nursing programs in favor of more concentrated support of BSN and graduate degree nurse training? Explain why you do or do not favor such action.
6. Why is educational mobility important for nurses? What approaches do you favor to achieve such mobility?
7. As a new doctoral graduate in nursing, what are the advantages and disadvantages for accepting a nursing faculty position?
8. Are faculty shortages a critical issue in nursing? Explain.
9. Why is it imperative that nursing education programs act as agents of change?
10. Give an example of a partnership between nursing education and nursing practice.

11. Explain the advantages and disadvantages of various modes of distance education for students and faculty.

 REFERENCES

Aiken, L. H. (1995). Transformation in the nursing workforce. *Nursing Outlook*, 43(5), 201–209.

Aiken, L., Gwyther, M. E., & Whelan, E. (1996). Federal support of graduate nursing education: Rationale and policy options. *Nursing Outlook*, 44, 11–17.

Aiken, L. H., & Salmon, M. E. (1994). Health care workforce priorities: What nursing should know. *Inquiry*, 31, 318–329.

American Association of Colleges of Nursing. (1998b). Essentials of baccalaureate education. Washington, DC: Author.

American Association of Colleges of Nursing. (1998b). Issue Bulletin: As RNs age, nursing schools seek to expand the pool of younger faculty. Washington, DC, Author.

American Association of Colleges of Nursing. (1996). Essentials of master's education for advanced practice nursing. Washington, DC: Author.

American Association of Colleges of Nursing. (1997, October 27). A vision of baccalaureate and graduate education: The next decade [On-line]. Available: http:www.aacn.nche.edu/publications.

American Association of Colleges of Nursing. (1999a). Educational mobility. *Journal of Professional Nursing*, 14(5), 314–316.

American Association of Colleges of Nursing. (1999b). *1997–1998 enrollment and graduations in baccalaureate and graduate programs in nursing*. Washington, DC: Author.

American Association of Colleges of Nursing. (1999c, February). *Talking points: While demand for RNs climbs, undergraduate nursing enrollments decline*. Washington, DC: Author.

American Association of Colleges of Nursing. (1999d, April). *Issue bulletin: Faculty shortages intensify the nation's nursing deficit*. Washington, DC: Author.

American Nurses' Association. (1965). *Educational preparation for nurse practitioners and assistants to nurses: A position paper*. New York: Author.

American Nurses' Association. (1983). *Education for nursing practice in the context of the 1980s*. St. Louis, MO: Author.

Banta, T. W. (1988). Promise and perils. In T. W. Banta (Ed.), *Implementing outcomes assessment: Promise and perils*. New directions for institutional research No. 59. San Francisco: Jossey-Bass.

Bellack, J. P., Gerrity, P., Moore, S. M., Novotny, J., Quinn, D., Norman, L., Harper, D. C. (1997). Taking aim at interdisciplinary education for continuous improvement in health care. *Nursing and Health Care Perspectives*, 18, (6) 308–315.

Buerhaus, P. I., & Auerbach, D. (1999). Slow growth in the United States of the number of minorities in the RN workforce. *Image: Journal of Nursing Scholarship*, 31, (2) 179–183.

Buerhaus, P. I. & Staiger, D. O. (1999). Trouble in the nurse labor market? Recent trends and future outlook. *Health Affairs*, 18(1), 214–222.

Drucker, P. F., (August 24, 1998). The next information revolution. *Forbes*, 47–57.

Hartshorn, J. C. (1998). Distance education in nursing: Strategies, successes, and challenges. In S. F. Viegas & K. Dunn (Eds.) *Telemedicine: Practicing in the information age* (pp. 167–174). Philadelphia: Lippincott-Raven.

Kalisch, P. A., & Kalisch, B. J. (1995). The advance of American nursing. (3rd Ed.). Philadelphia: Lippincott.

Kelly, L. Y. (1975). (3rd ed.) *Dimensions of professional nursing.* New York: Macmillan.

Lysaught, J. P. (1970). *An abstract for action. National Commission for the Study of Nursing and Nursing Education.* New York: McGraw-Hill.

McClelland, E., Aulwes, M. A., Bradley, P., Chapman, J. A., Crouse, P., Erickson, J. A., Kirkpatrick, S., Newell, M. C., Sellers, S. I., Strachota, E., & Zenor, B. (1997). The Iowa articulation story. *Nurse Educator, 22(22),* 19–24.

National Center for Education Statistics. (1995, February). *Pocket projections: Projections of education statistics to 2005.* Washington, DC: U.S. Department of Education.

National Commission on the Cost of Higher Education (1998, January 21). *Straight talk about college costs and prices.* Washington, DC: Author. Available: http://chronicle.com/data/focus.dir/data.dir/p121.98/costreport.htm.

Pew Health Professions Commission. (1995). *Critical challenges: Revitalizing the health professions for the twenty-first century.* San Francisco: UCSF Center for Health Professions.

Stamps, D. (1998). The for profit future of higher education. *Training.*

Thompson, C., & Bartles, J. E. (1999). Outcomes assessment: Implications for nursing education. *Journal of Professional Nursing,* 15(3), 170–178.

 SUGGESTED READING

Association of Governing Boards of Universities and Colleges. (1999). Ten public policy issues for higher education in 1999 and 2000 (AGB Public Policy Paper Series No. 99-1). Washington, DC: Author.

Barber, K., Wyatt, K., & Gergasi, F. (1999). On-line interactive evaluation and clinical instruction. *Nurse Educator,* 24(2), 37–40.

Buerhaus, P. I., & Auerbach, D. (1999). Slow growth in the United States in the number of minorities in the RN workforce. *Image,* 31, 179–183.

Bureau of the Census. Washington, DC: U.S. Department of Commerce; and Division of Nursing. (1996, March). *Advance notes from the National Sample Survey of Registered Nurses.* Washington, DC: U.S. Department of Health and Human Services.

Fagin, C. (1997, December 30). How nursing should respond to the third report of Pew Health Professions Commission [On-line]. Available: http:www.nursing-world.org/ojin/tpc5/tpc5_2.htm.

Viegas, S. F., & Dunn, K. (Eds). (1999). *Telemedicine: Practicing in the information age.* Philadelphia: Lippincott-Raven.

Chapter 8

The Nursing Labor Market: Demand, Supply, and Wages

Cyril F. Chang
Sylvia A. Price
Susan K. Pfoutz

OUTLINE

II. Nursing Salary and Employment: A Historical Overview
     A. Trends in Nursing Earnings
     B. Trends in Nursing Employment
III. Factors Affecting Nursing Salaries
     A. Experience
     B. Breaks in Service
     C. Education
     D. Settings and Specialty
     E. Higher Wages for Overtime, Nights, and Weekends
     F. Part-Time Nurses
     G. Union Membership and Geographic Location
IV. Demand Trends

(continued)

LEARNING OBJECTIVES

- Examine the nursing population and review the history of nursing earnings and employment.
- Examine the factors that determine nursing wages and salaries.
- Assess the future demand for the nursing labor force and analyze the possible effects of managed care.
- Examine major nursing labor supply trends.
- Assess emerging health-care trends that can affect the nursing labor market.
- Learn how labor markets work and how individual nurses can turn threats into opportunities.

The two previous chapters have provided the basis for understanding how the nursing labor market functions. Specifically, Chapter 6 presented a theoretical framework for the nursing labor market, and Chapter 7 focused on nursing education and government support for it. The emphasis of these two chapters was on how the nursing labor market reacts to changes in the supply and demand conditions of the health-care market as a whole. The purpose of this chapter is to examine current labor market conditions and review earnings and employment trends from the perspective of the individual nurse. The focus is on the effects of individual qualifications and work-setting characteristics on employment and salaries. It begins with a brief history of nursing earnings and employment. It then discusses the jobs that nurses perform and reviews salary and compensation trends. The chapter ends with a discussion of many common misconceptions about the nursing labor market and an overview of the job outlook for the near future.

 ## NURSING POPULATION

According to the National League for Nursing (NLN), there were 2.6 million registered nurses (RNs) in the United States in 1996 (NLN, 1997a). Of this total, about 59 percent were employed full time, 23.7 percent were employed part time, and 17.3 percent were not employed. The Bureau of Labor Statistics (1998) reports that among the employed RNs, two of three were employed in hospitals. The rest were employed in physicians' offices and clinics, home-health-care agencies, nursing homes, temporary help agencies, schools, managed care organizations, and government agencies.

Nurses work in a wide range of practice settings. The location of a practice setting is a critical aspect of any service.

Over the last 20 years, the number of nurses employed in health care increased substantially. The data in Table 8–1 show there were about 1.3 million active RNs in 1980. By 1996, the total had increased to more than 2.1 million, making RNs the largest group of health-care personnel in the American health-care system (National Center for Health Statistics, 1998). Not only has the number of RNs increased, but also the ratio of RNs to the general population has increased. In 1980, for example, there were 560 RNs per 100,000 people in the United States. By 1996, the RN-to-population ratio had risen to 798 per 100,000 people.

The increases in the number of nurses have in large part come from the country's nursing schools. Between 1970 and 1996, for example, the total number of nursing graduates increased from 43,103 to 94,757—a 120 percent increase in 26 years (National Center for Health Statistics, 1998). Most of the new nurses were graduates of the baccalaureate and associate degree nursing programs, as demonstrated by the statistical trends presented in Figure 8–1. In contrast, the number of graduates from diploma schools had declined.

Supply of employees is critical to providing a service.

In the mid-1990s, enrollments in basic RN programs fell for the first time in many years. From 1993 to 1996, according to a recent NLN report, the total number of nursing students fell by 32,000 students (NLN, 1997a). Among

TABLE 8–1. ACTIVE NURSING PERSONNEL IN THE UNITED STATES, 1980, 1990, AND 1996

	1980		1990		1996	
	Number	**%**	**Number**	**%**	**Number**	**%**
Registered nurses	1,272,900	100.0	1,789,600	100.0	2,115,700	100.0
Associate and diploma	908,300	71.4	1,107,300	61.9	1,235,000	58.4
Baccalaureate	297,300	23.3	549,000	30.7	673,200	31.8
Master's and doctorate	67,300	5.3	133,300	7.4	207,500	9.8
			RNs per 100,000 population			
Registered nurses	561		714		798	
Associate and diploma	400		442		466	
Baccalaureate	131		219		254	
Master's and doctorate	30		53		78	

Source: National Center for Health Statistics. (1998). *Health, United States, 1998.* Hyattsville, MD: U.S. Public Health Services, Table 103.

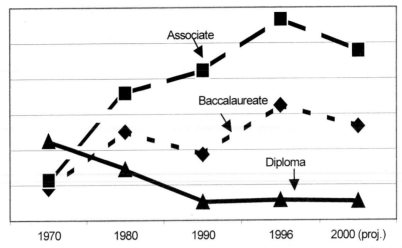

FIG. 8–1. Graduates of nursing schools. (From National Center for Health Statistics. (1998). *Health, United States, 1998.* Hyattsville, MD: U.S. Public Health Services, Table 106.)

the three basic RN programs, baccalaureate enrollments declined by 5.7 percent, associate degree enrollments fell by 9.6 percent, and diploma enrollments fell by 22.7 percent. In contrast, post-RN enrollments experienced a slight increase of 2 percent, from 47,000 in 1995 to 48,030 in 1996. The reduction in enrollment was greater for 1996 than previous years. The year also saw a decline in the total number of nursing graduates. Compared with 1995, for example, approximately 2,350 (or 2.4 percent) fewer students graduated in 1996 (NLN, 1997a). Given the recent decreases in enrollments in the basic nursing programs, this declining trend of nursing graduates could continue for the foreseeable future.

 NURSING SALARY AND EMPLOYMENT: A HISTORICAL OVERVIEW

Nurses play many important roles in health care. First, they provide direct care to help patients recover from their illnesses. Second, they are both educators and advocates, promoting health and preventing disease in communities where they live. Third, in their new roles as case managers, managed care gatekeepers, and health-plan managers and administrators, nurses manage the care plans of their patients directly and indirectly while assisting to keep the costs of health care down. However, they have not been paid well in the past for the work they did and the responsibilities that they were asked to bear.

Salary *is the money received by an employee for services rendered under a contract between an employer and employee.*

TRENDS IN NURSING EARNINGS

Nursing compensation has undergone radical changes in the last 40 years. In the 1950s and 1960s, nurses worked long hours and earned less than school teachers, the average factory workers, and even clerical workers such as secretaries (Kalisch & Kalisch, 1986; Wolfe, 1997). Pay and working conditions began to improve in the 1970s. However, substantial gains in compensation and working conditions were not made until the early 1990s, when nurses became more skilled in using collective bargaining as a strategy to improve salaries and work conditions. Wages and benefits were also boosted by periodic shortages of a nursing workforce.

Today, nurses' salaries and benefits compare favorably with those of teachers and other professionals with similar education and skills. For example, the average salary of full-time RNs was $42,071 in 1996. The average salary of full-time licensed practical nurses (LPNs) was $24,336. The salaries of advanced practice nurses such as nurse practitioners, nurse midwives, and nurse anesthetists have increased substantially in recent years (see Table 8–2).

RNs and LPNs have both experienced more gains in wages than have other occupations in recent years. Buerhaus and Staiger (1996) reported that from 1983 to 1991, RNs experienced notable gains in inflation-adjusted

TABLE 8–2. NURSING SALARIES, 1996

Type of Nurses	Average Annual Salary ($)
Full-time salaried licensed practical nurses	24,336
Full-time salaried registered nurses	42,071
Nurse practitioners	66,800
Nurse midwives	70,100
Nurse anesthetists	82,000

Sources: National League for Nursing. (1997). *National Nurses Week,* May 5–12, and Bureau of Labor Statistics. (1998). *Occupational Outlook Handbook, the 1998–99 edition.* Washington, DC: U.S. Department of Labor.

hourly wages, averaging nearly a 3 percent gain per year. In contrast, the average gain in inflation-adjusted wages in other occupations was only 2 percent or less. Similarly, LPN wages have grown steadily since the mid-1980s, albeit at a slower rate than RN wages. Conversely, nurse's aides experienced very little growth in wages, and their modest wage gains were comparable with most other occupations.

However, a new trend in nursing earnings has emerged. Based on a review of nine studies published between 1991 and 1996, Brewer (1997) noticed that the rate of wage increase has slowed since 1992. For example, Buerhaus and Staiger (1996) reported no growth in inflation-adjusted wages from 1992 to 1994. Similarly, Sachs and Spreier (1996) found a meager wage growth of 0.3 percent in 1996 after adjusting for inflation. Begany (1995) reported that RNs experienced a decrease of 1.0 percent in wages in 1995. Taken as a whole, the results of the nine studies suggest that since 1992, wage growth seems to have slowed and the average growth rate appears to be at or below the economy-wide inflation rate.

Wage increases are usually related to demand.

TRENDS IN NURSING EMPLOYMENT

Nursing has experienced impressive gains in employment in recent years. Buerhaus and Staiger (1996) reported that employment measured on a full-time equivalence (FTE) basis increased by 30 percent for RNs between 1983 and 1994. The rates of FTE growth for RNs and nurse's aides were nearly double that of all other occupations, which grew only 16 percent between 1983 and 1994. In contrast, the overall employment for LPNs has declined by about 10 percent.

Job prospects for RNs are good in the foreseeable future, according to the U.S. Department of Labor. The Bureau of Labor Statistics *Occupation Outlook Handbook* for 2000–2001 provided the following upbeat job outlook forecast: "Employment of registered nurses is expected to grow faster than the average for all occupations through the year 2008 and, because the occupation is large, many new jobs will result" (Bureau of Labor Statistics, 2000, p. 212). However, job growth for RNs will be uneven among the different major work settings. The Bureau of Labor Statistics (1998) has predicted, and most nursing experts agree, that employment in the hospital sector will grow more slowly than in the past. The Pew Health Professions Commission predicted in a 1995 report that up to 50 percent of hospitals and up to 60 percent of hospital beds would be lost. The commission also predicted that up to half of RN jobs in the hospitals across the country would be lost as a result of downsizing in the hospital industry.

The deceleration of employment for hospital-based nurses began in the early 1990s, as more jobs became available in nonhospital settings such as home health agencies, managed care organizations, government agencies, and a wide range of public and private community work settings. These downward trends in nursing employment were more pronounced in states with high rates of health maintence organization (HMO) enrollment, according to Buerhaus and Staiger (1996). In addition, the decline in the proportion of RNs working in hospitals was larger and occurred earlier in states with high HMO enrollment than in states with low HMO enrollment. A more recent examination also shows a deceleration in the growth of home-care nurses as managed care features are being applied to home care (Buerhaus & Staiger, 1999). However, managed care was not the only factor in the stagnation of earnings and employment. The recession in the early 1990s, major cutbacks in Medicaid and Medicare programs, and cost-cutting measures in hospitals to adjust to rising competition in the health industry also contributed to the slowing of job growth and of earnings increases for nurses.

 ## ECONOMIC ANALYSIS
NURSING SALARY AND EMPLOYMENT

The salary, workforce, and work-setting changes for professional nurses are evident in actual nursing situations. For example, a nurse who graduated in 1980 would have earned about $14,500 a year when first starting her or his career, and would have worked in a hospital as a staff nurse. After 5 to 10 years, this nurse would earn about $25,000 and would likely change her or his specialty, but would still be working in the hospital setting. By 1990, the nurse would have most likely transferred to home care, ambulatory care, or become a team leader or nurse manager in an acute care setting.

Competition in the marketplace often leads to cost-cutting and restructuring of businesses.

 ## FACTORS AFFECTING NURSING SALARIES

Individuals who wish to become registered nurses qualify for the licensing examination with one of three types of nursing educational programs: the 2-year associate degree, the 3-year diploma, or the 4-year baccalaureate degree. Do the starting salaries for RNs with different degrees differ significantly? Do nursing degrees significantly affect the subsequent salary progression of experienced RNs? What other individual and work-setting factors determine nurses' wages and benefits? These are important questions to individual nurses as they make career-choice decisions as to whether the additional years of education are worth the investment in time and money and whether and when to relocate in pursuit of career advancements and professional satisfaction.

Economists and nursing researchers have long been interested in the study of nursing salaries, benefits, and working conditions. They have examined the influences on nursing earnings and employment of such external forces as cutbacks in Medicaid and Medicare and reductions in federal and state support for nursing education (Pew Health Professions Commission, 1995; Brewer, 1997; Wolfe, 1997). They have also addressed a host of personal and work-setting factors that can significantly influence the number of nurses who get jobs and how much they can expect to earn. Unlike external market forces, which are mostly beyond the control of individual nurses, personal qualifications and the setting in which nurses work can be influenced by individual career-choice decisions. The effects of these personal factors and work-setting characteristics on nursing earnings are discussed in the following sections.

EXPERIENCE

A widely held belief in nursing is that nurses' earnings, like those of teachers, quickly level off after only a few years of increases. How true is this perception? According to the most recent biennial earnings survey conducted by the nursing journal RN, seniority as measured by years of uninterrupted nursing experience makes a significant difference in nurses' pay (Ventura, 1997). For example, nurses reported in the 1997 survey that those with at least 16 years of experience made an average of $21.90 an hour, nearly $6.00 more than those with less than 3 years' experience—a difference of 27 percent. On an annual basis, the most experienced nurses made 35 percent—about $16,410—more than those with the least experience.

BREAKS IN SERVICE

Whereas years of experience have a positive impact on nurses' benefits and salaries, breaks in service can have a significant negative impact. Breaks in service include frequent changes in employment state (e.g., from active to inactive status), long periods of unemployment, and part-time work. In a statistical investigation of the link between breaks in service and nursing earnings and employment, Ault and Rutman (1998) concluded that those who had switched employment state more than twice in the 1980s were penalized nearly 10 percent with respect to their 1989 wage rate. The nurses with breaks in their service record also experienced slower growth of wages, averaging 24 percent slower growth per year over a nurse's lifetime.

EDUCATION

Many studies have confirmed that a nurse's educational background has a relatively insignificant impact on wage rates (Buerhaus & Staiger, 1996; Brewer, 1997; Ventura, 1997; Ault & Rutman, 1998). Observed wage levels are similar whether the individual earned an associate, diploma, or baccalaureate degree. Most nurses reported that they received no financial incentive for having a bachelor of science in nursing (BSN) degree and that they were not rewarded financially for earning specialty certification (Ventura, 1997). Yet many nursing opportunities and roles require a BSN.

Nurses who have earned a postbaccalaureate degree, however, experience a higher return to a baccalaureate degree. This can be explained by the emerging trend of nurses with graduate degrees working in advanced practice managerial and supervisory positions and earning higher salaries than their peers who have earned only a basic nursing degree.

SETTINGS AND SPECIALTY

In the past, working in the acute care setting offered the highest pay among the various work settings in nursing. In recent years, many of the alternative settings, such as ambulatory care or health maintenance organizations, have been rapidly catching up with the acute care setting (Ventura, 1997). Meanwhile, home health and community nurses are not far behind the wage growth experienced by nurses working in the HMO and ambulatory care settings. These trends reflect the practice in health care of shifting patients from the costly inpatient settings to the less costly outpatient and alternative care settings.

Within the hospital setting, nursing specialty makes a substantial difference in earnings. A recent survey indicated that nurses in acute care and pediatric care earned the highest wages, at $20.30 per hour (Ventura, 1997). Those in intensive care units and cardiac care units also fared well, at an average of $19.45 an hour. The average hourly wage of all hospital nurses was $19.10.

HIGHER WAGES FOR OVERTIME, NIGHTS, AND WEEKENDS

Higher overtime pay is a traditional source of extra income for nurses. Nurses can also bolster their income by working night shifts and on weekends. Health care is an industry that operates on a 24-hour basis. To lure workers to work at night and on weekends, employers have traditionally paid more for these shifts. For example, full-time RNs who did overtime work averaged $6,000 extra pay per year to supplement their regular salaries (Ventura, 1997).

Opportunities to do overtime work have declined in recent years, however. For example, an RN survey shows that in 1997, only 75 percent of the surveyed nurses reported that they had worked overtime during the past 2 years, and they averaged about 4 hours of overtime work a week. These figures are much lower than the 95 percent of nurses who reported doing overtime work in the 1993 and 1995 surveys, when the average overtime was 5.5 hours and 4.5 hours per week, respectively (Ventura, 1997). Mergers, consolidations, and hospital closures have resulted in job losses and reduced need for overtime work.

Overtime work, weekend work, and night duties are less desirable than regular work during the day. Employers typically pay more to attract employees to fill these irregular time slots.

PART-TIME NURSES

Ventura (1997) reported that part-time nurses earned an average of $20.55 an hour in 1997—an increase of $1.35 or almost 7 percent from 1995. This was almost double the raise full-time nurses received over the same time period. Full-timers earned $1.45 less per hour than their part-time counterparts in 1997. The difference was $1.00 in 1995. Part-timers worked an average of 27 hours per week in 1997 compared with the 45 hours worked by full-timers. As a result, part-timers reported an annual income of $28,400, whereas the full-timers earned about $16,000 more in 1996. Some nurses trade the larger amount of free time and the ability to choose when to work that are the hallmarks of part-time employment for the higher income of full-time employment.

UNION MEMBERSHIP AND GEOGRAPHIC LOCATION

Only about 14 percent of surveyed RNs were union members in 1996 (Buerhaus & Staiger, 1999). This percentage has remained the same over the last 6 years. Union membership varies significantly across the different regions of the country. Less than 5 percent of the full-time and part-time RNs in the South Atlantic, mid-South, and Southwest reported that they belonged to a union. In contrast, 28 percent of the RNs in New England, 27 percent in the mid-Atlantic states, and 35 percent in the Far West reported that they were unionized.

Unionized RNs were paid better at $22.00 an hour, or $2.80 more than those not covered by a collective bargaining agreement. Their average annual income, at $46,225, was also $6,000 higher than the average annual income of nonunionized nurses. The Southern region continues to have the lowest wage rate—at $18.15—but nurses in that region received the largest raises. In contrast, nurses in the East earned $3.30 more per hour than their Southern counterparts and had the highest average annual salary ($46,120) but also had the smallest raises. The geographic differences in nursing salaries and wages are narrowing, perhaps reflecting differences in managed care penetration. Mobility and the greater availability of information may also have played a role in closing the geographic differences in salaries.

 ECONOMIC ANALYSIS
SUPPLY, DEMAND, AND WAGE CHANGE

A new graduate nurse in 1990 was typically offered three nursing positions, including some in specialties that were previously closed to new graduates, such as critical care. In addition, she or he might be offered a signup bonus of $1000; in some cases, the employee who recruited the new nurse might get a bonus as well.

Two years later, however, new graduates typically spent 3 months looking for a position and might have had to relocate to do so. Some new graduates even started working in nonnursing jobs before finding a nursing one. Wage increases that were commonplace in 1990 had all but disappeared by 1992 because of continued increases in nursing supply and slower growth of demand.

DEMAND TRENDS

Health-care delivery is undergoing radical changes in the United States. Gone forever are the practices of retrospective reimbursements by insurance companies for providers' services based on their cost. Cost-conscious health plans and insurance companies increasingly involve themselves in the management of the delivery process to ensure quality while attempting to keep costs down. In the process, many health-care services have shifted from the more costly inpatient setting to the outpatient setting. Meanwhile, attempts have been made to shift from a focus on sickness care to a proactive focus on wellness care and prevention services. These and other changes in how health care is delivered and paid for have had a profound impact on the demand for a nursing labor force.

> **Demand trends *in nursing are the historical patterns of the number of nurses hired at different points in time for the country as a whole or for different regions of the country.***

For example, nursing shortages were periodically reported in the late 1980s and early 1990s. Commentators frequently cited employers' inability to fill all their vacant nursing positions in certain geographic areas and in some of the specialties, such as critical care and the emergency department, as evidence of a shortage. The data presented in Table 8–1 clearly suggest that the number of nurses was increasing rapidly during this period. The observed "shortages" were primarily the result of the rapid increase in the demand for health care, which was causing employers to hire more nurses.

But as managed care enrollment grew in the 1990s and health insurance companies stepped up their cost-cutting efforts, the demand for health care began to decelerate. As a result, many hospitals laid off nurses or kept their vacant nursing positions unfilled. The rapid succession of nursing shortages and surpluses observed in the mid-1990s appears to have resulted from the wide swings in the demand for health care. These fluctuations quickly spilled over to the job markets as both employers and employees tried to cope with the changing market environment.

Despite the ups and downs in the labor market and the uncertainty that they have brought about, the demand for a nursing labor force will remain strong in the near future. The following is a list of labor demand trends that are likely to improve nursing pay and job prospects:

- The U.S. population continues to grow at a steady rate of about 1 percent per year, according to the U.S. Bureau of the Census (Day, 2000). By the year 2000, total population will reach 275 million. Based on the experiences from health planning, population growth is a major predictor of future demand for health care and a health-care workforce.

- The population, including nurses, is getting older. The median age of the U.S. population will rise from 34.3 in 1995 (the highest ever recorded) to 35.7 in 2000 (Brewer, 1997). By 2000, 12.6 percent of the general population will be 65 years or older. This trend is driven mostly by the aging of the population born during the baby boom period after World War II (1946 to 1964). Older individuals have more health problems and need more health care, especially long-term and geriatric care, than younger individuals.

- Technology is more complex, and this trend in all likelihood will continue in the 21st century. Unlike the cost-saving role that technology plays in the for-profit economy, complex technologies do not replace labor in health care. On the contrary, they usually require not only a greater amount of labor services but also the services of more skilled personnel to operate them. As nurses deepen their technological sophistication and become more productive—both in terms of how well they can perform a particular task and in terms of how many different tasks they can each perform—the demand for their services will likely increase.

- The large waves of teenagers, and the risky behaviors associated with those years, will likely drive up demand for health care (Buerhaus, 1998). Smoking, for example, has been firmly linked to a host of health-care problems when smokers grow older (Centers for Disease Control and Prevention [CDC], 1996). The health-care costs of smokers will be higher than those of nonsmokers (CDC, 1994).

- State governments are taking steps to expand Medicaid coverage for uninsured adults and children, reducing the ranks of the uninsured and increasing the overall demand for health care.

- Managed care enrollment is growing rapidly in both the public and the private sectors. Although managed care organizations use inpatient care less than traditional health plans do, their emphasis on prevention, wellness care, and case management are creating new job opportunities for nurses in both the traditional clinical settings and new managerial settings.

In summary, although uncertainty abounds in the short term, the employment outlook for nurses remains robust in the long term. Nurses who have the right skill set, especially state-of-the-art information technology skills, and are willing to adapt to changing environments will have many jobs available to them.

SUPPLY TRENDS

Employers draw their needed nursing workforce from three sources of supply: new graduates of nursing programs, previously inactive nurses (i.e., those who had earlier left the nursing profession for a variety of personal and professional reasons) who have reentered the labor market, and existing nurses working longer hours or irregular hours such as those involving night or weekend shifts. The next sections address the questions of how each of the three sources of labor supply affects wages and employment, and how these changes in employment and wages in turn affect the amounts of services that nurses are willing and able to supply.

TRENDS IN UNDERGRADUATE NURSING PROGRAMS

In 1996, there were 1508 nursing programs in the United States that prepared students to become RNs (see Table 8–3). Of this total, 109 programs offered a diploma degree, 876 offered an associate degree, and 523 offered a baccalaureate degree (National Center for Health Statistics, 1998). In addition to these programs, there were over 1000 nursing schools that prepare LPNs.

Over the last 20 years, the number of baccalaureate and associate nursing programs has continually increased, as demonstrated by Figure 8–2. For example, there were 697 associate programs in 1980 and 876 in 1996, a net increase of 179. In the same period, the number of baccalaureate programs increased by 147. In contrast, the number of diploma programs has declined steadily, with 202 of them closed between 1980 and 1996.

With fewer diploma schools training new nurses, the total number of graduates of these 3-year schools has declined by more than 60 percent between 1980 and 1996. However, based on the statistics provided in Table 8–3, increases in the number of graduates of associate and baccalaureate programs more than offset the decline in the number of diploma school graduates. The net increase in total nursing graduates who were prepared to become RNs was more than 25 percent over the period from 1980 to 1996. Will this trend continue?

Recent admission data suggest that the increase in nursing graduates is likely to slow because nursing schools of all types admitted fewer students in the last few years. For example, nursing schools began to experience a decline in enrollment beginning in the 1992–1993 academic year. This trend continued in the late 1990s and will result in slower increases in the number of graduates entering the job market (NLN, 1997a).

TABLE 8–3. NURSING GRADUATES AND NUMBER OF SCHOOLS IN THE UNITED STATES, 1980, 1990, AND 1996

	1980		1990		1996	
	Number	%	Number	%	Number	%
Nursing Graduates						
Registered nurses	75,523	100.0	66,088	100.0	94,757	100.0
Diploma	14,495	19.2	5,199	7.9	5,703	6.0
Associate	36,034	47.7	42,318	64.0	56,641	59.8
Baccalaureate	24,994	33.1	18,571	28.1	32,413	34.2
Licensed practical nurses	41,892	100.0	35,417	100.0	NA	NA
Nursing Schools						
Registered nurses	1,385	100.0	1,470	100.0	1,508	100.0
Diploma	311	22.5	152	10.3	109	7.2
Associate	697	50.3	829	56.4	876	58.1
Baccalaureate	377	27.2	489	33.3	523	34.7
Licensed practical nurses	1,299	100.0	1,154	100.0	NA	100.0

Source: National Center for Health Statistics. (1998). *Health, United States, 1998.* Hyattsville, MD: U.S. Public Health Services, Table 106.
NA = Data not available.

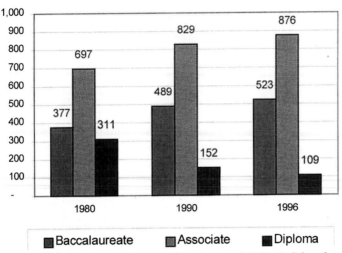

FIG. 8–2. Number of nursing schools, 1980, 1990, and 1996. Left bar, baccalaureate programs; middle bar, associate programs; right bar, diploma programs. (From National Center for Health Statistics. (1998). *Health, United States, 1998.* Hyattsville, MD: U.S. Public Health Services, Table 106.)

TRENDS IN GRADUATE NURSING PROGRAMS

In contrast to the recent declining trends in undergraduate enrollments, more nursing students are graduating at the master's level. In 1980, for example, 67,300 nurses, or 5.3 percent of the total active nursing personnel, were prepared at the master's or doctorate levels (see Table 8–1). In 1996, the number rose to 207,500, or 9.8 percent of the total. The number of master's programs has also risen in recent years. In 1995 alone, for example, 30 new master's programs were established (NLN, 1997a). Master's programs now total 306 in the United States. Geographically, the South has the highest concentration, with 94 master's programs. The lowest number of programs (47) are found in the West. New York and Pennsylvania continue to lead the states in the number of master's programs, with 26 and 25 programs, respectively.

Although the number of master's programs and their enrollment levels have risen dramatically, master's-prepared nurses as a group are still a relatively small part of the overall nursing workforce. The data in Table 8–1 suggest that less than 1 in every 10 RNs had earned a master's degree in 1996. Meanwhile, the demand for advanced practice nurses and other nurses with a master's degree has increased faster than the supply (NLN, 1997b). As a result, according to the American Association of Colleges of Nursing

(AACN, 1998), job placement rate for master's-prepared nursing graduates was among the highest of any degree levels at graduation (AACN, 1998), reflecting the health system's growing demand for registered nurses with advanced clinical skills.

Parallel to the rise in the number of master's programs was a steady increase in the number of doctoral nursing programs. In 1995, for example, there were a total of 64 doctoral programs, 4 more programs than in the previous year (NLN, 1997a). There have also been small enrollment increases in the doctoral programs, averaging about 26 students a year (Ault & Rutman, 1998). In fall 1996, the total number of doctoral students enrolled increased by 3.7 percent over the previous year and reached a total of 2954 students. However, relative to the number of nurses with doctoral degrees needed to conduct nursing research and teach future nurses, the total pool of such nurses is still too small, according to the AACN (Ault & Rutman, 1998).

 ECONOMIC ANALYSIS
DEMAND FOR ADVANCED PRACTICE NURSES

An experienced RN was laid off when the hospital where he worked merged with another hospital and downsized the psychiatric services department where he used to work. He went back to school to attend a graduate family nurse practitioner program. Within 2 years, and before graduation, he was offered three different positions—two in community health clinics and one in a hospital emergency department—at salary levels higher than what he was earning before.

This change in his situation can be easily explained by familiar economic principles. The demand for family nurse practitioners is increasing due to increased use of advanced practice nurses (APNs) in managed care. His experiences with acute care and psychiatric services made his APN skills even more valuable for emergency departments, where psychiatric problems are on the rise. The supply has not yet kept pace with the demand. Wages, as a result, have increased as employers compete to hire more APNs.

 WILL THERE BE A NURSING SHORTAGE?

Across the country, nurses are experiencing unprecedented changes in institutional staffing patterns. The trends to downsize hospitals and to make health-care providers more flexible and cost efficient have resulted in a number of major changes in work patterns. These include the following:

- More frequent floating of nurses from one unit or department to another
- Substitution of less expensive and lesser-trained personnel, such as LPNs and nurse's aides, for the more expensive and better-trained RNs
- Emphasis on cross-training of nursing and other personnel to make them more adaptable to the needs of their work environments

In the process, some layoffs of nurses have occurred because of elimination of departments, mergers of institutions, and other institutional changes. Meanwhile, growth in home health care and nonacute care has created new job opportunities and new roles for professional nurses. Amid all these changes, will there be a nursing shortage in the near future?

A labor shortage results when the demand for labor outstrips the supply. An increase in supply or a decrease in demand can eliminate a shortage.

ECONOMIC ANALYSIS
PROJECTING A BALANCE IN DEMAND AND SUPPLY

California has made a significant commitment to strategic planning for its nursing workforce. By analyzing supply and demand factors, nursing economists E. M. Lewis, K. R. Sechrist, and their colleagues who worked on a statewide workforce strategic committee were able to identify important labor trends and build a forecast model. They produced the following statements about California's nursing workforce for the period from 1995 to 1998 to assist in the workforce planning process for California (Lewis et al., 1997, p. 3–5):

- California's supply of nurses appears to be adequate for the demand.
- Demand for nurses is expected to increase negligibly.
- There are major shifts in the location of positions among employment sectors. A loss of nearly 4000 RN staff nurse positions is expected in acute care hospitals.
- The increasing demand for nurses in community and outpatient settings requires nurses with a different set of skills than those required in hospital settings.
- The current nursing workforce does not reflect the ethnic and racial group representation of California's population.
- California's nursing workforce is aging, with half the RNs who are working full time being over age 45 and 30 percent being over age 50.

The likelihood of having another nursing shortage in the near future depends on the strength of demand relative to the supply of nursing workforce. On the demand side, the demand for nurses is likely to remain strong, subject to wide swings caused by fluctuations in the market for general health care. The supply of nursing workforce comes from three sources, as discussed earlier. The first source, the supply of new nurses, was discussed in the previous sections. The two additional sources of nursing labor supply are nurses returning to the workforce and existing nurses who work longer hours.

Nationally, about 17 percent of the 2.5 million RNs are inactive (NLN, 1997a). The possibility of their return to work, together with the longer hours that existing nurses may provide under a sufficient set of incentives, can practically turn a nursing shortage to a surplus. Much can be learned by examining the factors that influence nurses' decisions to return to the workforce and to work a certain number of hours. Both of these decisions are related to the following three interrelated factors:

1. Wages in the nursing labor market
2. Job opportunities in other professions in which nurses can participate
3. The preferences of individual nurses concerning careers versus families

Nurses have very little influence over the second factor. The third factor is strictly personal. These personal preferences are difficult to predict and control. Thus, whether inactive nurses will return to work and existing ones will work longer hours will most likely depend on nurses' pay and working conditions. In other words, a shortage will not result if employers are willing to pay or make the necessary improvements in working conditions, or both.

> *Inactive nurses are a source of nursing supply. They can increase the supply if they return to the profession when pay or working conditions improve.*

In the long run, a factor that can potentially contribute to a nursing shortage is demographics. In 1996, the average age of all active nurses was 42.3 years and that of RNs was 44.3 years (Moses, 1996). By the year 2000, two-thirds of RNs will be over 40 years old (Aiken, 1995). Older nurses tend to work fewer hours and to move out of the hospital setting (Brewer, 1997). A large exodus of older nurses in 10 to 15 years because of retirement and health reasons could reduce the existing pool of available nurses. This makes a shortage a distinct possibility unless effective policy measures are taken to counterbalance the aging of the nursing population and the resulting reduction of the labor supply.

In brief, there appears to be a sufficient supply of nurses to provide the needed care as long as nursing educators and educational institutions maintain their current capacity to train and educate future nurses. But a nursing shortage is still possible if there is a serious unwillingness on the part of employers to pay adequately in today's tight labor market. Meanwhile, job opportunities elsewhere in the economy, the age composition of the nursing population, and nurses' own career and job-market preferences can also affect both the likelihood and severity of a nursing shortage.

 ## ECONOMIC ANALYSIS
DEMAND AND NURSING ROLES

The increased demand for nurses in many new and different settings has expanded the opportunities for nurses to develop many different roles. The situation of the Wilson family offers an interesting example. Laurel is a nurse who graduated from a diploma program in 1960. She has worked since that time as a part-time nurse at the local community hospital. When her husband was laid off from his factory job she needed to work additional hours. When he was making more money and had significant overtime, she would reduce her hours. At age 59, she has chosen to cut back to contingent status, working only 1 to 3 days per month.

Because of her enthusiasm, three of her children decided to enter nursing. Jennifer, the oldest, graduated from the same diploma program as her mother. Laurel's son, Gregory, aspired to have an expanded role in nursing and earn a salary conducive to a growing family. This goal was an incentive for him to enroll in a baccalaureate program at the state university. He was an excellent student and after graduation worked in the intensive care area. With this experience, he went back to school and graduated from a nurse anesthetist graduate program. He now earns $85,000 per year.

The youngest daughter, Kristin, has an ambition to succeed in health care. She was also an excellent student and graduated from the baccalaureate program at the state university. She worked at the university hospital for a while but felt constrained by the bureaucracy and limited opportunities for advancement. She decided to obtain an MBA from her alma mater. With this advanced business degree, she now owns her own case management company, which specializes in case management for Workman's Compensation participants and for elderly people who require services to remain in their homes. In this position, Kristin is independent and can use the skills from both her degrees to earn a respectable income.

With all her children out of school and successful, Laurel desired a more responsible position. That wish has led her to enroll in a BSN completion program. Her goal after graduation is to become a hospital case manager.

 LESSONS TO BE LEARNED

MYTHS

An important lesson that can be learned from this chapter is that there are many misconceptions about nurses' salaries and employment. These beliefs are either inconsistent with the predictions of economic theories or at odds with reality. Some of these myths are summarized and dispelled here.

Myth 1: Nurses Are Underpaid

For many years in the 1950s and 1960s, nurses were indeed underpaid compared with teachers and other female-dominated professions with similar educational requirements (Yett, 1975). Over the last 20 years, however, nurses have experienced impressive gains in salaries and fringe benefits, with full-time registered nurses earning an average salary of $42,071 in 1997.

Table 8–4 presents data comparing nurses' current salaries and compensation with those of several white-collar occupations such as teachers, administrative and managerial personnel, and clerical workers. According to the Bureau of Labor Statistics, nurses on average earned a total compensation (salary and benefits) of $28.59 per hour in 1998, an amount essentially the same as teachers' $28.82 per hour. The hourly compensation of nurses was lower than those of executive, administrative, and managerial personnel, but much higher than those of many white-collar professionals, such as technical workers and administrative support personnel.

Myth 2: Nurses Are Overworked Because They Are Taking Care of More Patients

As illustrated by the data in Table 8–5, hospital admissions have declined steadily since Medicare began to pay for hospital inpatient services by the Diagnosis Related Group (DRG) method in the early 1980s. The average hospital stay has also been shortened considerably during the same period. In contrast, the total number of personnel employed by community hospitals in the United States, including both RNs and LPNs, has increased.

TABLE 8–4. EMPLOYER HOURLY COSTS OF WHITE-COLLAR EMPLOYEES IN SELECT OCCUPATIONAL GROUPS, 1998

Occupational Group	Total Compensation per Hour ($)	Wages and Salaries per Hour ($)
White-collar occupations	23.84	17.52
Professional specialty and technical	31.56	23.34
Nurses	28.59	20.88
Elementary and secondary school teachers	28.82	21.38
Technical	23.96	17.34
Executive, administrative, and managerial	34.39	24.85
Administrative support, including clerical	16.09	11.47

Source: Bureau of Labor Statistics. (1998, March) *Employment cost trends.* Washington, DC: U.S. Department of Labor, Table 2.

TABLE 8–5. HOSPITAL ADMISSIONS AND LEVELS OF STAFFING, 1980, 1990, AND 1996

	1980	1990	1996
Hospital admissions (1000s)	36,143	31,181	31,099
Length of stay (days)	9.9	9.1	7.5
No. of persons employed in hospitals (1000s)	4,036	4,690	5,041
No. of RNs employed in hospitals (1000s)	629*	810	1,313
No. of LPNs employed in hospitals (1000s)	234*	168	224

Sources: National Center for Health Statistics. (1992, 1998) *Health, United States.* Hyattsville, MD: U.S. Public Health Services; Bureau of Labor Statistics. (1998). *Occupational outlook handbook, the 1998–99 edition,* Washington, DC: U.S. Department of Labor.
    *1981 data.

Thus, the perception that each nurse is taking care of more patients cannot be supported by available data. Because hospitals contain sicker patients who have greater needs for care, more sophisticated information systems that adjust nurse-patient ratios are critically needed.

Myth 3: Nursing Is a Dead-End Profession

For years, nursing and teaching were the two large professions in which salaries peaked after a few years of employment and few opportunities existed for career advancement. Although this perception may still be true for the teaching profession, the situation has improved for the nursing profession. In addition to working in hospitals and clinics, nurses today can find employment opportunities in a wide range of job settings, including human resources management, occupational or industrial health, home health agencies, nursing homes, public health agencies, and managed care organizations. Master's-prepared nurses can pursue careers as advanced practice nurses in primary care specialties such as women's health, primary adult health, pediatrics, geriatrics, and psycho-emotional health services. Nurses are performing increasingly larger and more direct roles in the new and changing managed care environment, either providing patient care or managing the care delivery for a high number of patients (Porter-O'Grady, 1997).

Myth 4: There Is a Nursing Shortage

Repeated claims of a nursing shortage have been made in the past 40 years. The earlier alarms about a shortage of nursing personnel and the concerns over the expected adverse consequences of not having enough nurses to provide patient care prompted the U.S. Congress to enact legislation to support nursing education (see Chapter 7). In recent years, accounts of a nursing shortage in hospital intensive care units, emergency departments, operating rooms, and obstetric units have been repeatedly reported in trade and professional journals and the mass media. Do we really have a nursing shortage? Is a shortage on the way?

Peter Buerhaus, a noted researcher on nursing labor economics issues, has recently expressed the view that strong demand for health care coupled with a declining trend in nursing school enrollments may indeed cause a tightening of the labor market for nurses (Buerhaus, 1998). However, in the increasingly more competitive health-care market, hospitals and other employers will offer higher salaries or other innovative incentives to recruit nurses. Those who do not do so, according to Buerhaus, may not be able to compete and will be out of the market. Higher wages and benefits will induce more nurses to work overtime and part-time nurses to work full time, thereby increasing the amount of nursing labor supplied. Higher wages and benefits will signal future and potential nurses to prepare themselves to enter the profession. In sum, short-term imbalances between demand and supply in a dynamic labor market are normal and inevitable. But as the health-care market becomes more competitive, market-driven corrections in wages and benefits will serve as an automatic adjustment mechanism to bring the forces of supply and demand into balance.

RISKS AND OPPORTUNITIES

The nursing profession is currently in a state of flux. After many years of steady gains in employment and compensation in the late 1980s and early 1990s, nurses are losing ground in some work settings, such as the hospital sector. Meanwhile, fewer students are enrolling in nursing programs and the total number of nursing programs has slightly decreased. This is the time for a careful examination of both current and emerging health-care market trends and how they may affect the nursing profession. To assist in this discussion, the National League for Nursing has suggested the following roles or role expansions for nurses (NLN, 1997b):

- *Clinical pathway developer.* Nurses will take a lead role in developing clinical pathways and protocols to standardize the cost-efficient management of high-quality patient care in all settings.
- *Care coordinator.* Experiments in skill mix will focus on nurses as care coordinators and team leaders, with direct care increasingly provided by a variety of lesser-trained caregivers and support staff.
- *Ambulatory care provider.* Declining inpatient demand and reengineering will drive some 15 to 25 percent of hospital-based nurses into nonacute and ambulatory care settings by the year 2000.
- *Case manager.* Case management to reduce costs and integrate clinical and preventive services will become an increasingly important management responsibility for which nurses are uniquely well qualified.
- *Gatekeeper.* Advanced practice nurses may be independent gatekeepers in tomorrow's integrated delivery networks.
- *Primary care provider.* Nurses will take a lead role in primary care, helping to alleviate the shortage of primary care providers.
- *Advanced practitioner.* Advanced practice nurses can provide patient care at a lower cost than physicians (with equal or superior quality) for many categories of primary care, urgent care, and chronically ill patients.
- *Enrolled population manager.* Advanced practice nurses working on a primary care team can expand the capacity of a health-care team to manage an enrolled population in an HMO setting.

- *Chronic-care provider.* Nurses will manage patients who are chronically ill or need ongoing monitoring. Obstetrics, arthritis, and pediatrics are likely services for nurse management.
- *Manager of high-risk patients.* Nurses will take the lead in providing case management for high-risk patients, using sophisticated patient management tools and information systems to coordinate and control the care of high-risk enrollees.
- *Health promoter.* Nurse-led initiatives in health promotion and prevention will be essential under capitation, in order to keep patients as healthy as possible, treat them early, and use as few resources as necessary.
- *Entrepreneur.* Increasingly, nurses will be starting businesses to provide services within large managed care systems, such as services to at-risk families or managing employee assistance programs.

SUMMARY

The job market for nursing continues to experience uncertainty and changes. In the next decade, with fewer nursing graduates entering the job market and with existing nurses getting older, the short-term outlook for nursing employment and wages appears to be good. The increased emphasis on quality, efficiency, and cost has also provided nurses with a rare opportunity to gain more responsibilities in providing patient care and making policy changes that affect the allocation of health-care resources. To realize meaningful gains for the profession, both current and future nurses need to be aware of the trends and required skills so that nurses will have the necessary tools to engage in the roles needed in the health-care system of the 21st century.

DISCUSSION QUESTIONS

1. How much are full-time RNs, LPNs, and nurse's aides paid annually in your market area? Are they paid well compared with other professionals with similar educational background and training?
2. Why were nurses paid less than other professionals with similar education and training in the 1950s and 1960s? What are the major institutional and economic factors that caused nurses' salaries and benefits to increase faster than the average worker in other industries?
3. Discuss the new roles that nurses can expect to play and the skills that are required to perform well in the new health-care environment.

4. Assess the demand for a nursing workforce in the near future. Back up your assessment with your observations about the demand for health care, growth of managed care, and other major trends in health-care delivery and financing that you think are relevant.
5. Will there be a nursing shortage? If a shortage were to develop, what would be the likely demand-side and supply-side causes?
6. Assess the following statement: "A nursing shortage has more to do with a shortage of willingness to pay than with a shortage of graduates from nursing schools."

 REFERENCES

Aiken, H. L. (1995). Transformation of the workforce. *Nursing Outlook*, 43(3), 201–209.

American Association of Colleges of Nursing. (1998). *1996–97 enrollment and graduations in baccalaureate and graduate programs in nursing*. Washington, DC: Author.

Ault, D. E., & Rutman, G. L. (1998). Factors affecting levels and growth rates in the wage rates of women: Evidence from nursing. *Applied Economics*, 30(6), 727–739.

Begany, T. (1995). 1995 earnings survey: The news is mixed. RN, 58(10), 49–54, 56.

Brewer, C. S. (1997). Through the looking glass: The labor market for registered nurses in the 21st century. *Nursing and Health Care Perspectives*, 1(5), 260–268.

Buerhaus, P. I. (1998). Is a nursing shortage on the way? *Nursing*, 28(8), 34–35.

Buerhaus, P. I., & Staiger, D. O. (1996). Managed care and the nurse workforce. *Journal of the American Medical Association*, 276(18), 1487–1493.

Buerhaus, P. I., & Staiger, D. O. (1999). Trouble in the nurse labor market? Recent trends and future outlook. *Health Affairs*, 18(1), 214–222.

Bureau of Labor Statistics. (2000). *Occupational outlook handbook, the 2000–2001 edition*. Washington, DC: U.S. Department of Labor.

Bureau of the Census. (2000). Population Projections of the United States by Age, Race, Hispanic Origin, and Nativity: 1999 to 2000 [On-line]. Available: http://www.census.gov:80/population/www/projections/popproj.html.

Centers for Disease Control and Prevention. (1994). Medical-care expenditures attributable to cigarette smoking, United States, 1993. MMWR *Morbidity and Mortality Weekly Report*, 43(26), 469–472.

Centers for Disease Control and Prevention. (1996). Projected smoking-related deaths among youth, United States. MMWR *Morbidity and Mortality Weekly Report*, 45(44), 971–974.

Kalisch, P., & Kalisch, B. (1986). *Advancement of American nursing*. Boston: Little, Brown.

Lewis E. M., Sechrist, K. R., Schultz, M. A., & Keating, S. B. (1997). California strategic planning committee for nursing: Experiences and challenges. *Journal of Nursing Administration*, 27(3), 3–5.

Moses, E. (1996). *Advance notes I and II: From the National Sample Survey of Registered Nurses*. Rockville, MD: Health Resources Services Administration, Bureau of Health Professions.

National Center for Health Statistics. (1998). *Health, United States, 1998*. Hyattsville, MD: U.S. Public Health Service.

National League for Nursing. (1997a). *The final report of the Commission on a Workforce for a Restructured Health Care System. Part 3, Nursing supply and demand*. Washington, DC: Author.

National League of Nursing. (1997b). *The final report of the Commission on a Workforce for a Restructured Health Care System. Part 1, Executive summary*. Washington, DC: Author.

Pew Health Professions Commission. (1995). *Critical challenges: Revitalizing the health professions for the twenty-first century*. San Francisco: UCSF Center for the Health Professions.

Porter-O'Grady, T. (1997). Over the horizon: The future of the advanced practice nurse. *Nursing Administration Quarterly*, 21(4), 1–11.

Sachs, R. H., & Spreier, S. W. (1996). Reward ceremonies: The 1996 Hay compensation survey. *Hospitals and Health Networks*, 70(2), 26–43.

Ventura, M. J. (1997). The 1997 earnings survey: Slow gains, high earnings. RN, 60(10), 40–47.

Wolfe, M. N. (1997). Nursing compensation: A historical review. *Hospital Topics*, 75(2), 27–30.

Yett, D. E. (1975). *An economic analysis of the nurse shortage*. Lexington, MA: Lexington Books.

 # SUGGESTED READING

Bozell, J. (1999). *Anatomy of a job search: A nurse's guide to finding and landing the job you want*. Springhouse, PA: Springhouse Publishing.

Case, B. (1997). *Career planning for nurses*. Albany, NY: Delmar.

Herman, J., & Young, S. W. (1998). Forecasting the nursing workforce in a dynamic health care market. *Nursing Economics*, 16(4), 170–181.

Krall, L., & Prus, M. J. (1995). Institutional changes in hospital nursing. *Journal of Economic Issues*, 29(1), 67–93.

Miller, M. A. (1997). Nursing pay in private industry. *Compensation and Working Conditions*, 2(1), 11–23.

Morris, S. (1997). *Health economics for nurses: An introductory guide*. Upper Saddle River, NJ: Prentice Hall.

Part III

The Nursing Service Market

This part of the book explores how economic conditions and changes in health-care systems affect the work that nurses do. In recent years, policy makers and nursing leaders have worked closely to create a more community-based health-care system. This movement to a system of community-centered services provides career opportunities in a variety of new settings for nurses at various levels of preparation and licensure. New and expanded opportunities also exist for nurses to pursue entrepreneurial ventures. Even in existing health-care settings, nurses are presented with new role options for contributing to individual patient care. The opportunities are limited only by nurses' creativity and vision.

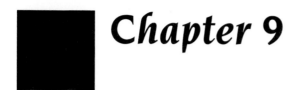

Chapter 9

Opportunities in the Health-Care Market

Kathy L. Beck
Susan K. Pfoutz

LEARNING OBJECTIVES

■ Describe economic changes in health care that affect nursing employment.

■ Identify and examine practice opportunities in a variety of settings in which nurses work.

■ Describe settings that have shown a significant increase in the percentage of nurses providing care.

■ Describe future opportunities within the discussed settings.

 ## CHANGES IN HEALTH-CARE DELIVERY

This chapter describes changes in health-care delivery that affect employment opportunities for registered nurses. A major trend is movement from acute care to community-based settings. The new locus of health-care delivery may threaten positions traditionally held by nurses, but it simultaneously creates new options. This chapter highlights opportunities available in a spectrum of health-care settings where nurses can apply their knowledge of health promotion, maintenance, and restoration to a variety of client populations. Examples of innovative nursing practices in a variety of settings are also presented. Changes in nursing roles and the settings where nurses work reflect:

- New technologies that facilitate outpatient or community-based treatment
- Evolving mechanisms for financing health care with a focus on reducing costs
- Alternative organizational models for health-care delivery

The evolution of health-care delivery emphasizes new models of delivery and provision of services in the appropriate setting. Trends include decreasing the number of employees, reapportioning tasks, merging facilities, decreasing the number of acute care beds, closing acute care facilities, and changing practice methodologies. Assignment of personnel is designed to maximize the skills of each group of employees, facilitate communication among workers, and coordinate services among members of the health-care team.

Prior to World War II, health care was predominately practiced in the patient's home. However, as health-care technology increased, care became more oriented to the acute care setting. Today, the largest proportion of health care is practiced in the hospital (Jacox, 1997). However, the pendulum has slowly begun to shift away from the acute care setting once again. In fact, the Pew Health Professions Commission (1995) has projected that up to half of the nation's hospitals will close, resulting in a loss of approximately 60 percent of the hospital beds by 2005.

The evolution of work settings for nursing has paralleled that of health-care delivery. The number of registered nurses (Malone & Marullo, 1997):

- Has increased from 1,662,382 in 1980 to 2,558,874 in 1996.
- Is projected to continue to increase 25 percent from the 1996 level by 2005 for working nurses.
- Is projected to decline in acute care settings. This is demonstrated by a 6 percent decline in the number of registered nurses (RNs) practicing in acute care from 1992 to 1994, representing 63.8 percent of working registered nurses. The proportion continued to decline to 60 percent of all nurses in 1996. The number of registered nurses practicing in acute care settings is predicted to continue to decrease to 57.4 percent by 2005.

Nursing will be the fifth-fastest-growing occupation in the United States if the numbers of working nurses increase as predicted (Malone & Marullo, 1997).

 ## NURSING EMPLOYMENT OPPORTUNITIES

The number of registered nurses is increasing and is projected to continue to increase; however, the percentage of nurses who work in acute care settings is decreasing. Where are registered nurses working? Two settings with the largest increases in registered nurses are community-based home care and long-term care. Other community-based opportunities for nursing employment include public health, occupational health, school health, ambulatory care, hospice care, parish health, and correctional nursing. Nurses also undertake entrepreneurial ventures or work in agencies providing and regulating nursing education. Preparing nurses for these employment opportunities will increase the demand for nursing education and for qualified faculty to teach in nursing programs. Institutions of higher education and the needs for nursing faculty are analyzed in Chapter 7. These diverse settings provide a wide variety of challenges and opportunities for nurses.

ACUTE CARE

The current trends demonstrate some decrease in employment of nurses in hospital or acute care settings. However, almost two-thirds of nurses remain employed in the acute care setting. The increased severity of patient illness and number of comorbid conditions seen in hospitals has led to an increase in the ratio of nurses to patients. Although there has been somewhat diminished growth in the number of hospital nurses since 1988, the ratio of nurses has increased from 50 to 102 per 100 hospitalized patients (Aiken & Salmon, 1994; Aiken, 1995). The number of hospital days has declined drastically: There were 55 million fewer hospital days in 1994 compared with 10 years previously. The shortened hospital stays for patients require nursing care and patient education to be concentrated into a shorter period. These data suggest an ongoing demand for hospital nurses. However, nurses will require a higher level of expertise in training and skills for working in the acute care setting because of the increasing severity of illness of the hospitalized patient.

Indirect Care Roles for Nurses

Although the number of nurses employed in acute care settings is decreasing, there are new opportunities for nurses to contribute in different ways to support the care of patients. Roles that support patient care include case management, infection control, resource procurement, information science, and education. In each of these roles, nurses use their clinical and organizational expertise to support delivery of care that achieves positive health outcomes, prepares patients and families for discharge, prevents complications, and can be evaluated for its economic outcomes.

The changing roles for nurses in the acute care setting are the result of increased severity of illness in hospitalized patients and shorter stays. The ratio of nurses to patients is increasing as nurses contribute to care delivery in both direct and indirect care roles.

Advanced Practice Nursing

Advanced practice nurses provide clinical leadership in the delivery of care in acute care settings. The clinical specialist role provides an opportunity for nurses to use advanced clinical knowledge to consult with other nurses on care delivery, educate staff on best care practices, develop systems of care delivery, and influence the quality of care provided. Acute care nurse practitioners use their advanced clinical knowledge to provide complex physical care to hospitalized patients, often substituting for medical residents. Thus, these specialists use their nursing expertise to enhance patient care in the acute care setting (see Chapter 10).

Acute care nurse practitioners can substitute for medical residents by providing care that is within residents' scope of practice, of comparable quality, and of equal or lower cost.

 ## ECONOMIC ANALYSIS
NURSE MIDWIVES IN THE ACUTE CARE SETTING

A body of research literature has demonstrated the comparability of nurse midwifery care to physician care (Office of Technology Assessment (OTA), 1986). The cost of educating a nurse midwife was $16,800 in 1990, compared with $86,100 for physicians. In addition to the savings associated with the difference in cost of education, the differences in salary can lead to cost savings for institutions that use midwives rather than obstetricians.

The following example describes the evolution of the use of midwives in a large medical center. A nurse midwifery service was developed at a large level 3 health center in 1987. The goals of this service were to provide health care to adolescent clients from the outpatient department, participate in the education of medical students, and attract some private insurance clients. This center soon merged with a level 2 facility. All obstetric clients were assessed and triaged to either a low-risk or a high-risk unit, where care would be provided by midwives or medical residents, respectively. Another change resulting from the merger was lack of physician or resident coverage in the birth center.

With an increased volume of deliveries and limited potential for providing physician coverage, the decision was made to have nurse midwives cover the birth center as well as perform emergency procedures and births when physicians could not be present. Within a year the service recruited five additional nurse midwives and three more in the second year because of the volume of service.

Although there were philosophical differences between the physician and nurse midwifery care, this model demonstrated the ability of nurse midwives to replace residents in an inpatient facility at an affordable cost. This practice model was discontinued when the low-risk and high-risk units merged; however, experience demonstrated that the use of advanced practice nurses in a large obstetrical service was accompanied by growth in the number of persons seeking care (Ament & Hanson, 1998).

HOME HEALTH CARE

The setting with the greatest growth in percentage of total registered nurses employed is the care of the patient in his or her own home. The percentage of registered nurses providing care in home health is expected to rise from 5.95 percent in 1994 to 10.8 percent by 2005, with an average annual increase of 7.0 percent. The number of registered nurses working in home health is expected to increase by 127 percent between 1994 and 2005, with an annual increase of 11.55 percent.

Home-health-care agencies have grown from 5676 agencies in 1989 to 10,027 in 1996 (Bureau of Labor Statistics, 1994; Keepnews, 1998; Malone & Marullo, 1997). Table 9–1 demonstrates the changing number and types of Medicare-certified home-care agencies since 1967. Hospital-based and freestanding proprietary agencies have demonstrated the largest rate of growth (National Association for Home Care [NAHC], 2000). Despite this dramatic increase in home health care, home-care services still represent only 3 percent of personal health-care expenditures. In 1996 home-care services represented 8.9 percent of total Medicare payments and 7.8 percent of Medicaid payments. The Medicare percentage dropped to 6.1 percent in 1998 and continues to decline because of the effects of the Balanced Budget Agreement. By the end of 1999 the total number of home care agencies has declined to 7747, a loss of 2697 agencies since 1997 (NAHC, 2000).

Home-care services are financed by a variety of sources. However, Figure 9–1 demonstrates that Medicare still represents the largest source of reimbursement, accounting for 40 percent of the home-care services provided. Medicaid funds another quarter of the care, for a total governmental proportion of almost three-quarters of all home-care services provided. The re-

TABLE 9–1. NUMBER OF MEDICARE-CERTIFIED HOME-CARE AGENCIES

Year	VNA	Public	Proprietary	Hospital	Total
1967	549	939	0	133	1,753
1975	525	1,228	47	273	2,242
1985	514	1,205	1,943	1,277	5,983
1995	575	1,182	3,951	2,470	9,120
1996	576	1,177	4,658	2,634	10,027
1997	553	1,149	5,024	2,698	10,444
1998	460	968	3,414	2,356	8,086
1999	452	918	3,192	2,300	7,747

Source: Health Care Financing Administration, Center for Information Systems, Health Standards and Quality Bureau, 2000.
VNA = Visiting Nurses Association.

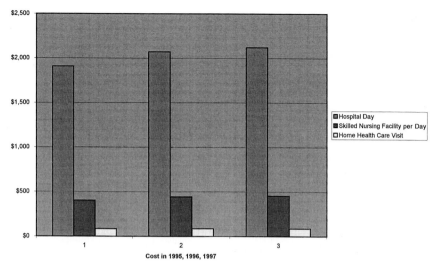

FIG. 9–1. Comparative cost of service per hospital day, skilled nursing facility per day, and home-health-care visit in 1995, 1996, and 1997.

mainder of home-care services is paid for out of pocket by recipients (23 percent) or by private insurance (NAHC, 1999). This distribution of financial burden is the reason the Health Care Financing Administration (HCFA) plays such a major role in the policy development and related reimbursement of home-health agencies.

History

Home-care agencies have been providing care to patients in their homes since the 1880s. The current demand for home-care services is supported by the approximately 7 million patients who receive care in their homes (NAHC, 1999, 2000). According to the American Nurses Association (1998), home-health-care nursing "is holistic and is focused on the individual client, integrating family/caregiver, environmental, and community resources to promote an optimal level of client well-being." Daley and Miller (1996) found that home health nurses synthesize data about the individual, family, and environment to provide seamless, complex care.

In 1992, 10 percent of working registered nurses practiced in home-care settings. Of those working in home health, 35 percent had baccalaureate degrees (American Nurses Association [ANA], 1997). Although the number of employees in home care has been small, this figure almost doubled between 1991 and 1996, from 344,000 to 666,000 (NAHC, 1997). The rapid growth in home-care employees demonstrates how the increased demand for services has increased employment opportunities.

Economic Implications

The cost effectiveness of home care has been examined for those receiving care following a hospital stay as well as for persons with a functional or cognitive disability. Table 9–2 describes the cost savings of home care compared with hospital care (NAHC, 1999). Although the length of service may vary, the table clearly shows that it is less expensive to maintain an individual at home with home care than to pay for extended care or hospital services. However, additional services may be required to maintain people in their homes. As the length of stay in the acute care setting continues to decrease and admission criteria to the inpatient setting become more stringent, the amount of care and complexity of services provided in the home will continue to increase and evolve.

The comparative cost per day of home health care versus hospital care demonstrates a lower cost of service for home health care.

Attempts to limit the total cost of health-care expenditures have been described throughout the text. Similar efforts are affecting the home-care industry as well. The HCFA is developing a prospective payment system to be implemented in the near future. In the meantime, an interim payment system has been implemented to limit costs of services. Agencies will be paid the lowest of the actual allowable cost, aggregate cost per visit, or the aggregate cost per beneficiary. A computerized record system from HCFA called Outcome and Assessment Information Set (OASIS), which incorporates a uniform data set for home care and hospice care, is also being man-

---

TABLE 9–2. COMPARISON OF HOSPITAL, SKILLED NURSING FACILITY, AND HOME HEALTH MEDICARE CHARGES, 1995–1997

Source of Care	1995	1996	1997
Hospital charges per day	$1909	$2071	$2121
Skilled nursing facility charges per day	$ 401	$ 443	$ 454
Home-health charges per visit	$ 84	$ 86	$ 88

Sources: The 1995 and 1996 hospital and skilled nursing facility Medicare charge data are from the annual statistical supplement to the Social Security Bulletin, Social Security Administration (December, 1997).

Note: Additional years are projected using consumer price index forecasts from the Bureau of Labor Statistics' Web site (http://stats.bls.gov/) and "The Economic and Budget Outlook: Fiscal Years 1999–2008," Congressional Budget Office Web site (http://www.cbo.gov/) (January, 1998).

dated to monitor service delivery, quality of care, and outcomes (NAHC, 1999).

The NAHC reports that as many as 2697 home-health agencies had closed by fall 1999 because of these new regulations and limitations in re-imbursement. To limit the devastating impact on agencies and avoid disruption of services, legislation was passed to increase the cost per visit, increase the per beneficiary limit, delay the cost limitation, and delay the prospective payment system until October 1, 2000 (NAHC, 2000).

Use of Advanced Practice Nurses in Home Care

Adult health, geriatric, and mental health nurse practitioners have the potential to provide primary care and case management services to assist the elderly and mentally ill to remain in their homes by managing risks and preventing disability. The outcomes of these home-care services include maintenance or improvement of functional status, disease management, limitation of costs related to hospitalization and nursing-home use, improved patient quality of life, and reduction of caregiver burden. For the mentally ill, home-care services have resulted in a decreased time in institutions and decreased costs per year. For nurse practitioner services to become more available in home care, there is a need for teaching programs in home care (Mitty & Mezey, 1998).

Current information and developments regarding home care and hospice care can be located at the National Association of Home Care Web site (see Appendix B).

HOSPICE CARE

Hospice care is a setting that provides practice opportunities for nurses interested in end-of-life care. The hospice movement views dying as a natural part of life that can occur in the home setting.

History

The place where patients die has followed the evolution of health care. Initially, dying occurred in the home but moved to the acute care setting as technology to keep patients alive increased. More patients are now choosing to die in their homes, in comfort and with their families. Hospice care provides palliative care, with the major focus being on assisting the patient and family to cope with death through a multidisciplinary team approach (Segal, 1985).

The history of the hospice movement began in the United States in 1963 with Dr. Saunders's address at Yale University (Segal, 1985). Implementation began in 1974 with the opening of Hospice, Incorporated. The first hospice in the United States, the Connecticut Hospice, began services in March 1974 (Segal, 1985). Dr. Elizabeth Kubler-Ross's book *On Death and Dying* (1969), which urged caregivers and families to deal with the dying by using compassion and providing relief for pain, supported the concepts of hospice care. The growth of the hospice philosophy is demonstrated by the existence of almost 3000 hospice organizations in the United States as of 1997 (NAHC, 2000).

Congress passed legislation in 1982 (PL 97–248) creating Medicare hospice benefits. Medicare beneficiaries are eligible for hospice services when they are terminally ill with a life expectancy of 6 months or less. A result of the Balanced Budget Act of 1997, the hospice benefit within Medicare includes an initial 90-day period, a subsequent 90-day period, and unlimited subsequent 60-day benefit periods as long as the person remains certified as terminally ill at the beginning of the benefit period (NAHC, 2000).

Demand for Hospice Services

Hospice benefits in 1996 amounted to $1.98 billion, which was only 1 percent of the Medicare budget. There is an aggregate cap amount for each hospice agency; this amount is adjusted annually for inflation or deflation. In October 1996, the cap amount was $13,974. Managed care organizations negotiate a specified fee for care of each patient. Each contract specifies the approved providers and access to specialty care (NAHC, 2000).

The history of the hospice movement demonstrates a growth in demand for hospice services derived from growing acceptance of these services. Hospice participation in Medicare has grown to 2274 agencies in 1997 (NAHC, 2000). Hospice care is used by a variety of recipients, mostly over the age of 55.

The demand for hospice services is increasing, as evidenced by the increasing number of patients served and the number of agencies providing hospice services.

Economic Implications

Hospice care has also proved to be more cost effective than providing the same care in an inpatient, acute care setting. NAHC (1997) reported on two hospice outcome studies. The first was a study conducted by Abt Associates in 1988 that concluded that Medicare saved $1.26 for every dollar spent on hospice care. This data reflected the first 3 years of Medicare's hospice ex-

TABLE 9–3. COMPARISON OF HOSPITAL, SKILLED NURSING FACILITY, AND HOSPICE MEDICARE CHARGES, 1995–1997

Source of Care	1995	1996	1997
Hospital charges per day	$1909	$2071	$2121
Skilled nursing facility charges per day	$ 401	$ 443	$ 454
Hospice charges per covered day of care	$ 103	$ 105	$ 108

Source: Health Care Financing Administration.

perience. These savings were particularly prominent in the last month of life. The second, more recent study was published in 1995 by the National Hospice Organization and confirmed the former findings. This study reported that Medicare beneficiaries enrolled in hospice care cost Medicare $2884 for services in the last month of life (NAHC, 1997). Table 9–3 illustrates the per-day cost comparison among hospital care, skilled nursing care, and hospice care.

The cost of hospice care per day is less than that of hospital care or extended care.

Hospice care as part of the home-health setting has continued to grow rapidly and should continue to grow with the evolution of society's feelings about death and dying, the increase in the elderly population and in the number of persons with aquired immunodeficiency syndrome (AIDS), and the increasing cost of health care. The effectiveness of this holistic manner of treatment has been demonstrated. Current hospice information can be obtained from the NAHC Web site (see Appendix B).

EXTENDED CARE

The setting with the second greatest growth in percentage of total registered nurses employed is extended-care facilities. Extended-care facilities include basic and skilled nursing facilities. More recently, extended-care facilities have been referred to as providing *subacute care.* The percentage of working registered nurses providing care in a nursing-home or extended-care setting is expected to rise from 5.8 percent in 1994 to 8.2 percent by 2005 (Bureau of Labor Statistics, 1994; Malone & Marullo, 1997; Keepnews, 1998). Seven percent of registered nurses working in 1992 practiced in nursing homes and facilities for the developmentally disabled (Bureau of Labor

Statistics, 1994), and more than 45 percent of these RNs held diplomas in nursing (ANA, 1997). The increased need for extended care results from an aging population and the trend of early hospital discharges.

Nursing homes provide subacute, skilled care to geriatric patients and patients with special needs. Since 1995, some health-care organizations have realized that postacute care is a desirable alternative to continued care in acute care facilities. Because the reimbursement for hospital services for elderly people is determined by a prospective payment that is determined by diagnosis, subacute care provides a less costly alternative for providing needed services. This funding shift fueled a proliferation of both hospital-based and freestanding nursing homes (Stahl, 1997).

The need for registered nurses to care for patients in the nursing-home and subacute care settings will continue to grow as the population ages and as the need for cost-effective, postacute, skilled care increases.

Economic Implications

Although nursing-home care is less expensive than hospital care, as demonstrated in Tables 9–2 and 9–3, extended care is still expensive, with costs for skilled nursing facilities averaging $13,620 per month (Social Security Bulletin, 1997). Basic extended care is less expensive but costs $5000 per month, or $60,000 per year. Less costly alternatives to long-term placement in extended-care facilities are appealing. Once family resources are depleted, Medicaid based on public funds is responsible for these costs.

PUBLIC HEALTH AND COMMUNITY HEALTH NURSING

The public heath and community health settings include health departments, nonprofit agencies, and other community-based agencies. The Public Health Nursing Section of the American Public Health Association (1996) defines public health nursing as "the practice of promoting and protecting the health of populations using knowledge from nursing, social, and public health sciences" (p. 1). The American Nurses Association (1986) defines community health as "a synthesis of nursing practice and public health practice applied to and promoting and preserving the health of populations" (p. 1).

Supply of Registered Nurses

In 1992, 10 percent of registered nurse jobs were in public or community health settings and more than 35 percent of those nurses held a baccalaureate degree in nursing (ANA, 1997). The registered nurses employed in these settings represent the "largest group of health professionals upholding the public infrastructure in local communities" (Zerwekh, 1993, p. 1676). By 1996, the percentage of working registered nurses employed in public health settings had already increased to 13 percent, a 3 percent increase over the 1992 proportion. This setting is expected to continue to experience growth, with shortages expected particularly in case manager and school nursing roles (Hoffman, 1997; Keepnews, 1998; Stewart, 1998).

History

In the United States, public health nursing traces its foundation to Lillian Wald, who established the Henry Street Settlement in the Lower East Side of New York in 1893 with her colleague Mary Brewster to address the health needs of immigrant families. Initially, financial assistance was sought from wealthy benefactors. Later the funding for public health projects was expanded by seeking public funding for school health programs from the Commissioner of Health in New York City in 1902 and for home visiting to policyholders from the Metropolitan Life Insurance Company in 1909. The settlement house grew and became the New York Visiting Nurse Service. Lillian Wald and her colleagues were also active in advocacy for political changes that affected the health of various communities, such as creating the Children's Bureau in 1912. Their effectiveness in creating political change was especially remarkable because women did not have the right to vote until 1920 (Swanson & Nies, 1997).

Current models of public health nursing practice are based on the work of these pioneers. This practice focuses on aggregates rather than the individual, and on prevention rather than treatment of illness. Public health nurses examine the determinants of health—biological or hereditary factors, environmental factors, health behavior, and health services and technology—to determine appropriate action. With this focus on a broad concept of health, public health nurses provide community prevention activities, advocacy for political change, and services to those who would otherwise not receive care (White, 1982; Kruss et al., 1997).

In 1988, the Institute of Medicine published a document describing the core functions of public health, which apply to public health nursing as well (Institute of Medicine, 1988; Conley, 1995). These functions relate to the practice of population-focused care. Conley (1995) described how the Washington State Health Department applied these core functions:

1. Community assessment, the first core function, involves examination of the strengths and weaknesses of the community in order to develop priorities for activities to improve health.

2. The second core function is policy development, which includes facilitating the development of plans to address the health priorities previously identified, recommending specific actions to address needs, increasing the awareness of policy makers concerning factors that affect community health, and advocating for target populations' needs.
3. Lastly, assurance is a core function involving evaluation of community goal attainment, examination of program implementation, collaboration with the community to reduce barriers to services, facilitation of strategies to meet the needs of high-risk families, and assisting the community to implement plans.

These core public health functions do not specifically include the provision of direct care but rather focus on the assessment and facilitation of needed services within the community. Such activities require nurses to increase their skills in community assessment, work with interdisciplinary teams, and collaborate with community leaders and groups. Debate continues regarding whether public health services should include direct health care to populations without access to other services. These core functions are stimulating public health nursing to develop community partnerships, contract with various organizations to provide services, and examine new ways to improve the health of the community.

Economic Implications

Public health nursing, as part of the larger public health community, is challenged to sell the value of prevention on a community level. Demonstrating cost effectiveness requires that the cost of health problems prevented be less than the cost of the service provided. Collaboration and interdisciplinary practice are designed to decrease the costs of duplication of service and to improve efficiency.

The cost effectiveness of health promotion and prevention activities is demonstrated when the activities can prevent costly illness care.

✕ ECONOMIC ANALYSIS
✕ COST EFFECTIVENESS OF HEALTH PROMOTION

The Women, Infants, and Children (WIC) program was established in cooperation with the Department of Agriculture to provide pregnant and lactating women and children younger than 5 years with supplemental food. Families who are earning up to 185 percent of the poverty level are eligible for this program. Once enrolled in the program, families receive coupons for appropriate healthy foods that can be redeemed at participating merchants. In addition to the food supplements, families receive nutritional counseling, assessment of child growth and anemia, and referrals to other appropriate services by public health nurses and nutritionists. WIC increases its impact by improving family participation in well-child care and age-appropriate immunization services.

This program has been recognized as contributing to the decreasing proportion of low-birth-weight infants. Cost savings result from elimination of the use of neonatal intensive care services. The nutritional value of the foods also contributes to the health of the infants after birth. It has been estimated that every dollar spent on WIC saves $2 to $4 in health-care costs. (Nutrition News, 1999).

Another value of public health programs is providing screening programs for community residents of all ages, which allows for case finding. This activity follows the philosophy that early identification of problems facilitates less invasive treatment and the best health outcomes. Community-level screening has been a tradition in community health practice across the life span.

Case finding of deviations from health facilitates treatment early in the disease process, which results in lower costs and better health outcomes.

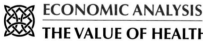

ECONOMIC ANALYSIS
THE VALUE OF HEALTH FAIRS

As part of their community assessment, local health departments prioritize the needs of their community and the resources of their agency. In the case of a rural health department, the demographic characteristics of the county show that there are many young families who lack health insurance and have not obtained the state low-cost insurance for their children. There are also many older farm families who do not have supplemental Medicare insurance to pay for medications and preventive services.

In August the public health department sponsors a back-to-school health fair. At this event there are many booths sponsored by local agencies that provide information for parents and children. Knowing that mortality and morbidity for children are often due to accidents, particularly farm accidents, several booths address safety. Fire safety, poison control, bike safety, and car safety for children are presented. A nurse practitioner is available to provide back-to-school physical exams if needed. Immunizations and lead screening are available to children who need them. A computer is available to check the state immunization registry so that appropriate immunizations are given. Parents are counseled on ways to complete immunizations after the fair if more than one dose is needed. Representatives from the state insurance program are available so parents can determine whether they are eligible and can apply. Several agencies that address chronic illness in children are also present to inform families of their services. Along with the services, many fun activities are provided for children.

After school resumes, the adult health promotion staff plan for services to the elderly population. A senior health fair is planned. At this fair the following events are scheduled: influenza and pneumonia immunization, hearing screening, vision acuity and glaucoma screening, and some basic laboratory tests (provided for a nominal fee). Staff members from other local agencies providing services to seniors have booths with information that describe their services. Local agencies that provide screening services have coupons for such services as mammography, PSA tests for prostate screening, and more complete vision testing.

These health fairs provide a mechanism for the health department to provide preventive services, screen for age-appropriate problems, and link residents to services in their community.

OCCUPATIONAL HEALTH

Occupational health is another community-based setting in which demand for nurses is increasing. Occupational health practice is concerned with the health of the working population, including the control and prevention of occupational diseases. Depending on the employer, the services may also be extended to the family of the worker.

History

In the United States, occupational health nursing began after the Industrial Revolution, when nurses began to care for coal miners and their families.

The state of Vermont organized the first official occupational health nurses in 1895, focusing on the employees of the Vermont Marble Company. The first organized industrial nursing movement began in 1915 in Boston (Swanson & Nies, 1997). In 1977, nurses practicing in this area began to call themselves occupational health nurses instead of industrial health nurses. The professional organization changed its name from the American Association of Industrial Nurses to the American Association of Occupational Health Nursing (AAOHN).

Recent congressional legislation solidified the need for nurses practicing in this setting (Silberstein, 1985). In 1992, 1994, and 1996, 1 percent of the working registered nurses were providing nursing care to the working population (ANA, 1997). The registered nurse workforce in this setting has remained steady over the last several years, with no foreseeable changes in the future.

Practice and Nursing Demand

The AAOHN developed a conceptual model of occupational health nursing that describes this field as providing care to workers, including health promotion and care for acute, chronic, and emergent health concerns. Occupational health nurses also monitor and manage disabilities following injury or illness. This practice also includes maintenance of a safe work environment, development of policy, research, and assurance of compliance with a wide variety of regulations, including those of the Occupational Safety and Health Administration (OSHA). The model also reflects the impact on occupational health nursing of population and economic trends, the legislative context of regulation, and a corporate environment (Swanson & Nies, 1997; American Association of Occupational Health Nursing, 1999).

A prominent occupational health nursing function is the assessment and management of actual or potential environmental hazards and the reduction of risk related to exposures to physical, chemical, or biological agents. Many local, state, and federal agencies exist to regulate environmentally hazardous agents and enforce regulations on their use. Occupational nurses participate in the assessment, policy development, and management of environmental health issues (Rogers & Cohn, 1998). Many sources include psychosocial hazards and violence as workplace hazards. Occupational health nurses also conduct research to promote the use of protective equipment mandated in the workplace. For example, research has addressed the use of protective equipment related to noise in the occupational setting (Lusk & Kelemen, 1995).

ECONOMIC ANALYSIS
CASE MANAGEMENT OF OCCUPATIONAL ILLNESS

Case management of worker injury, disability, and illness facilitates increased worker health and a faster return to work, which limits the cost of health care and of lost work. Illness management has a group focus. The goals include improvement of self-care, coordination of services, assessment of providers and treatments, and development of effective treatment plans. This process involves a collaboration with employees, families, employers, health-care providers, and insurance providers to streamline health care.

Case management continues from the acute phase, which often involves hospital care, to coordination of care, which often involves an outpatient phase, and to dealing with any potential sequelae of the health concern in the shortest amount of time. These activities all have economic implications for reducing the cost of illness or injury care and increasing worker productivity (Dees & Anderson, 1996). Companies are particularly concerned when workers are receiving Workmen's Compensation, making the illness or injury job related.

Case management in occupational health is directed to the early detection and treatment of illness and injury to promote early recovery, decreased health-care costs, and early return to work.

Economic Implications

Occupational health nursing has great economic impact. Identification of physical, biological, and psychosocial hazards in the workplace provides the opportunity to decrease exposure and prevent harm to workers. Cost savings result from decreased health costs and limited lost time for the worker. Additional savings occur when occupational health and safety standards can be maintained, preventing penalties from OSHA because of failure to comply with regulations.

Direct care services for workers assist workers to remain healthy when possible, to identify illness early, and to receive appropriate care to manage the illness or injury. The benefits to the worker relate to maintenance of better health and reduced health costs. The employer benefits include decreased health costs and time lost from work.

Current issues in occupational health nursing can be found on the AAOHN Web site (see Appendix B).

SCHOOL HEALTH

School nursing was established to promote and protect the health of school-aged children. In the United States, school health services have been present since the last portion of the 19th century. In 1902 the New York City schools hired the first school nurse to improve school attendance by follow-up of communicable disease. These services spread rapidly to other cities and other parts of the country. Policies were influenced by state executives, enacted legislation, and judicial actions (Swanson & Nies, 1997). School programs have evolved to include a wide variety of activities, such as the following:

- Health promotion and teaching
- Assessment and management of acute and chronic illness
- Interdisciplinary planning for students with special needs
- Screening programs
- School-based clinics

Many U.S. policies have been directed to promoting the success and health of school-aged children. National educational goals for all children were set forth in Public Act 103–227 in 1994. In addition, the secretaries of Health and Human Services and of Education have identified barriers affecting children's success. These policy statements and goals affect the environment for school nursing by identifying goals for students and barriers that limit achieving those goals (Swanson & Nies, 1997).

Practice

The activities of professional organizations are important to the achievement of national health goals for school-aged children. The nurse who practices in this setting is likely to belong to or work with a variety of professional organizations that support school health, including the following:

- American Nurses Association
- American Public Health Association
- American School Health Association
- National Association of Pediatric Nurses

- National Association of State School Nurse Consultants
- National League for Nursing
- National School Health Education Association

Brainerd (1998) reported on the progress toward meeting the goals established in 1994 by a coalition of agencies to improve school health nursing. Seven key needs in school health were identified:

1. Definition and advancement of the role of the school nurse
2. Implementation of school health nursing standards
3. Attention to legal and ethical concerns
4. Efforts to inform policy makers about current school health nursing services
5. Provision of more appropriate orientation and ongoing preparation for school nurses
6. Conduct of school health nursing research
7. Securing of adequate funding for school health nursing services

Demand and Supply of School Health Nurses

The demand for school nursing services is supported by policy statements and goals set forth by public policy groups and professional organizations that define a need to address the health requirements of preschool to adolescent children. Specialized planning and services are mandated for children with special health needs.

However, both private and public school districts are constrained by limited financial resources. These constraints result in each school district setting its own priorities for desired school health services and obtaining funds to support them.

Economic Implications

The potential economic value of school health nursing involves improving the health of school-aged children. When children are identified and referred for care early, cost savings are realized. Health promotion also results in decreased use of health services. A decrease in the incidence of vaccine-preventable diseases results from surveillance and referral of children who do not have complete immunizations. Interdisciplinary planning and coordination for students with special needs assists in improving their overall well-being and ability to learn as well as providing more comprehensive management of their conditions.

✦ ECONOMIC ANALYSIS
THE VALUE OF SCHOOL NURSING

Although many school districts have been reluctant to invest in school nurses, a small school district with six elementary schools, two middle schools, and one high school has chosen to hire two school nurses. One nurse manages school health needs at the elementary schools; the other manages school health for the middle and high schools. Both nurses have experience as public health nurses, so they meet with the teachers, administrators, and parents in the district to assess the district school health needs. The following five school health priorities are identified, along with plans for meeting them:

1. Immunizations
   - The nurses arranged assistance to develop a computerized database that recorded all children's immunization data and provided reminders at the beginning of each school year.
   - The nurses worked with local health-care providers to establish an immunization clinic so that children could receive hepatitis B and chicken pox vaccinations, which are not mandatory now but soon will be.
2. Communicable disease management
   - The nurses maintain a schedule so that they can be reached at any time with questions about communicable disease.
   - The nurses have worked with local pediatricians and the health department to identify resources for care and appropriate reporting mechanisms for the school.
3. Interdisciplinary team planning
   - Using the schedule, nurses plan to assess special education students for their nursing needs and to participate in the team planning sessions.
   - The nurses maintain contact with local pediatricians to keep communication among the school, family, and health-care provider current.
4. Medication administration
   - Because nurses cannot be at each school when medications are given, the nurses meet with teachers and the designated person who will administer medication to provide medication teaching.
   - The nurses contact each family and health-care provider to gain information about the child's health needs and medication changes.

5. Comprehensive health education
   - The nurses realized that this program cannot be established immediately, so they established a health committee composed of teachers, administrators, parents, and some students. This committee discusses school health education needs.
   - The nurses examine existing school health curricula for committee review.
   - The nurses contact local agencies for existing teaching materials.
   - The nurses establish a 2-year time frame to assess, develop, and gain approval of a school health curriculum. The goal is to have 20 lessons per grade that can be taught by teachers as well as nurses.

This plan demonstrates the value that nurses can bring to school health promotion and illness management. The goal is to prevent as much illness and injury as possible and to manage existing child health problems. Students with identified illnesses are less likely to miss a large number of school days.

Although this plan seems idealistic, some level of school nursing is mandated for special education students, so the program could be used to meet other needs as well.

PARISH NURSING

Communities of faith and other religious organizations have been involved with healing for more than 2000 years. Yet the modern use of congregation-based practice dates to the 1980s. Religious leaders recognize the value of this ministry as compatible with the faith community's mission of healing and promotion of well-being. The value of parish nursing includes its potential for reaching individuals, families, and groups within an established, trusted community. Health promotion activities include the psychosocial and spiritual components of health provided in the context of their own religious community (Miskelly, 1995; Shank, Weis, & Matheus, 1996; Weis, Matheus, & Shank, 1997).

Practice

Parish nursing involves the promotion of wellness by a parish nurse who is part of the ministerial team of the congregation, providing a holistic approach to the physical, emotional, and spiritual needs of the congregation members. The amount of these services varies, but many parish nurses work 16 to 20 hours per week. Education for this role varies from informal continuing education and literature to formal educational experiences

(Miskelly, 1995; Shank, Weis, & Matheus, 1996; Weis, Matheus, & Shank, 1997). The parish nurse is a resource person and consultant to individuals for health promotion, health counseling, advocacy, and community referrals. In addition to the individual focus, Miskelly (1995) describes a vision of the parish nurse as a community health nurse whose community is the congregation.

Several models exist for this practice. The institutional volunteer model involves a nurse who volunteers her time but has a relationship with the parish and a health-care institution, which provide some assistance. A second model is the congregationally paid model, in which the congregation pays for the nurse's services. Finally, the congregational volunteer model involves a nurse who is directly associated with the congregation but provides services as a volunteer (Miskelly, 1995).

Demand

The demand for parish nursing has been stimulated by an increasing focus on health concerns ranging from health promotion to disease management and by fragmentation within the health-care system, emphasis on self-care, limited access to services because of high cost, and the need to address people within a community as well as in institutional settings. The National Parish Nurse Resource Center in Park Ridge, Illinois, estimated that over 2000 nurses function as parish nurses (Miskelly, 1995).

ECONOMIC ANALYSIS
PARISH NURSING AND CARDIOVASCULAR WELLNESS

Marylane Wade Koch

Because parish nurses work within their faith communities as educators, benefits for both the individual and the community at large can occur. Susan is a 48-year-old, recently divorced woman employed full time in a management job as well as being a mother to two children, aged 3 and 13. She knows she should care for herself, but often her personal health needs seem to come last on the list. Her mother has congestive heart disease. Susan knows that many of her own behaviors are less than heart healthy.

Last month, the parish nurse at her church set up a health fair with free screenings for cholesterol and blood pressure. The fair had some fun activities for children as well, so Susan attended. She left with educational materials and information from her health screenings, which indicated elevated cholesterol level and blood pressure. These screening values concerned her because she knew she had made lifestyle choices that were not heart healthy and she had a family history of heart disease.

Spiritually, Susan has always believed her body was God's temple and that she was a steward of her health, a gift from God. She also knew she was responsible for providing for her children and needed to be healthy. After the fair, she took her screening values to her doctor for review. He said her elevated blood pressure and cholesterol could possibly be controlled by a change in her diet, exercise, and stress management. Where was she to get the help and support for such change? The doctor asked her to return in 6 months for a reevaluation, at which time medication intervention might be an alternative.

Susan contacted the parish nurse and asked for an appointment to discuss her health concerns. The nurse, Linda, met with Susan and helped her develop a plan to address her health concerns. Susan was invited to an exercise session that used dance and 1960s music, something Susan enjoyed, and offered childcare for participants. She met with a dietitian, a volunteer to the health ministry of the church, who showed her how to prepare healthy, low-fat meals twice a month and freeze them for easy access after work. Linda offered to take Susan's blood pressure weekly on Sunday mornings and monitor changes.

The following month, Linda met with Susan to talk about stress management in her life. Linda told her about classes the church offered on topics such as living with and loving your teenager, caring for aging parents, and managing finances. These classes differed from similar ones at the community college because they included meaningful scripture and prayer support. Susan added one class each month to her schedule. Susan started having a short devotion with her children at breakfast and started their day with prayer.

Linda calls Susan intermittently to check on her and offer prayer and support. Linda gave Susan educational information on hormones and heart disease, because Susan was perimenopausal. Susan started attending a divorce support group at church as well. When Susan returned to her doctor, her cholesterol level and blood pressure had decreased. The doctor opted for no medical intervention at that time and scheduled Susan for a follow-up in another year.

The cost implications of the interventions by the parish nurse are many. The cost of cardiovascular disease and stroke in the United States in 1999 was estimated at $286.5 billion. This sum included both direct costs, such as hospitalizations, physician visits, medications, home care, and durable medical equipment, as well as indirect costs such as lost productivity because of resulting morbidity and mortality (American Heart Association, 1999a). In 1994, 309,000 of the 688,000 outpatient surgical cardiovascular procedures performed in the United States were on women. Of these women, 175,000 had a cardiac catheterization, at an average cost of $10,880. A coronary artery bypass cost about $44,820, and a percutaneous transluminal coronary bypass cost $20,370 (American Heart Association, 1999b).

A study by researchers at Northwestern University Medical School showed that people with low risk of heart disease during middle age needed less hospital care in later years (News America Digital Publishing, 1999). Risk factors included high blood pressure, high cholesterol, smoking, previous heart attack, diabetes, or an abnormal heartbeat. Women in the study cost Medicare less than half as much as an at-risk woman. The majority of the savings were associated with three preventable or controllable risk factors: smoking, high blood pressure, and high cholesterol. Dr. Valentin Fuster, president of the American Heart Association, stated that the drugs and lifestyle changes needed to control high blood pressure and high cholesterol are cheap compared with the cost of one heart attack. Thus, the parish nurse's interventions had a high economic value.

CORRECTIONAL HEALTH

The population of prisoners has drastically increased, with the current numbers of incarcerated persons being the highest in data collection history. Prison health is a major issue because courts have ruled that provision of adequate health care by correctional facilities is part of inmates' constitutional rights under the Eighth and Fourteenth Amendments. It is estimated that more than 1.6 million persons compose the prison population in the United States (Maeve, 1997). The demand for correctional health nurses is thus high.

Practice

Mortality and morbidity data suggest that higher rates of disease and disability exist in prisoners regardless of their age. Infectious diseases, health consequences of drug abuse, seizure disorders, mental health problems, trauma, and chronic health problems are among the health challenges of inmates (Droes, 1994). Specific infectious disease concerns for this population include tuberculosis and human immunodeficiency virus (HIV) infection.

Kassof (1995) describes the challenges of working with women inmates, many of whom are dually diagnosed with mental illness and substance abuse. Many women have also experienced varying forms of emotional and sexual abuse. Provision of mental health treatment services that address these concerns can decrease the rate of return to prison. The responsibilities of correctional health nurses include primary prevention of illness and infectious disease in the corrections environment. Treatment and rehabilitation of existing health concerns are also important to this nursing specialty.

As prisoners grow older, chronic illnesses become a greater concern. In 1995 there were 55,000 state and federal inmates aged 50 years and older. These numbers are estimated to continue growing (Clark, 1999). Legislation mandating minimum sentencing and a policy of "three strikes and you're out" will result in an increase in elderly prisoners. The needs of these elderly inmates have implications for nursing services, mental health services, and the physical environment of the prison. Aging prisoners present special concerns because they are a unique subculture isolated from the wider society in a total institutional environment having its own rules and mores. The prison experience affects social support of family life, self-concept, traditional work roles, personal choices, possessions, and privacy (LaMere, Smyer, & Gragert, 1996). Smyer, Gragert, and LaMere (1997) describe three types of elderly prisoners who have different attitudes concerning adjustment and fear of violence:

1. Persons who are convicted after the age of 50 and have special adjustment and fear issues
2. Persons who are over 50 and have been in prison on and off during their lives and thus have fewer adjustment concerns
3. Persons who have aged in prison and have few skills for returning to the community

Elderly prisoners require assessment and intervention to prevent illness and disease, address existing chronic health problems, promote adjustment to the prison environment, and prepare them for community release programs when possible.

Droes (1994) examined the special challenges of correctional health nursing in both jail and prison settings. Structural considerations included security issues, inadequate facilities for the purposes desired, and limited staffing. Nurses provide both inpatient and ambulatory care services while managing the health-care unit. The perceptions of custody staffs regarding correctional health care span a continuum from toleration to viewing it as assisting in their work. Nurses in the study had varying views of their practice, from a narrower perspective on treating specific illness to a broader one that included public health and social-psychological roles.

Economic Implications

Correctional health nursing provides the opportunity to assess inmates for physical and psychological problems. Correct identification and appropriate treatment can lead to decreased health-care costs. With increased numbers of prisoners being sentenced for extended periods, if not life in prison, the health-care management of these individuals is a social cost. Prevention of illness and appropriate disease management can reduce the overall costs of care.

AMBULATORY CARE

Ambulatory health care is a setting that includes physicians' offices, free-standing clinics, minor medical clinics, health maintenance organizations (HMOs), and mixed professional practice groups.

Practice

Ambulatory health nursing focuses on systematic assessment, diagnosis of acute illness, and preventive care for patients and families. The nurse practicing in this setting functions independently and must be self-directed.

History

Ambulatory care can be traced back as far as 1786, when the first dispensary was established in Philadelphia, and 1893, when New York City opened milk stations to teach mothers about infant feedings (Daugherty & Buchanan, 1985).

Supply of Registered Nurses

In 1992, almost 8 percent of employed registered nurses worked in ambulatory care settings and just over 40 percent of these were diploma graduates (ANA, 1997). By 1996, the percentage of registered nurses practicing in ambulatory care settings had increased to 8.5 percent (Keepnews, 1998). This percentage should continue to increase with the rapid growth of outpatient care facilities.

Ambulatory Care Clinics and Health Maintenance Organizations

As is the case in acute care settings, ambulatory care provides a mixture of direct and indirect care roles for nurses. The direct care roles for nurses in ambulatory care settings are determined both by the nurse's educational preparation and the organization of the setting. Nurses can provide a variety of direct care services, including history taking, health assessment, preventive and well-person care, and management of acute and chronic illness. Client and caregiver education are also important to health maintenance and illness management. Nurses provide a wide range of educational services to individuals, families, groups, and other staff members.

The goal of cost containment provides opportunities for nurses who have a comprehensive understanding of the health-care system to provide the following services: identifying information needs such as documentation and patient education, redesigning and managing the delivery of care, and coordinating the provision of service with insurance companies and other agencies. Integrated health-care systems and HMOs also hire nurses to make decisions regarding which services will be reimbursed and to coordinate the provision of services so that care is received in the least costly environment possible.

Nurse-Managed Centers

A subspecialty of ambulatory care nursing is that of the nurse-managed center (NMC). Nurse-managed centers date to the early settlement houses of 100 years ago, an example being Lillian Wald's House on Henry Street. This phenomenon has grown since the emergence of nurse practitioners in the 1960s. An estimated 250 NMCs were operating by 1990. A study of NMCs demonstrates that many are new, less than 5 years old. Types of NMCs include community clinics, centers affiliated with hospitals or other agencies (e.g., HMOs or schools of nursing), and private nursing practices. Services offered within a nurse-managed center include acute care and illness management by nurse practitioners, and community health nursing services such as health education, health promotion, research, and case management (Yoder, 1996). Obtaining funding for NMCs is difficult. NMCs have used funding from contracts, fees, third-party reimbursement, charitable funding, and grants.

Nurse-managed centers have the ability to deliver holistic services within the community at an efficient cost. A community assessment is important to determine the need for NMC services. The assessment should include analysis of the community's needs and the ability of a particular center to address those needs before the decision is made to create an NMC (Yoder, 1996).

ECONOMIC ANALYSIS
EVOLUTION OF A NURSE-MANAGED CENTER

A community health nursing faculty member at a large university established a site for undergraduate community health nursing students in one apartment in the married student housing complex. Students developed a variety of health-education and health-promotion services at this site, such as nutrition education, prenatal classes, a parenting support group, and related home visits. One group of special interest included married foreign students with families. Working with foreign students provided an opportunity to develop skills working with culturally diverse groups. Many cultural practices are exhibited in childbirth and parenting.

As the site developed, more students and families participated in the center's activities. Nurse practitioner students were invited to become a part of the center. With advanced practice nursing students and faculty services available, the center expanded to a more comprehensive primary care clinic. The clinic then initiated negotiations to become eligible for reimbursement from the university-based health maintenance organization. Reimbursement allowed the center to become self-sufficient.

NURSE-OWNED BUSINESSES

Registered nurses are creative professionals who can assume the role of entrepreneur. *Entrepreneurs* are people who assume the risks associated with a freestanding business. Services provided in these businesses cover a broad spectrum from consultative services to health-care organization and leadership and from development of health-care products (such as computer software) to educational services or assessment, referral, and case management for specific populations. Gerre Lamb defines a nurse entrepreneur as "someone who identifies a patient need and envisions how nursing can respond to that need in an effective way and then formulates and executes a plan to meet the need. . . . It's looking for opportunities and really seizing the moment" (Simpson, 1997, p. 24). The role of entrepreneur is explored further in Chapter 10.

Nurse-owned businesses are created by individuals who use their nursing expertise to create a solution to some patient or other health-care need and who assume a financial risk to implement their vision.

Supply and Demand

As health care becomes more complex and regulatory compliance more challenging, nurse entrepreneurs and those with a venturesome spirit will become even more in demand. Nurses with a wide variety of expertise and interests will create solutions to emerging health-care issues. There is no specific training for becoming a nurse entrepreneur. Table 9–4 describes a wide range of services that can be addressed by nurse entrepreneurs.

TABLE 9–4. EXAMPLES OF NURSING BUSINESSES

Nursing Arena	Service Provided
Clinical practice	Nurse practitioner in private practice
	Gerontology resource and referral
	Provision of foot care in the community
	Wellness programs in community sites and businesses
	Employee assistance programs
	Maternal child services: childbirth preparation, lactation consultation, parenting
	Nurse-managed clinics
	Anesthesia, pain management
	End-of-life care
Consultation	Quality management
	Infection control
	Publishing, nurse editors
	Ethical issues and systems of review
Management	Quality management
	System design and reorganization
	Information science and information systems
	Accreditation
Case management	Focus on specific client populations, such as:
	Workmen's Compensation
	Elderly
	Substance abuse in general populations, professionals
Education	Continuing education
	Client populations: diabetic education, maternal child health, etc.
	Orientation to specific new ideas or technologies
Research	Create integrative reviews of the literature or research
	Identify funding sources
	Contract to conduct research on specified problem
	Consult on the conduct of the implementation of research
	Create practice guidelines

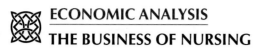

ECONOMIC ANALYSIS
THE BUSINESS OF NURSING

Tom Renkes

While working as a nurse manager in a major health-care center in the late 1980s, I saw nurses observing business decisions in health care rather than making their own business decisions. Each committee meeting would touch on agendas and issues, with the result depending on some executive making the decision. After watching this for years, I decided things might be done differently if given the right tools.

Indications of a changing health-care environment have been obvious from the end of the 1970s. The questions kept nagging me: Why can most of the business world change on a dime and be successful but health care cannot? Where are the health-care professionals, particularly nurses, in all this decision making? With so many nursing layoffs in health care, who's controlling our destiny as professionals?

It took two fishing trips and one week back at work for me to decide that things could be done differently. In reviewing functions that needed attention at several health centers and managed care companies, the following were the most evident: licensing and accreditation of facilities, quality management programs, and credentialing of professionals. Once these priorities were set, I made numerous business calls to colleagues for support in providing needed skills and referring clients. I then contacted a business attorney and accountant. Finally, I developed marketing strategies for product, price, promotion, and distribution of what was to become a new nursing business venture.

The *product* was consultation services that provided assistance for health-care agency needs—most often licensing and credentialing of facilities, quality management, or professional credentialing. Frequently the clinical areas involved were substance abuse and mental health. These system problems require demanding work that usually involved overtime, stress, and distraction from revenue production for full-time employees.

The *price* was set low by a business philosophy committed to limiting the impact on fees directed at patients and clients. Business expenses could be kept to a minimum by working swiftly and efficiently, using office space in the home, and making just enough money to maintain our current lifestyle.

Promotion involved utilization of a large network of colleagues and previous contacts. Word-of-mouth advertising allowed for a more selective process of accepting or rejecting business. In starting a new business, too rapid growth can cause rapid disintegration of services. That is the death knell to a business succeeding from a customer service perspective. The mantra became: "Only as good as your last paycheck." There was no reserve revenue to back the slow times, and no banks willing to open lines of credit. Everything depended on how well the service was provided that day. *Distribution* was the easiest part. I would travel to extend the range of my services and to achieve a quick response to client needs.

What I had to do next was retire at the age of 31 and hope for the best. Astounding as it was, within 2 months I was making twice as much money as I had been making as a middle manager. At the same time I saved business costs for the health employers who hired me as a consultant because my rates were cheaper than the cost of the full-time employees needed to perform the same functions. I was also beginning to subcontract with colleagues, adding services and providing those colleagues with additional income. I frequently had educational contracts for personnel credentialing, and I was busiest of all with HMO credentialing contracts.

Keys to success included attention to detail in all areas, provision of extra services to get the job done, and a commitment to achieving a positive impact on the organization, not just getting the plan on paper or achieving a credential. Greatest of all was the fact that I was controlling my destiny by keeping up with health-care changes in business journals and by constant contact with other health-care professionals. Over the last 9 years, there have been some failures and mistakes, but never a thought of giving up; rather, I learned from those mistakes. In time the original business grew by obtaining new contracts, employees, and consultants. The business also assisted some employees to finish school, assume new positions, and own a business.

Nurses need to be aware of all the opportunities available to them in the health-care marketplace. Employment provides one avenue, but there is immense satisfaction in creating and controlling your own destiny.

SUMMARY

As health care moves from care in the acute care setting to community-based services, nursing must prepare itself for these changes. Sheila Ryan (1997) said it best when she said, "along with these changes will come the cessation of our stale obsession with counting content and process(es) based on disease models of caretaking for institutionalized sick individuals." As a profession, nursing must be ready to make changes in educational preparation, market nursing services to the public, exhibit an entrepreneurial spirit, and embrace the changes in health care in order for nurses to be the leaders rather than the followers in the evolution of health care. Nursing is "essential for these new practice futures" (Ryan, 1997). In summary, as health care continues to become more diverse, registered nurses will be in greater demand than ever before, their roles will continue to expand, and the settings that registered nurses work in will become more diversified.

DISCUSSION QUESTIONS

1. Discuss the movement in health care away from care of the patient in the home to the acute care setting and back again.
2. Discuss the impact of community based care on the settings where nurses work.
3. Describe two settings that have had the most significant growth in the percentage of working registered nurses. Describe these two settings.
4. List the range of practice settings where registered nurses are employed.

 REFERENCES

Aiken, L. (1995). Transformation of the nursing workforce. *Nursing Outlook*, 43(5) 201–209.

Aiken, L., & Salmon, M. (1994). Health care workforce priorities: What nursing should know. *Inquiry*, 31(3), 318–329.

Ament, L. A., & Hanson, L. (1998). A model for the future: Certified nurse-midwives replace residents and house staff in hospitals. *Nursing and Health Care Perspectives*, 19(3), 106.

American Association of Occupational Health Nurses (AAOHN) [On-line]. Available: www.AAOHN.org.

American Heart Association. (1999a). Economic costs of cardiovascular diseases [On-line]. Available: http://www.americanheart.org/statistics/10econom.html.

American Heart Association. (1999b). Medical procedures, facilities, and costs [On-line]. Available: http://www.americanheart.org/statistics/09medicl.html.

American Nurses Association. (1986). *Standards of community health nursing practice*. Kansas City, MO: Author.

American Nurses Association. (1997). Nursing facts: Today's registered nurses—numbers and demographics [On-line]. Available: http://www.nursingword.org/readroom/fsdemogr.htm.

American Nurses Association. (1998). *Home health nurse: Description of practice.* [On-line]. Available: http://www.nursingworld.org/ancc/generist/gb3.htm.

American Public Health Association (1996). The definition and role of public health nursing: A statement of the APHA public health nursing section, March 1996 Update. Washington, DC: Author.

Brainard, E. (1998). School health nursing services progress review: Report of 1996 national meeting. *Journal of School Health, 68*(1), 12–17.

Bureau of Labor Statistics, U.S. Department of Labor. (1994). *National industry-occupational matrix: Employment by industry and occupation. 1994 and projected 2005 alternatives: Registered nurses.* Washington, DC: U.S. Government Printing Office.

Clark, M. J. (1999). Care of clients in corrections settings. In M. J. Clark, *Nursing in the community: Dimensions of community health nursing* (pp. 685–701). Stamford, CT: Appleton & Lange.

Conley, E. (1995). Public health nursing within core public health functions: "Back to the Future." *Journal of Public Health Management Practice, 1*(3), 1–8.

Daley, B., & Miller, M. (1996). Defining home health care nursing: Implications for continuing nursing education. *Journal of Continuing Education in Nursing, 27*(5), 228–237.

Daugherty, L., & Buchanan, G. (1985). Nursing role in ambulatory care. In L. Jarvis (Ed.), *Community health nursing: Keeping the public healthy* (2nd ed.). Philadelphia: FA Davis.

Dees, J. P., & Anderson, N. L. (1996). Case management: A management system for quality and cost effective outcomes. *AAOHN Journal, 44*(8), 385–390.

Droes, N. S. (1994). Correctional nursing practice. *Journal of Community Health Nursing, 11*(4), 201–210.

Hoffman, L. (1997). Market demand for case managers soar. *Case Management Advisor, Salary Survey/Supplement,* 1–4.

Institute of Medicine, The National Academy of Science. (1988). *The future of public health.* Washington, DC: National Academy Press.

Jacox, A. (1997, December 30). Determinates of who does what in health care [On-line]. *Online Journal of Issues in Nursing.* Available: http://www.nursingworld.org/ojin/tpc5/tpc5_1.htm.

Keepnews, D. (1998, May/June). The National Sample Survey of Registered nurses: What does it tell us? *American Nurse, 30*(3), 10.

Kruss, T., Proulx-Girouard, L., Lovitt, S., Katz, C. B., & Kennelly, P. (1997). A public health nursing model. *Public Health Nursing,* Vol. 14, 81–91.

Kubler-Ross, E. (1969). *On death and dying: What the dying have to teach doctors, nurses, clergy and their own families.* New York: Macmillan.

LaMere, S., Smyer, T., & Gragert, M. (1996). The aging inmate. *Journal of Psychosocial Nursing, 34*(4), 25–30.

Lusk, S. L., & Kelemen, M. J. (1995). Predicting use of hearing protection: A preliminary study. *Public Health Nursing, 10*(3), 189–196.

Maeve, M. K. (1997). Nursing practice with incarcerated women: Caring within mandated alienation. *Issues in Mental Health Nursing, 18,* 495–510.

Malone, B., & Marullo, G. (1997). Workforce trends among U.S. registered nurses: A report for the International Council of Nurses ICN Workforce Forum [On-line]. Available: http://www.nursingworld.org/readroom/usworder.htm.

Miskelly, S. (1995). A parish nursing model: Applying the community health nursing process in a church community. *Journal of Community Health Nursing, 12*(1), 1–14.

Mitty, E., & Mezey, M. (1998). Integrating advanced practice nurses in home care: Recommendations for a teaching home care program. *Nursing and Health Care Perspectives, 19*(6), 264–270.

National Association for Home Care. (2000, March). *Basic statistics about home care 2000.* [On-line]: http://www.nahc.org/Consumers/hcstats.htm.

News America Digital Publishing. (1999). Heart disease risk in middle age predicts Medicare costs later [On-line]. Available: http://www.foxmarketwire.com/wires/1014/f_ap_1014_34.sml.

Office of Technology Assessment (1986). Physicians assistants and certified nurse midwives: A policy analysis. Washington, DC: U.S. Government Printing Office.

Pew Health Professions Commission. (1995). *Critical challenges: Revitalizing the health care professions for the twenty-first century.* San Francisco: UCSF Center for the Health Professions.

Public Health Nursing Section, American Public Health Association (1996). *The definition and role of public health nursing in the delivery of health care.* Washington, DC: Author.

Rogers, B. (1990). Occupational health nursing practice, education, and research. Challenges for the future. AAOHN Journal, 38(11), 536–543.

Rogers, B., & Cohn, A. R. (1998). Expanding horizons: Integrating environmental health in occupational health nursing. AAOHN Journal, 46(1), 9–13.

Ryan, S. (1997, August 20). Accreditation for the future: A director's perspective [On-line]. *Online Journal of Issues in Nursing.* Available: http://www.nursingworld.org/ojin/tpc4/tpc4_3.htm.

Segal, B. (1985). Nursing role in hospice care. In L. Jarvis (Ed.), *Community health nursing: Keeping the public healthy* (2nd ed.). Philadelphia: FA Davis.

Shank, M. J., Weis, D., & Matheus, R. (1996). Parish nursing: Ministry of healing. *Geriatric Nursing,* 17(1), 11–13.

Silberstein, C. (1985). Nursing role in occupational health. In L. Jarvis (Ed.), *Community health nursing: Keeping the public healthy* (2nd ed.). Philadelphia: FA Davis.

Simpson, R. (1997). Technology and the potential for entrepreneurship. *Nursing Management,* 28(10), 24–25.

Smyer, T., Gragert, M. D., & LaMere, S. (1997). Stay safe! Stay healthy! Surviving old age in prison. *Journal of Psychosocial Nursing,* 35(9), 10–17.

Social Security Administration (1999). *Social Security Bulletin Annual Statistical Supplement 1999.* Washington, DC: Social Security Administration Office of Research, Evaluation, and Statistics, pp. 311–330.

Stahl, D. (1997). Managed care trends: The effect on subacute care. *Nursing Management,* 28(3), 17–21.

Stewart, M. (1998, May/June). School nurse: Who is caring for our nation's children? *American Nurse,* 30(3), p. 13.

Swanson, J. M., & Nies, M. (1997). *Community health nursing: Promoting the health of aggregates* (2nd ed.). Philadelphia: WB Saunders.

USDA Study finds most WIC babies getting nutrients, Moms aren't. (1999). *Nutrition Week,* XXVII, 1–4.

Weis, D., Matheus, R., & Shank, M. J. (1997). Health care delivery in faith communities: The parish nurse model. *Public Health Nursing,* 14(6), 368–372.

White, M. S. (1982). Construct for public health nursing. *Nursing Outlook,* 30, 527–530.

Yoder, M. K. (1996). Starting a nurse-managed center for older adults: The needs assessment process. *Geriatric Nursing,* 17(1), 14–19.

Zerwekh, J. (1993). Doing to the people: Public health nursing today and tomorrow [Commentary]. *American Journal of Public Health,* 83(12), 1676–1678.

 ## SUGGESTED READING

Dienemann, J. A. (Ed.). (1998). *Nursing administration: Managing patient care.* Stamford, CT: Appleton & Lange.

Cherry, B., & Jacob, S. R. (1999). *Contemporary nursing: Issues, trends, and management.* St. Louis: Mosby.

Holman, E. J., & Branstetter, E. (1997). An academic nursing clinic's financial survival. *Nursing Economics,* 15(5), 248–252.

Kalina, C. M. (1998). Linking resources to process in disability management. AAOHN Journal, 46(8), 385–390.

Kanter, R. B. (1989). *When giants learn to dance.* New York: Simon & Schuster.

Kassof, M. (1995). Viewpoint: Prison mental health program makes a difference. *Michigan Nurse,* 68(11), 13.

Kosinski, M. (1998). Effective outcomes management in occupational and environmental health. AAOHN Journal, 46(10), 500–509.

Nunnery, R. K. (1997). *Advancing your career: Concepts of professional nursing.* Philadelphia: FA Davis.

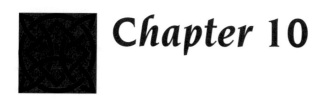

Chapter 10

Evolving Roles and Professional Practice Models for Nursing

Sylvia A. Price
Loraine Frank-Lightfoot

LEARNING OBJECTIVES

- ▪ Describe the implications of the Pew Health Professions Commission report for health-care practitioners.
- ▪ Describe advanced practice nursing.
- ▪ Compare and contrast the roles of nurses as advanced practice nurses, entrepreneurs or intrapreneurs, unlicensed assistive personnel coordinators, and case managers.
- ▪ Describe and analyze the research on unlicensed assistive personnel practice.
- ▪ Describe the role of the nursing case manager.
- ▪ Discuss the importance of collaboration in nursing practice.
- ▪ Analyze the case management and collaborative practice models and their impact on the cost effectiveness of patient care.
- ▪ Describe nurses' role in the health-care system of the 21st century.

The previous chapters have described the forces affecting the cost of health-care delivery, the nursing labor market, and the settings where nurses work. This chapter focuses on the economic implications of evolving roles and professional practice models for nursing in the 21st century. Nurses should have a significant role in redesigning the health-care system to effectively utilize economic resources and coordinate services appropriately. The survival of health-care organizations within our society is dependent on evolving nursing roles that help facilities respond appropriately to the forces of change, which include changing patterns of health-care delivery, advances in science and technology, and cost-containment strategies.

IMPLICATIONS OF THE PEW REPORT FOR HEALTH PROFESSIONALS

The Pew Health Professions Commission (1995) stressed that most of the public- and private-sector demands for reform are being driven by the perception that health care is consuming too much of our nation's resources.

Therefore, practitioners must be responsible for providing cost-effective and appropriate care. The system that is emerging will demand cost reductions; health professionals will choose either to participate in this process or abdicate it to nonclinicians. The latter choice would not be in the best interests of the nation's health. It seems evident from this report that knowledgeable health-care professionals are best qualified to use limited resources to maximize favorable clinical outcomes.

The commission further stated that it is essential for health professionals to be competent and willing to manage the cost of care. They must be prepared to practice in managed care and integrated systems. The practitioner in the 21st century must be knowledgeable and apply increasingly complex technologies not only in an appropriate but also in a cost-effective manner in order to balance clinical and system demands.

Because nurses constitute the largest group of health-care professionals, they are in a unique position to implement innovative and cost-effective roles in their arenas of practice. They have a significant role in the provision of cost-effective, high-quality client care.

Health care is consuming too much of our nation's resources.

 ## ROLES AND OPPORTUNITIES FOR NURSES

The roles of nurses continue to expand, reflecting the changes in the health-care delivery system. These roles include advanced practice nurse (APN), clinical nurse specialist (CNS), nurse practitioner (NP), case manager, unlicensed assistive personnel coordinator, certified registered nurse anesthetist (CRNA), certified nurse midwife (CNM), and nurse entrepreneur or intrapreneur. It is essential to clarify the competencies required in these nursing roles, not only as they exist today but as they are projected to evolve. Once expectations are ascertained, education and experience need to be determined to provide for congruence between the individual and the role.

Advanced practice nurses require specific educational preparation and certification to practice in their particular roles.

NURSES IN ADVANCED PRACTICE

The roles of APNs, including NPs, CNSs, CRNAs, and CNMs, have been evolving over many years. This evolution has increased in momentum with the emphasis on health-care reform. The field of primary care has experienced a reawakening in recent years. Despite intense challenges and competition, primary care NPs in adult, child, and family nursing are not only surviving but also thriving. As in all health professions, the current practice of NPs has evolved from that of the NPs who pioneered the primary care role (Brown, 1996). The rapid changes in society and the health-care system over the past decade have sparked dialogue about how best to conceptualize and label the advanced practice domains of NPs and CNSs (Elder & Bullough, 1990).

APNs acknowledge the similarities among the advanced practice roles while stressing the strengths, contributions, and individuality of each role. Advanced practice roles share the foundation of a nursing perspective in the care of individuals and families. Table 10–1 describes many nursing roles, including the possible settings and growth potential for each.

Studies on the role of advanced practice nurses emphasize economic outcomes as well as patient outcomes. For example, the cost effectiveness of neonatal nurse practitioners (NNPs) was investigated in a retrospective study (Bissinger et al., 1997). The researchers conducted a record review in a 36-bed neonatal intensive care unit at a health science center in the southeastern United States. The quality and cost of care given by NNPs and medical house staff were compared. The researchers posed the following question: Is there a difference in length of stay (LOS), days on ventilator, days on oxygen, mortality, morbidity, and cost of care when infants weighing between 500 and 1250 grams are cared for by NNPs versus medical house staff?

The analysis demonstrated that the two groups of infants had similar sample characteristics, suggesting comparable levels of health. Although the groups cared for by NNPs or by medical house staff did not differ significantly in the quality-of-care parameters of LOS, ventilator days, days on oxygen, morbidity, and mortality, the NNP-managed infants experienced a mean LOS that was 14 days shorter and a mean number of days on oxygen that was 11 days shorter.

The cost of care was significantly different for the two provider groups, with the average cost of care per patient for the NNP-treated group being $88,932 and for the physician-treated group being $107,171. A Quality of Care Index demonstrated similar quality of care by the NNPs and the physicians. A cost-effectiveness ratio was calculated by dividing the mean cost of care by the Quality of Care Index score to determine the cost required for achieving a specified level of quality. The cost-effectiveness ratio was $105,070 for the physician group and $88,051 for the NNP group. This analysis reveals that the cost for providing essentially the same quality of care to neonates was approximately $18,240 less per infant with the NNP providers.

TABLE 10–1. SUMMARY OF NURSING ROLE DESCRIPTIONS

Nursing Role	Description	Educational Preparation	Setting of Practice	Client Population	Growth Potential
Nurse practitioner (NP)	RN with advanced education in a specialized clinical area who can practice independently	MSN/MS is currently required for certification exam.	Inpatient settings: extended care, acute care, critical care, emergency care Ambulatory care Community settings	Life span: infants to elderly and families. Wellness to illness, including acute and chronic illness. Acute care, adult, emergency, family, gerontology, neonatal, occupational health, pediatric, psychiatric, school, women's health.	Varies by region and specialty. Some areas are approaching saturation.
Clinical nurse specialist (CNS)	RN with advanced education in a specific clinical area who provides advanced care and consults with others in care provision and systems of care	MSN/MS is currently required for certification exam.	Inpatient settings predominate: extended care, acute care, critical care, emergency care Ambulatory care Some community settings	Life span: infants to elderly. Wellness to illness, including acute and chronic illness. Additional focus is groups and systems.	Varies by region and specialty. Shortage in acute care.
Certified registered nurse anesthetist (CRNA)	RN with advanced education in administering and monitoring the delivery of anesthesia and analgesia	MS/MSN; few certificate programs remain. 24–36 months of study required for certification.	Inpatient: acute care, operating rooms, ambulatory surgery, intrapartum units, other pain management settings	Life span: infants to elderly. Clinical issues: surgical anesthesia, intrapartum pain management oncology and other pain management.	Continued demand, with many opportunities for general or specialty practice throughout the United States.

TABLE 10–1. (CONTINUED)

Nursing Role	Description	Educational Preparation	Setting of Practice	Client Population	Growth Potential
Certified nurse midwife (CNM)	RN with advanced education for gynecological and maternity care plus care during labor and birth	MSN/MS is currently required for certification exam.	Inpatient and ambulatory obstetrical and gynecological services, community	Women: adolescent and older; newborns.	Opportunities for varied aspects of practice.
Nurse Manager	RN with advanced educational preparation who integrates clinical and management skills as leader, manager, change agent, corporate thinker throughout the organization	RN with BSN or MSN preferred.	Any health care agency unit, division, or organizational level in acute, critical, emergency, extended, ambulatory, or community care	Across the life span from infant to elderly. Across the illness to wellness continuum. Individual, family, and community level of care.	Positions and responsibilities change as health care evolves. Other patient care activities may be included. Design may vary, but skills remain in demand.
Case Manager	Continuous monitoring and evaluation of client care through interdisciplinary teams and standardized plans	RN with BSN or MSN preferred	Any health care agency unit or division. Acute, critical, emergency, extended, ambulatory, or community care	Across the life span and the illness to wellness continuum. Individual, family, and community level of care	Form of case management varies, but coordination of resources and processes of care remains.

TABLE 10–1. (CONTINUED)

Nursing Role	Description	Educational Preparation	Setting of Practice	Client Population	Growth Potential
Entrepreneur/ Intrapreneur	Nurse who develops a new idea, service, or organization to meet a health care or other need.	RN with creativity. Specific education is helpful but not required	Any health care agency or unit. Acute, critical, emergency, extended, ambulatory, or community care or management level.	Address any health care issue of individual, family or community. Client can also be health care organization or policy body.	With technology and system changes, the need for individual and organizational innovation accelerates.
Staff Nurse	Direct care provider. Includes supervision of others, provision & coordination of care	RN: AD to MS nurse	Any health care agency or unit. Acute, critical, emergency, extended, ambulatory, or community care	Across the life span and the illness to wellness continuum includes individual, family, community level of care.	New skills: supervision of UAP, interdisciplinary plan, resource management

249

The researchers imply that the differences in total cost are related to the shorter LOS for the NNP patient group. The continuous presence of the NNP throughout a neonate's hospitalization provides greater coordination of care than a larger number of rotating physician house officers who may care for each infant. Neonatal NPs also contribute knowledge of nursing-care needs and excellent communication skills that facilitate a coordinated effort by the team of care providers. This coordination of care may result in earlier discharges, and hence lower costs due to shorter LOSs.

The CNS role also has a positive affect on cost containment, as described in the accompanying economic analysis.

ECONOMIC ANALYSIS
CLINICAL NURSE SPECIALISTS HAVE ECONOMIC IMPACT

Naylor and associates (1994) explored the effects on elderly cardiac patients and their primary caregivers of comprehensive discharge planning by CNSs. While the patients were hospitalized, CNSs visited patients at least every 48 hours during their hospitalization and were available by telephone throughout their stay and for 2 weeks after discharge. In addition, CNSs initiated at least two telephone contacts to patients and caregivers during the first 2 weeks after hospital discharge.

Results indicated that from hospital discharge to 6 weeks after discharge, patients in the intervention group had fewer readmissions, fewer total days rehospitalized, lower readmission charges, and lower charges for health-care services. It is interesting to note that although there were significant reductions in health-care costs and in hospital readmissions, the effects of the intervention rapidly decreased after a certain time. Telephone follow-up was very effective for up to 6 weeks postdischarge, but was not strong enough to have an effect 6 to 12 weeks postdischarge. CNSs are now visiting patients in their homes. Will this intervention improve patient outcomes over a long period after discharge?

Building on previous research and using a randomized clinical trial, Naylor and colleagues (1999) examined the impact of discharge planning and follow-up by CNSs or gerontological APNs during and following hospitalization for a group of at-risk elders. This randomized clinical trial sought to examine the impact of comprehensive APN intervention on patient health outcomes, service utilization, and health-care cost.

The sample consisted of 363 patients who were over age 65, were admitted to the hospital with one of the specified medical or surgical conditions, spoke English, and were alert. Once eligibility was determined and consent obtained, subjects were randomly assigned to either the APN discharge planning group (the treatment group) or the routine care group (the comparison group). Outcome indicators included hospital readmissions, recurrence or exacerbation of cause of hospitalization, comorbidities, or new health problems. Variables studied were time to first hospital readmission, mean length of new hospitalization, number of unscheduled acute care visits, cost of hospital readmission, functional status, depression, and patient satisfaction.

Analysis demonstrated that the two groups of subjects were similar on sample characteristics, indicating the comparability of the groups at the beginning of the study. Both groups had similar attrition (30 percent for the treatment group versus 26 percent for the comparison group). Hospital readmission was more likely for the control group (37.1 percent, representing 760 hospital days) than the treatment group (20.3 percent, representing 270 hospital days) ($p < .01$). In addition, more of the control group had multiple readmisssions (14.5 percent versus 6.2 percent, $p = .01$). In numeric terms, by 24 weeks the treatment group had 49 hospital readmissions whereas the control group had 107. The number of hospital days for readmissions was significantly greater for the control group. The time between hospital discharge and the first readmission was significantly longer for the treatment group. These hospitalizations related to previous conditions (60.3 percent), comorbidity-related conditions (22.4 percent), and new conditions (17.3 percent). The treatment group had significantly fewer hospitalizations for the initial condition, and somewhat less for comorbidities and new health problems.

Other outcomes that were not significantly different between the two treatment groups were mean functional status, depression, and patient satisfaction (very high). The number of visits in the home by nurses, therapists, social workers, and home-health aides did not differ for the two groups, nor did home visit costs differ. At 24 weeks, the aggregate acute health-care costs were approximately twice as much for the control group as for the treatment group ($p < .001$). Group costs were $1,238,928 for the control group and $642,595 for the APN group, representing an individual cost of $6,661 versus $3,630.

This study demonstrated that APNs who provided intensive discharge planning and home follow-up to high-risk elders were able to lengthen the time to the first hospital admission, reduce the number of readmissions, and decrease cost. This study is also significant in that participants did not represent a single diagnostic condition but a variety of common diagnoses. The management protocol addressed the primary health problem, other diagnoses, and other health and social concerns. Home-care services in and of themselves were not sufficient for improved outcomes: One in two of the patients receiving home care was readmitted whereas one in five of the APN-managed patients was readmitted. This study supports the expertise of gerontologically prepared APNs.

ENTREPRENEUR AND INTRAPRENEUR

Entrepreneurs often leave the employment of others and start a business of their own. Drucker (1985) notes, "Entrepreneurs always search for change, respond to it, and exploit it as an opportunity" (p. 21). He posits innovation as the specific tool of entrepreneurs; it is a means by which they exploit change as an opportunity for a different business or different service. Entrepreneurs in nursing are a diverse group. They function in a variety of roles, such as serving as a consultant to a drug rehabilitation center or providing preventive and clinical services to clients. They also have created businesses that provide skilled nursing services for temporary staffing of hospitals and extended-care facilities, corporate employee health programs, management training, and elder care services.

In contrast, an *intrapreneur* is an individual responsible for creating innovations *within* an organization. Hollander, Allen, and Mechanic (1992) emphasized that the intrapreneur is the intracorporate entrepreneur. Intrapreneurs work to turn their ideas into reality. Within the organization this individual may have access to the financial resources that are necessary to support an idea or innovation.

Intrapreneurs are creative and self-directive people who nurture entrepreneurial activities within the organization in which they are employed. They work with staff and direct their talents toward the goals of the organization.

Use of intrapreneurs is a cost-effective way to achieve new program development goals within the nursing department of a hospital or in a home-care setting. For example, nurse intrapreneurs can assist their organizations to respond to changes and opportunities that are evident in health care today. It is imperative that these organizations foster a culture that supports the nurse intrapreneur who has an innovative approach for improving patient-care outcomes.

ECONOMIC ANALYSIS
VALUE OF A NURSE INTRAPRENUER

A nurse intraprenuer in a medical unit at a large university hospital developed an innovative approach for managing medically stable geriatric patients, especially those who were to be transferred to an extended-care facility. This nurse developed a proposal for a unit referred to as the "Continuity of Care" unit. The unit was opened and is functioning cost effectively while providing high-quality care for this patient group (Hollander, Allen, & Mechanic, 1992).

Further examples of nurse-owned and nurse-managed businesses can be found in Chapter 9 and in Simms, Price, and Ervin, *The Professional Practice of Nursing Administration* (2000).

SUPERVISING UNLICENSED ASSISTIVE PERSONNEL

A role currently being incorporated into health-care institutions is that of unlicensed assistive personnel (UAP). The related nursing role is as coordinators or supervisors of UAP in the clinical setting, because UAP always work under the supervision of a registered nurse (RN).

The use of UAP in areas in which RNs and licensed practical nurses (LPNs) would have been appropriate in the past is an example of substitution. Unlicensed assistive personnel function in an assistive role in providing patient-care activities as delegated by and under the supervision of a registered nurse.

Cost containment is one of the major reasons for implementing a UAP model of care. This model raises the issue of the appropriate use of UAP as adjuncts and not as replacements for the registered nurse.

Assistive personnel were used in hospitals in the past, especially during the nursing shortages of World Wars I and II. Hospitals employed assistive personnel, and later practical nurses, when practice patterns such as functional and team nursing were in vogue. In the early 1970s an interest in all-RN staffs was apparent (Milstead, 1993; Kalisch & Kalisch, 1995), which resulted in a shift to a higher ratio of registered nurses.

The nursing shortage delayed this trend in the late 1980s and resulted in changes in staffing patterns evident in the 1990s. Aiken (1995) reports that hospital inpatient nurse employment between 1988 and 1992 increased only 6 percent, which constitutes the lowest growth rate of any patient-care setting. Many hospitals are reducing registered nurses as a proportion of total nursing personnel and are increasing the employment of UAP.

There is a great deal of uncertainty or concern about the role of UAP in patient care. A major issue is the fact that at present, there are no guidelines regarding preparation for the role. Programs designed for UAP in hospitals vary in both content and length. For example, a study done in multiple states found that most UAP were not provided training for activities of daily living (ADL) and supportive tasks, but did receive from 1 to 6 weeks' training for technical tasks, much of which was on-the-job training. The study also indicated that nurse managers thought UAP education should be more comprehensive and complete (Salmond, 1995). In long-term settings, however, specific guidelines have been established under the Omnibus Reconciliation Act, which identifies curriculum and program length for certified nursing assistants in an extended-care facility.

Another major issue is the regulation of UAP. The Joint Commission on Accreditation of Healthcare Organizations requires that UAP demonstrate competence and that the health-care facility employing these individuals must validate their competence in a specific skill area. Koch and Esmon (1998) emphasize that some providers believe that regulation of UAP will help to ensure safe patient care through standardization of training and utilization, whereas others oppose it because they are concerned that regulation will create another "legitimate occupation" that is more readily substituted for the RN. Shoffner (1997) stresses that there is insufficient research to clearly demonstrate that patient care is compromised by the use of UAP. Numerous anecdotal reports indicate that a decrease in professional nursing care and an increase in unlicensed personnel providing care are detrimental to the patient.

The use of UAP is an example of the economic principle of substitution (see Chapter 6), in which a different role is developed in place of a previous one. In this case the attempt is to save money by putting cheaper UAP in place of an RN. However, a cost-benefit analysis needs to be conducted because any decrease in quality could actually increase costs (see Chapter 14).

The focus on UAP has fostered research studying the effects of UAP as adjuncts that will complement but not replace RNs. Bernreuter and Cardona (1997a, 1997b) surveyed and critiqued studies related to unlicensed assistive personnel from 1975 to 1997. In studies that were related to staffing pattern changes, they found extensive use of UAP. In California, 94 of 102 general hospitals used UAP primarily in bedside care. Only 3 percent of the

UAP were supervised consistently by the same RN (Barter, McLaughlin, & Thomas, 1994).

Productivity is a critical economic element in the use of UAP. Does the presence of this type of worker increase or decrease the workload of the RN? Salmond's (1995) study of orthopedic units in 31 states found that the workloads of staff nurses were not decreased by the use of UAP. Thirty percent of the staff nurses believed their workload was increased by the use of UAP. Eighty percent of the UAP performed supportive tasks, such as activities of daily living, intake and output, weights, and vital signs. Fifty percent or more performed more technical tasks, such as placing the patient on and off continuous passive motion machines, applying immobilization devices, and setting up and applying traction. Only 25 percent performed pin care on orthopedic patients, collected and tested urine specimens, or checked tube patency.

Neidlinger and associates (1993) studied the job composition on two experimental units where UAP were integrated into the staffing and on two control units in a 560-bed university medical center. This study reported excessive nonproductive time associated with UAP. A study by Lengacher and coworkers (1996) described a partnership between the RN and multiskilled worker on two medical/surgical units, one a pilot unit and the other a control unit. Productivity was measured by time spent in documentation and by salary cost. The actual cost per patient day was greater in the UAP unit for both documentation and salary costs. Blegen, Goode, and Reed (1998) demonstrated that, controlling for severity of patient illness, there was a negative relationship between the percentage of RN staff and three of the quality indicators (medication errors, decubiti, and patient falls) from the ANA Report Card. These studies are summarized in Table 10–2.

Research on unlicensed assistive personnel does not provide conclusive findings. A more standardized methodology of evaluating the impact of unlicensed personnel on health care is required. Manuel and Alster (1995) describe some of the factors that may affect these outcomes: cost of time of training UAP, cost of additional documentation time, limited ability of nurses to supervise UAP, and the manner in which additional nursing time is assigned. The integrative review of UAP research conducted by Bernreuter and Cardona (1997a, 1997b) demonstrated a consideration of quality outcomes, perceptions of patient and nurse satisfaction, and cost.

Additional research on UAP needs to focus on the following:

- Practice patterns that describe the roles and mix of professional nurses and assistive personnel
- Type of unit or setting
- Comparable financial outcomes, such as cost per patient day for care and number of hours per day of total care for each type of staff

TABLE 10–2. UNLICENSED ASSISTIVE PERSONNEL RESEARCH

Authors	Setting	Variables	Cost Outcomes	Conclusions
Blegen, Goode, & Reed (1998)	Relate % patient-care hours by RN staff to outcomes in university medical center.	Medication errors Patient falls Skin breakdown Patient and family complaints Infections Deaths	Controlling for acuity, % of RN staff hours was negatively related to medication errors, decubiti, and complaints. Total hours of care provided were related to decubiti, mortality, medication errors.	The relationship between % RN hours of total staffing to outcomes was curvilinear. Above 87.5% RN hours, adverse outcomes also increased.
Lengacher et al. (1996)	Test partners in patient care (PIPC) model that used experimental design to test use of multiskilled (UAP) workers in med–surg units compared with traditional aides.	Cost per patient day Decreased documentation time Patient and provider satisfaction Quality of care Role of nurse Partnership	Significantly higher actual unit salaries/patient day on UAP units. Significant increase in documentation time on units with UAP. Actual unit salaries per patient day were higher on UAP unit before and after introduction of UAP. Actual supply costs increased on the UAP unit.	Costs and time in documentation could improve. Differences in units and staff mix could result in differences.
Neidlinger et al. (1993)	560-bed university medical center. Experimental and control units with assistants used as nurse's aides.	Use of temp staff Personnel cost/ patient day Quality = audit Patient and nurse satisfaction	Both units decreased registry cost 73% and 61%. Control units cost more before and after. Audit quality decreased. Experimental units had greater cost increases. Patient satisfaction was equal or slightly higher.	Work sampling showed nurses devoted more time to treatment procedures and assessment. Assistive personnel focused on hygiene. Nurses were satisfied with job satisfaction decreased. Some demonstrated beginning of acceptance.

256

- Documentation time, supervision time, and training time, with related costs

Bernreuter and Cardona (1997a, 1997b) concluded that use of such standard measures would assist in comparison of research and build a more consistent body of evidence.

The accompanying economic analysis depicts factors that are important in the implementation of the UAP role.

 ## ECONOMIC ANALYSIS
IMPACT OF UNLICENSED ASSISTIVE PERSONNEL IN HOSPITAL PRACTICE

A clinical manager is employed on a medical/surgical unit at Parker Hospital, a community hospital that has recently been acquired by Big City Integrated Health System. Systemwide analysis shows that Parker Hospital has a high ratio of RN staff to patients and of RN hours to the total hours of care provided per day. The patient care management team is planning to increase the use of UAP. The hospital has always used some assistive personnel for personal care, transportation, and taking of vital signs. In their expanded role, UAP will now do more procedures, including oxygen level testing, skin assessments, simple dressings, and several other similar procedures.

The plan begins in October, with all UAP required to take 10 half-day classes to teach them the new tasks they will perform as well as their documentation and reporting responsibilities. The manager is pleased with progress until the RNs on the unit report that they have never supervised assistants doing more complex tasks, are not comfortable delegating such tasks, and are unclear regarding their legal responsibilities. The manager takes this information back to the management team, and an additional series of five 3-hour sessions are developed for the RNs to prepare them for their part in this new system. In the beginning of November, the new staffing plan goes into effect.

Reading through the monthly reports for October through January, the clinical manager notes that:

- Nurses have reported an average of 40 hours more per week in overtime costs.
- Unit costs exceeded the amount budgeted for the training of the UAP and nursing staff.

- Assistive staff have been off duty an average of 10 shifts more per month than the previous average.
- Staffing costs per patient day in the months since the innovation are approximately the same (within $25 per patient day) as the period before the program implementation.

The initial evaluation by the staff is mixed. Nurses appreciate having additional hands for care, but they are stressed and dissatisfied at having more patients to care for and less time to spend evaluating, teaching, and preparing patients and families for discharge. Although there are no data to support it, nurses feel the quality of care has somehow declined. They are also still not comfortable with delegation. The assistive staff is mixed in their evaluations as well. They like having additional responsibilities, but they do not like having extensive supervision of their work.

An economic consultant is hired to evaluate the change. He recommends collecting data on not only the input (nursing salaries) but the output (quality care, patient and nurse satisfaction, patient length of stay, and patient readmissions).

NURSE CASE MANAGER

Nurse case managers coordinate the resources needed for clients along the continuum of health care. Case managers are members of an interdisciplinary team who assume responsibility for assessing patient outcomes. Tahan (1997) emphasizes that to be successful in their role, nurse case managers need to have certain skills for carrying out their clinical, managerial, and business responsibilities. They need to be clinically astute and skilled both in coordinating patients' discharge planning and in teaching patients and families. Case managers should be highly skilled in communication, negotiation, contracting, teamwork, delegation, and conducting meetings. It is crucial that they also have skills in financial analysis, financial reimbursement procedures, marketing, and customer relations.

Sandra Lowery, RN, past president of the New England Case Management Society, stated that the case manager is "uniquely qualified to maximize outcomes while monitoring costs" (Hesselgrave, 1997, p. 5). She notes that case managers have a key role in seeing that incentives between providers and payers are aligned toward continuity of care. "You can't control costs and effective use of health services if you exercise restrictive access to care by simply eliminating line-item services," states Lowery. "Good outcomes have to mean more than what happens next week—that's a Band-Aid approach. Quality care and appropriate intervention at the outset of diagnosis is the most effective strategy to maximize quality of life and minimize costs over the long term" (Hesselgrave, 1997, p. 5).

 ## PROFESSIONAL PRACTICE MODELS

The professional practice models discussed in this section depict various methods of delivering nursing care. The models emphasize the diversity of nursing personnel used in the delivery of health care, the coordination of services provided, and the outcomes of nursing care.

TEAM NURSING

The philosophy of team nursing emerged because of nursing shortages and technological advances after World War II. The Committee on the Functions of Nursing recommended that nursing should be organized using a team approach to patient care. A research study to assess whether the quality of nursing care could be enhanced by a team approach was initiated at Teachers College, Columbia University, directed by Eleanor Lambertsen (1958). The study revealed that team nursing was an efficient and cost-effective way to administer nursing care. Lambertsen described team nursing as a patient-centered philosophy of nursing care.

Team nursing is based on the belief that when the activities and efforts of diversified nursing personnel are coordinated by a professional nurse, the group's effort for the patient will surpass what can be done individually. The early proponents of team nursing believed that the nurse who assumes the leadership role of the team should be prepared at the baccalaureate level. Sherman (1990) emphasizes that this was not a feasible recommendation in the 1950s because of the scarcity of baccalaureate-prepared nurses. She implies there were problems with different conceptualizations of team nursing. For example, despite its introduction as a philosophy of nursing care, there was more emphasis on method than on outcome. Inexperienced nurses were placed in leadership roles with inadequate support and poorly trained staff. Just as case managers should be clinically and educationally well prepared, so too should nursing team leaders.

The idea of team nursing is that the patient is included in planning care and that the team leader is accountable for the nursing care given by team members. The team is responsible for the total care given to an assigned group of patients. The team leader assesses patient-care needs and plans nursing care assignments; team members must accept the leadership and supervision of the team leader. Effective communication is thus necessary for continuity of care. To be effective as a nursing care delivery model, team nursing must provide an approach for meeting patient-care needs while effectively and efficiently using health-care resources.

PRIMARY NURSING

Primary nursing was introduced in the 1960s as a planning and delivery system for comprehensive nursing care. The nursing philosophy is that one nurse is operationally responsible for the planning and delivery of care to a specific group of patients from admission to discharge. Nurses are responsible and accountable for patient-care outcomes. Proponents support this concept because it reflects nursing autonomy, authority, and accountability. The tenets of primary nursing include coordination of services, continuity, and quality of care. Manthey (1980) stressed that decentralized decision making is the organizational theory that provides the foundation for primary nursing; that is, authority is allocated at the level of action.

The primary nurse has 24-hour responsibility and accountability for care planning and is expected to act independently in planning and evaluating nursing care. The primary nurse communicates with other health-care personnel, provides direct patient care, and is responsible for patient-care outcomes. Cohen and Cesta (1997) emphasize that this delivery system is assuming characteristics of other patient-care models and is evolving into a prototype that can be adapted to alternative delivery models of nursing care.

CASE MANAGEMENT

Case management is a professional practice model for identifying resources and utilizing them efficiently and effectively in the provision of client-centered health care. It integrates the accountability and expertise of primary nursing with the collaborative effort of team nursing. Case management processes aim to achieve a link between the quality of care for a specific diagnosis and the cost associated with that care. The intent of this delivery model is to manage the use, quality, and cost of health-care resources needed for the patient's illness episode.

Autonomy, accountability, and authority are the essential components of a professional practice model.

Case Management in the Community

Case management can occur within acute care agencies or in the community. Rogers, Riordan, and Swindle (1991) emphasized that case management is an effective strategy for community settings because it allows the client easier access to a health-care system that is often complicated, fragmented, and confusing. Another advantage in the community setting is that case management provides nurses with increased autonomy and authority over their practice.

⊗ ECONOMIC ANALYSIS
CASE MANAGEMENT IN THE COMMUNITY

Joanne is a home-health nurse who has worked in a large metropolitan agency for 10 years and has formed a network of relationships with individuals and agencies that serve as referral sources for her clients. Currently, she is visiting and serving as case manager for Mr. John Jackson, a 78-year-old man with diabetes, a leg ulcer, and cataracts, who lives with his elderly wife in a rural area in Michigan.

Joanne initially focused her assessment on the client's physical needs. However, it became apparent that family problems were overwhelming the physical ones. For example, Mr. Jackson's 17-year-old granddaughter is living with them because she is unmarried and pregnant. The Jacksons cannot focus on themselves until they can obtain prenatal care for their granddaughter. Joanne refers the family to the AddCare program, which provides Medicaid insurance for pregnant women, and to Women, Infants, and Children (WIC), which will provide nutritious food for the granddaughter during pregnancy.

The Jacksons are also having difficulty getting to his primary care physician's office because he is unable to drive with his leg ulcer and cataracts. Mrs. Jackson does not drive. Joanne contacts the Area Agency on Aging and arranges transportation to the health-care provider.

Joanne learns that Mr. Jackson is not taking his prescribed treatment because his medications and medical supplies, including dressings for his leg ulcer, cost $400 per month. His Medicare does not pay for medications, and he does not have supplemental health insurance. She contacts a local program that assists seniors with unreimbursed medication costs. She then contacts the ophthalmologist to schedule an appointment for cataract surgery and has this office coordinate care with Mr. Jackson's primary care physician.

The coordination handled by this home-care nurse assists the family to remain independent in their home, increases continuity of care, and facilitates healing of the leg ulcer within the agency's targeted number of home visits for clients with diabetes. Joanne was able to achieve these outcomes by acting as a case manager. She also documented care with the new Medicare-required OASIS (Outcome and Assessment

Information Set) documentation system, which is moving toward prospective payment of services. Her case management role helped coordinate services to prevent costly complications, and her documentation helped set up a system of reimbursement for health-care services.

Cost Effectiveness of Nursing Case Management Models

Cohen (1991) described a classic investigation assessing the cost effectiveness of a nursing case management (NCM) model in a large acute care hospital setting. The model incorporated a team nursing approach using various skill levels of nursing personnel. Critical paths and NCM plans were used to monitor patient care. The study measured the effects of an NCM model on length of stay of patients hospitalized for cesarean section. It also assessed the cost of delivering care to this patient group. A quasi-experimental design compared the experimental group (using a case management model) with a control unit (using a conventional mode of patient-care delivery).

In this study, patient length of stay was designated as a measure of nursing workload, patient resource utilization, and cost effectiveness. A significant reduction of inpatient LOS was noted on the experimental unit, which reported a mean LOS of 4.86 days compared with 6.02 days on the control unit. Length of stay thus declined by 1.16 days (19 percent) between the experimental and control groups.

Direct nursing care encompassed all patient-assignable activity performed by the RN, LPN, and nursing assistant. The total number of aggregate direct nursing hours (including all professionals) was significantly higher for the experimental group (mean of 16.84 hours) than the control group (mean of 12.28 hours).

The extent to which the NCM model contributed to the cost effectiveness of patient care was investigated relative to resource utilization, charges generated by patient case, personnel skill mix costs, direct care costs, and total average cost of the NCM model. The data analysis revealed a decrease in resource use, charges, and expenditures for inpatients on the experimental unit. The experimental group charged an average of $5147.05 per case compared with the control group charges of $6198.90 per case.

The costs of direct nursing care were also higher for the professional skill mix in the control group ($389.89 per case) compared with the experimental unit ($266.64 per case). The average cost per patient case was lower for the case management group compared with the conventional practice group. A savings of $930.40 per patient case was realized between the experimental and control groups.

Cohen emphasizes that NCM provides the framework in which to collect data on the resources needed and used for delivery of patient care. These data can define the parameters and relative use of resources for patient-care services in an attempt to approximate costs.

Outcomes of Case Management

Huggins and Lehman (1997) described three studies conducted over a 3-year period at Carondelet St. Mary's Hospital. The purpose of these studies was to compare NCM outcomes regarding resources and service costs. The Carondelet nurse case management practice model improves quality of care in a cost-effective way. Nursing services are carried out in the community, in client homes, and in both community health center and parish nursing sites. The goal of these services is to provide coordination, health assessment, education, and discharge plan evaluation for clients who are at high risk for readmission to hospitals (e.g., elderly people over 60 years old, those with limited family support, the chronically ill, those with a high probability of physiologic instability, those who qualified for home health care for a short period of time and chose to remain at home, and those who consistently used the emergency department for immediate health-care needs).

The initial study done by Papenhausen in 1995 measured the effect of NCM intervention on client outcomes (perceived severity of illness, general self-efficacy, life quality, and self-help abilities) (Pappenhausen, 1995, 1996). The data revealed a decrease in severity of illness and a slight increase in self-help; that is, clients exhibited a decrease in perceived physical disability, reported fewer symptoms, and had improved management of symptom distress. This study demonstrated that NCM practice was associated with changes in client outcomes, and that clients perceived these changes.

In 1996, the data collected by Papenhausen was used to examine the cost of NCM service. NCM service time was defined as time involved in providing direct and indirect service to clients during the first 3 months in the program. Direct service was determined by the actual time spent in a home visit or physician office visit with the client. Indirect service costs included materials, office space, and organizational overhead. Cost was determined from organizational data on salaries and benefits of nurse case managers added to the costs of direct and indirect services. The average nurse case manager's salary was $21.14 per hour. Additional dollars for federally required organizational benefits were added to the base salary, bringing the total to $27.27. An analysis of indirect service (travel and documentation) and direct services (assessment, teaching, supporting, direct care, exploring alternatives, and other interventions) increased the hourly rate of NCM service to approximately $41.00.

In 1997, a second analysis of the previous Papenhausen data compared costs for a 6-month period before initiating NCM services with costs for a 6-month period after NCM services were begun for a sample of 53 clients. There were 236 encounters before the NCM model was implemented and 128 after, for a total of 364. Of these encounters, 144 were for inpatient services, 99 for outpatient services, and 121 for emergency department care. The data in this present study indicated an average utilization cost prior to NCM of $1651.73 per patient per month. The average utilization cost after the implementation of NCM was $475.14 per patient per month. In 1996, the average utilization cost of NCM services was $157.06 per patient per month; thus, the total cost per patient per month with NCM services was $632.20, resulting in a 61.7 percent reduction in costs.

Papenhausen (1995) suggests that the most plausible explanation for the differences in outcomes was the effectiveness of assessment and monitoring interventions and of educational interventions. These interventions increased the patients' compliance with the therapeutic regimen, identified and treated disease early, and assisted clients to effectively manage their own chronic illnesses.

COLLABORATIVE MODELS

Collaboration is the key to the success for nurses in their new roles, whether they are APNs, entrepreneurs or intrapreneurs, supervisors of unlicensed assistive personnel, or case managers. All these roles require extensive collaboration with others. Baggs and Schmitt (1990) define collaboration as nurses and physicians cooperatively working together, sharing responsibility for problem areas, and making decisions to formulate and carry out plans for patient care.

Collaboration, which includes cooperation and sharing, is essential to new nursing practice roles.

Coeling (1998) stresses that another factor that affects collaboration is the communication style, or manner of speaking, one uses when speaking to another person. Collaboration encompasses the back-and-forth communication between two or more persons. Coeling and Wilcox (1994) asked both nurses and physicians what would facilitate communication between them. Nurses reported that improved relationships with physicians would best facilitate their communications, whereas physicians stated that the most important factor was nurses providing more factual data in an organized manner. The authors note that it is important not only to develop appropriate communication styles but also to know what is important to the professional with whom you are speaking at the moment and to be able to adapt your manner of speaking to the needs and preferences of that particular individual. If health-care organizations are to remain viable in the age of managed care, collaboration among clinicians is imperative.

This process of communication and collaboration is the basis of successful performance improvement projects that move beyond a basic tweaking of the system. Collaborative projects bring about real and dramatic change in the way in which health-care practitioners provide care for patients. The collaborative process must involve all disciplines that affect the care of the target group of patients and their families. For example, a collaborative project for open heart patients would include participants from the preoperative, intraoperative, and postoperative phases, as well as representatives from the laboratory and from the respiratory therapy, pharmacy, cardiac rehabilitation, and posthospital care providers. The goal of the collaborative process is to provide better care to patients at a lower cost.

The first task in successful collaboration is bringing all participants together to listen to each other and identify areas for improvement. For the collaborative process to work, the goals and the purpose of the project must clearly be outlined. Broad goals for collaboration may be set prior to assembling the target group so that they have a guideline from which to work; however, participants must have control over the identification of specific initiatives and goals. The group must have the power and authority to make change. The changes need not be dramatic or spectacular, and they need not involve all participants.

In order to implement a change, at least one clinician must adapt his or her practice. The results and data should be shared in a format that is easily accessible and straightforward. A bulletin board in the unit that displays graphs and data regarding the change is an example of a communication strategy. The bulletin board must identify the goal(s) of the change, and the data must be current and show trends. In arenas related to physician practice, a physician champion is essential to facilitate the process. Through these types of identification and performance improvement processes, clinicians can make changes and improvements in their practice in a rapid manner.

Lewin (1951) described change as a three-step process that involved unfreezing, changing, and refreezing. Unfreezing means rethinking the existing equilibrium or present situation and agreeing that the status quo is not gratifying. It is in this stage that motivation for change occurs. The group must first make a diagnosis of the problem. Active participation in the identification of the problem and the generation of alternate solutions helps to modify attitudes. In the change stage, the emphasis is on moving to a new level of equilibrium. The actual change or moving requires that new responses be developed based on collected information. Refreezing stabilizes the change. The involved individuals in this stage integrate new concepts into their own value system that are congruent with the individual's existing self-concept and values. Reinforcement of the new behavior is essential to a successful implementation of the change.

To implement a true collaborative process, all parties must approach the change process with an open mind. Hidden agendas and the surface appearance of collaboration while continuing the same processes as before will quickly eliminate any hope of bringing about real change. Goals for the process must be clearly and succinctly identified, and they must make sense to those participating. The rationale for change must be definable and seen by all as an important factor affecting the care of their patients. The rationale for change must be significant enough to influence clinicians to change their practice.

Throughout the change process, the advantages of collaboration must be identified and defined. The need for collaboration is illustrated in the accompanying economic analysis, which deals with cardiac surgery. The practice of cardiac surgery is extensively studied because it has high volume, cost, risk, and customer expectations. Surgeons find themselves evaluated in all aspects of their performance, from the duration of surgery and number of complications to the number of days their patients remain in the hospital. Are these identifiers and qualifiers important in providing care to patients? They are important in identifying excellent performers to both insurance companies and consumers. Physicians and open heart programs that are unable to show average or better statistics will find themselves and their programs eliminated from managed care contracts and fighting for survival. Despite the pressures from managed care and insurers, let us not forget the real reason clinicians are in practice—to care for patients in the best possible manner. Measuring the performance of individual practitioners and programs allows consumers to choose better programs. This ultimately benefits patients.

How can collaboration help? Collaboration, with its process of listening to those who have a role in care, cooperating within this group, and sharing ideas and information, provides an avenue for practitioners to improve the care they provide to patients by incorporating ideas from all involved parties. This process can improve the ultimate product delivered: patient outcomes. Additionally, collaboration offers a means to decrease costs to the provider in a thoughtful and rational manner. Ultimately, the product is an improved patient outcome at a lower cost. The accompanying economic analysis is an example of a collaborative practice model in a hospital setting in which nurses in many different roles collaborated with other health professionals to bring about change that resulted in quality patient care and cost savings.

ECONOMIC ANALYSIS
THE VALUE OF COLLABORATIVE PRACTICE

Akron General Medical Center (AGMC) is a midsized (537-bed) teaching and tertiary referral center. The hospital performs an average of over 700 open heart surgical procedures per year. The medical center is facing many challenges related to managed care, including the demand for increased performance, that is, high-quality outcomes at a lower cost. In searching for ways to meet these continued challenges, Akron General has emphasized collaboration between health-care providers in examining and changing practice patterns. The following case study illustrates a collaborative practice model as well as the quality outcomes and financial savings resulting from collaboration.

In 1993, the administration of AGMC formed an interdisciplinary group to evaluate the performance of the cardiac surgery program. This interdisciplinary group included all cardiac surgeons, the nursing directors of the cardiac surgery unit (CSU) and telemetry unit, and representatives from anesthesia, respiratory therapy, administration, social services, and cardiac rehabilitation. This group was charged with evaluating current practices at AGMC compared with those at hospitals across the country. The interdisciplinary group recommended the following changes:

- Shorter-acting anesthetic agents, allowing earlier weaning and extubation from ventilatory support.
- Less cooling during the surgical procedure, allowing patients to come to the CSU warmer. This decreases the incidence of bleeding and arrhythmias and produces a patient who is more hemodynamically stable and requires lower doses of vasopressors.
- Increased patient activity, beginning after the patients are transferred from the CSU.

To assist in the implementation of these changes in practice, a cardiovascular case manager was hired. These initial changes were moderately successful. By the end of 1994, the anesthesiologists had changed practice and were using shorter-acting drugs for anesthesia. CSU staff nurses were administering smaller but more frequent doses of morphine. These changes allowed patients to be extubated within 8 to 12 hours of surgery, rather than the 12 to 18 hours required previously. Because patients were brought to the CSU warmer, there was a decrease in use of vasopressors and an increase in hemodynamic stability. The nurses in cardiac rehabilitation refined their walking program, which began on the second postoperative day, to increase activity.

During the period from 1995 through 1997, changes in practice continued to be initiated. Examples of these changes included the following:

- End tidal CO_2 monitoring was instituted postoperatively, giving the staff nurse at the bedside a mechanism for evaluating the effect of weaning a patient from ventilatory support without requiring an arterial blood gas (ABG) measurement.
- The extubation protocol included end tidal CO_2 monitoring and pulse oximetry and allowed the nurses in the CSU to perform all the weaning via an established policy and procedure. The duration of intubation decreased from 14.1 hours in 1994 to 10.1 hours in 1996.
- The protocol allowed the staff nurse to use fewer ABGs to wean patients. The number of ABGs from the day of surgery to the first postoperative day decreased from 8 to 4.5, with a savings of $104 per patient.
- The rapid weaning and extubating facilitated earlier ambulation and activity while the patient was still in the CSU.

These changes were difficult to quantify in terms of cost savings. AGMC could determine charges, but not actual costs. Length of stay decreased for coronary arterty bypass graft (CABG) both with and without catheterization. From 1994 through 1996, CABG with catheterization showed a decline of 2.6 days in LOS, a 21 percent reduction. For this same time period, CABG without catheterization showed a decline of 2.5 days in LOS, or a 25 percent reduction. Based on the average cost per patient day on a telemetry floor, this decrease in LOS resulted in a cost savings of $1650 per patient undergoing CABG without catheterization and $1716 per patient undergoing CABG with catheterization.

Prior to 1996, the unit's standing orders specified routine laboratory tests. The nurses and the physicians established new guidelines for the minimum required laboratory tests and discretionary parameters for laboratory testing. These changes in policy regarding laboratory tests resulted in a 13 percent decrease in laboratory testing from 1995 to 1997.

In August 1996, the multidisciplinary group decided to begin a trial of transferring a select group of patients (16 percent in 1996 and 26 percent in 1997) from the CSU to the telemetry floor on the first postoperative day rather than the routine second postoperative day. Cost savings of $619 resulted for every patient transferred on the first postoperative day as opposed to the second day.

In 1998, AGMC participated in a national collaborative process related to open heart surgery. VHA sponsored this collaborative process, which provided the opportunity to network with peers from 16 hospitals throughout the country that perform open heart surgical procedures.

The purpose of the collaboration was to improve outcomes and reduce costs in cardiac surgery.

Each of the participating teams in the collaborative effort consisted of an interdisciplinary group of representatives. The team using a performance improvement model focused on making changes that decreased LOS and cost while improving or having a neutral impact on patient outcomes. For example, one of AGMC's goals was to decrease extubation times such that 80 percent of first-time CABG patients would be extubated within 6 hours after surgery.

The case manager, CSU nursing director, and anesthesiologist met to discuss changes required to facilitate patient readiness for extubation. Factors identified as affecting length of intubation were examined for a typical month. These investigations included tracking all possible sedating medications given preoperatively, intraoperatively, and postoperatively; assessing the patient's respiratory status; and noting the length of surgery, the length of stay in the CSU, and the overall length of stay.

The following areas for change in practice were identified for achieving a shorter duration of intubation:

- Changes in anesthetic agents
- Changes in postoperative medication administration by the nursing staff (smaller doses of narcotic administered more frequently)
- Increased staff comfort with and dependence on end tidal CO_2 and pulse oximetry monitoring in making ventilator changes
- Increased vigilance in treating hypertensive patients as early as the condition was recognized

The goals of the team, including more rapid extubation, were discussed with the staff of the CSU and the anesthesia department. The data from the 1-month chart review were presented to both of these staffs. The day after the anesthesia group discussed the changes in practice for weaning and extubating, all anesthesia staff enacted the changes. This rapid change was a challenge to the nursing staff caring for the patients postoperatively. As individual nurses gained experience and confidence in caring for these rapidly weaned and extubated patients, they shared their experience and knowledge with their peers.

By the end of February, AGMC experienced a 32 percent decrease in the duration of intubation for patients undergoing a first-time CABG, from 8.8 to 6.0 hours. Fifty-six percent of patients were extubated within 6 hours of the completion of their surgery. This collaborative process between the CSU and anesthesia staff continued as the process for weaning and extubation of patients was further refined. By May, 71 percent of first-time CABG patients were extubated within 6 hours and the rapid weaning and extubation process had been expanded to include all open heart patients. The patients ready for transfer on the first postoperative day increased from an average of 26 percent to 45 percent within the first 3 months of the early extubation changes. Recent data indicate that the duration of intubation has stabilized at 4.67 hours for all patients, with 85 percent of all patients extubated within 6 hours of surgery. An average of 50 to 55 percent of all patients are transferred to a telemetry unit on the first postoperative day.

Patient activity has dramatically increased as a result of the changes made in weaning and extubation. All patients dangle and are up to a chair on the day of surgery. During 1997, only 86 percent of patients met this level of activity. Currently, 63 percent of patients ambulate in the hallway of the unit on the day of surgery, as opposed to 36 percent in 1997. Along with the earlier activity, AGMC has seen an increased number of patients transferred on the first postoperative day, and the rate of pneumonia has dropped to an all-time low in this population of patients. As part of this process, the number of ABGs drawn has decreased to three during the day of surgery, resulting in a cost savings of $45 per patient.

Overall costs and LOSs have shown a dramatic decrease since the implementation of the program. To evaluate the cost savings and decrease in LOS, data from June through September for both 1997 and 1998 were compared. For CABG with catheterization there has been a decrease in LOS of 1.6 days. This represents a decrease in cost of 9 percent. Cost savings for these same time periods for CABG without catheterization are currently being estimated. It is expected that the savings will be similar. The collaborative group is continuing to work to improve the care of the patients and examine new opportunities for cost savings. The willingness and commitment of the staff have improved patient care while decreasing costs.

SUMMARY

Health care is constantly changing because of factors such as increased competition in the marketplace, limited health-care resources, and governmental rules and regulations. Payers and consumers are demanding high-quality health care at an affordable price. Nursing roles are evolving, and innovative new roles are being designed. Nurses now focus on prevention, effectively manage the health and illness conditions of their clients, deliver cost-effective care, and emphasize the behavioral aspects of health care.

Because nursing is the focal point in interdisciplinary care, nurses must demonstrate a leadership role. It is nurses who have accepted the responsibility to ensure that each patient is comprehensively assessed and that plans of care are formulated, implemented, and evaluated. This is an exciting adventure and an opportunity for nurses to assume leadership roles in the planning and provision of care in the health-care enterprises of the 21st century.

The Pew Commission (1995) implies that there is a concern that the nation's enormous investment in health care is not producing the level of return expected. The health-care industry now realizes the necessity of doing more high-quality work less expensively and more appropriately. "Using resources more efficiently will require better design, and more efficient and effective leadership and management. In a market-driven system, public accountability will have to extend to the issues of over-utilization and under-utilization" (p. xv).

Professional nurses are in a pivotal position for making a difference in the delivery of patient care. It is imperative that these clinicians and educators work together to prepare nurses who will meet tomorrow's challenges by collaborating with professionals representing the many health-care disciplines in the 21st century. As case examples have demonstrated, collaborative practice works toward improving outcomes while reducing costs.

DISCUSSION QUESTIONS

1. What is the significance of the Pew Health Professions Commission's report concerning the competencies of practitioners in future health-care systems?
2. What are the roles of entrepreneur and intraprenueur nurses?
3. What are the nursing issues related to the use of unlicensed assistive personnel? Describe and analyze the research on UAP practice.
4. What are the essential components of the role of the nursing case manager?
5. What impact does case management as a delivery model have on cost effectiveness for patient care?
6. Give some examples of how nurses provide quality health care at an affordable cost.
7. Why is collaborative practice necessary in the provision of cost-effective health care?

8. What do you envision as nurses' roles in the health-care system of the 21st century?

 REFERENCES

Aiken, L. (1995). Transformation of the nursing workforce. *Nursing Outlook*, 43(5), 201–209.

Baggs, J., & Schmitt, M. (1990). Collaboration between nurses and physicians. *Image: Journal of Nursing Scholarship*, 20(3), 145–149.

Barter, M., McLaughlin, G., & Thomas, S. (1994). Use of unlicensed personnel by hospitals. *Nursing Economics*, 12(2), 822–887.

Bernreuter, M., & Cardona, S. (1997a). Survey and critique of studies related to unlicensed assistive personnel from 1975 to 1997, Part 1. *Journal of Nursing Administration*, 27(6), 24–29.

Bernreuter, M., & Cardona, S. (1997b). Survey and critique of studies related to unlicensed assistive personnel from 1975 to 1997, Part 2. *Journal of Nursing Administration*, 27(7), 49–55.

Bissinger, R. L., Allred, C. A., Arford, P. H., & Bellig, L. L. (1997). A cost-effectiveness analysis of neonatal nurse practitioners. *Nursing Economics*, 15(2), 92–99.

Blegen, M., Goode, C., & Reed, L. (1998). Nurse staffing and patient outcomes. *Nursing Research*, 47(1), 43–50.

Brown, M. (1996). Primary care nurse practitioners: Do not blend the colors in the rainbow of advanced practice nursing [On-line]. *Online Journal of Issues in Nursing*. Available: http://www.nursingworld/ojin/tpc1/tpc1_6.htm.

Coeling, H. (1998). Collaboration in practice. In S. Price, M. Koch, & S. Bassett, *Health care resource management: Present and future challenges* (pp. 185–202). St. Louis: Mosby.

Coeling, H., & Wilcox, J. (1994). Steps to collaboration. *Nursing Administration Quarterly*, 18(4), 44–55.

Cohen, E. (1991). Nursing case management: Does it pay? *Journal of Nursing Administration*, 21(4), 20–25.

Cohen, E., & Cesta, T. (1997). *Nursing case management: From concept to evaluation* (2nd ed.). St. Louis: Mosby.

Drucker, P. (1985). *Innovation and enterpreneurship*. New York: Harper & Row.

Elder, R., & Bullough, B. (1990). Nurse practitioners and clinical nurse specialists: Are the roles merging? *Clinical Nurse Specialist*, 4(2), 78–84.

Hesselgrave, B. (1997). The case for case management. *Medical Utilization Management*, 25(8), 5–8.

Hollander, S., Allen, K., & Mechanic, J. (1992). The intrapreneurial nursing department: Nature and nurture. *Nursing Economics*, 10(1), 5–14.

Huggins, D., & Lehman, K. (1997). Reducing costs through case management. *Nursing Management* 28(12), 34–37.

Kalisch, P., & Kalisch, B. (1995). *The advance of American nursing* (3rd ed.). Philadelphia: JB Lippincott.

Koch, R., & Esmon, D. (1998). Work redesign: Rethinking resource utilization. In S. Price, M. Koch, & S. Bassett, *Health care resource management: Present and future challenges* (pp. 65–74). St. Louis: Mosby.

Lambertsen, E. (1958). *Education for nursing leadership*. Philadelphia: JB Lippincott.

Lengacher, C., Mabe, P. R., Heinemann, D., VanCott, M. L., Swymer, S., & Kent, K. (1996). Effects of the PIPC model on outcome measures of productivity and costs. *Nursing Economics*, 14(4), 205–211, 238.

Lewin, K. (1951). *Field theory in social science: Selected theoretical papers*. New York: Harper & Row.

Manthey, M. (1980). A theoretical framework for primary nursing. *Journal of Nursing Administration*, 10(4), 11–15.

Manuel, P., & Alster, K. (1995). Unlicensed personnel: No cure for the ailing health care system. *Nursing and Health Care*, 15(1), 18–21.

Milstead, J. (1993). Delegation: A critical skill for the orthopaedic nurse. *Orthopedic Nursing*, 12(3), 44–46.

Naylor, M. D., Brooten, D., Jones, R., Lavizzo-Mourey, R., Mezey, M., & Pauly, M. (1999). Comprehensive discharge planning and home follow-up of hospitalized elders: A randomized clinical trial. *Journal of the American Medical Association*, 281(7), 613–620.

Naylor, M. D, Brooten, D., Jones, R., Lavizzo-Mourey, R., & Pauly, M. (1994). Comprehensive discharge planning for the hospitalized elderly: A randomized clinical trial. *Annals of Internal Medicine*, 120(12), 999–1006.

Neidlinger, S., Bostrom, J., Stricker, A., Hild, J., & Zhang, J. (1993). Incorporating nursing assistive personnel into a nursing professional practice model. *Journal of Nursing Administration*, 23(3), 29–37.

Papenhausen, J. L. (1996). Discovery and achieving clinical outcomes. In E. Cohen, *Nurse case management in the 21st century* (pp. 257–268). St. Louis: Mosby.

Papenhausen, J. L. (1995). *The effects of nursing case management on perceived severity of illness, enabling skill, self-help, and life quality in chronically ill older adults.* Unpublished doctoral dissertation, University of Texas, Austin.

Pew Health Professions Commission. (1995). *Critical challenges: Revitalizing the health professions for the twenty-first century.* San Francisco: UCSF Center for the Health Professions.

Rogers, M., Riordan, J., Swindle, D. (1991). Community-based nursing case management pays off. *Nursing Management*, 22(3), 30.

Salmond, S. (1995). Models of care using unlicensed assistive personnel. Part II. Perceived effectiveness. *Orthopedic Nursing*, 14(6), 47–58.

Sherman R. (1990). Team nursing revisited. *Journal of Nursing Administration*, 20(11), 43–46.

Shoffner, D. (1997). Who's behind the mask? UAP unveiled. *Tennessee Nurse*, 60(2), 13.

Simms, L., Price, S., & Ervin, N. (2000). *The professional practice of nursing administration.* Albany, NY: Delmar Publishers.

Tahan, H. (1997). The role of the nurse case manager. In E. Cohen & T. Cesta (Eds.), *Nursing case management: From concept to evaluation* (2nd ed., pp 197–209). St. Louis: Mosby.

 SUGGESTED READING

Cherry, B., & Jacob, S. R. (1999). *Contemporary nursing: Issues, trends, and management.* St. Louis: Mosby.

Fagin, C. (1992). Collaboration between nurses and physicians: No longer a choice. *Academic Medicine*, 67(5), 295–303.

Nunnery, R. K. (1997). *Advancing your career: Concepts of professional nursing.* Philadelphia: FA Davis.

Puertz, B. E., & Kelly Thomas, K. J. (1998). What's your niche? Starting a new venture. In J. A. Dienemann (Ed.), *Nursing administration: Managing patient care* (pp. 225–264). Stamford, CT: Appleton & Lange.

Scott, J. G., Sochalski, J., & Aiken, L. (1999). Review of magnet hospital research: Implications for nursing practice. *Journal of Nursing Administration*, 29(1), 9–19.

Tappen, R. M. (1995). *Nursing leadership and management: Concepts and practice.* Philadelphia: FA Davis.

Chapter 11

Nursing in the Global Environment

Cyril F. Chang
Lillian M. Simms

LEARNING OBJECTIVES

■ Learn about the interconnections between health care and the national and international economic environments.
■ Develop a greater awareness of the global aspects of nursing education and research.
■ Present specific examples of job opportunities in the global environment.
■ Discuss the importance of sharing nursing values around the world.
■ Understand the significance of taking a proactive approach to career choice and professional development.
■ Introduce a set of marketing tools needed to excel in the global environment.

Nurses' jobs, earnings, and even career decisions can be affected directly or indirectly by the events happening outside the clinical world of nursing. For example, the American economy has experienced about 10 years of uninterrupted prosperity. This long period of continued economic expansion has sustained the growth of national health-care spending and boosted the creation of many new types of jobs for professional nurses. Moreover, the U.S. domestic economy has become increasingly interwoven with the rest of the world. How well our economy is doing both affects and is affected by what is happening in the rest of the world.

It is increasingly important for nurses and other health-care workers to be knowledgeable about the complex and sometimes bewildering world of international economics. Changes in the economies of Canada, Europe, Russia, Mexico, countries of the Pacific Rim region, and many other trading partners of the United States affect the American economy. Major global economic factors are shown in Figure 11–1. This chapter explores nursing in the global environment with a focus on the current and emerging economic trends that can affect the nursing profession.

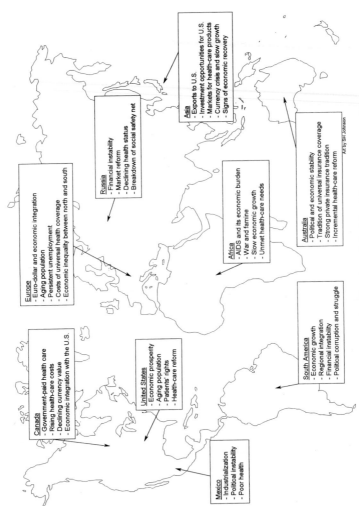

FIG. 11–1. Major international trends affecting global health-care economics.

Canada
- Government-paid health care
- Rising health-care costs
- Declining currency value
- Economic integration with the U.S.

United States
- Economic prosperity
- Aging population
- Patients' rights
- Health-care reform

Mexico
- Industrialization
- Political instability
- Poor health

Europe
- Euro-dollar and economic integration
- Aging population
- Persistent unemployment
- Costs of universal health coverage
- Economic inequality between north and south

Russia
- Financial instability
- Market reform
- Declining health status
- Breakdown of social safety net

Asia
- Exports to U.S.
- Investment opportunities for U.S.
- Markets for health-care products
- Currency crisis and slow growth
- Signs of economic recovery

Africa
- AIDS and its economic burden
- War and famine
- Slow economic growth
- Unmet health-care needs

Australia
- Political and economic stability
- Tradition of universal insurance coverage
- Strong private insurance tradition
- Incremental health-care reform

South America
- Economic growth
- Regional integration
- Financial instability
- Political corruption and struggle

Art by Sri Johnson

THE AMERICAN ECONOMY IN RETROSPECT

Understanding the global economy requires an appreciation of changes in the American economy. Periods of recession and recovery have influenced and will continue to influence health care in the United States.

THE RECESSION IN THE 1970S

In the mid-1970s, the American economy suffered a severe setback. This economic recession was mainly caused by a productivity slowdown in American industries and by a series of oil shocks triggered by the embargo of crude oil to major industrialized countries by the Organization of Petroleum Exporting Countries (OPEC). OPEC is an international cartel organized by major oil-producing countries to coordinate the production and sale of crude oil in the world oil market. A *cartel* is a group of sellers behaving like a monopoly to raise prices and profits. When countries or multinational firms behave like a monopoly, they are called *international cartels*.

A cartel *consists of a group of sellers behaving like a monopoly to raise prices and profits.*

The direct results of OPEC countries' limiting the supply of oil to the rest of the world were rising costs of industrial production and a worldwide recession. This oil-triggered recession of the mid- and late 1970s not only cost many Americans their jobs and income but also severely strained the health-care system. For example, the recession made the already troublesome twin problems of high health-care costs and large numbers of uninsured and underinsured people more difficult to manage.

Recession *is a decline in gross domestic product for at least two consecutive quarters.*

RECOVERY

In 1981, the domestic economy began to bounce back because of the policies of the Federal Reserve System and the Reagan administration. However, during the recovery period of 1982 to 1990, inflation rates remained high by historical standards and the economy suffered from another problem—large and growing federal budget deficits.

Since 1992, however, the American economy has entered a period of un-interrupted true prosperity with mild inflation and low unemployment. The real gross domestic product (GDP) grew at an average rate of 3 percent during this period. Productivity grew at an annual rate of 1.5 percent, and the unemployment rate had declined to 4.5 percent by the end of 1998 (White House, 1999). Inflation, which had troubled the United States for the last 20 years, has slowed to a low annual rate of 3 percent. Three major factors contributed to this longest period of continued economic expansion in recent history:

1. Increased use of cutting-edge technologies in manufacturing
2. Efficiency-raising and cost-cutting measures in management
3. Effective corporate strategies for working with employees and their labor unions

In this environment of rising income and low unemployment, prosperity lessened the urgency of solving our health-care problems and it became easier to deal with health-care issues at the governmental level. Tax revenues have increased because of the prosperous economy, and a budget surplus has stimulated interest in shoring up Social Security and Medicare. However, the influence of costly technologies and the health-care demands of an aging population with chronic illnesses have created an unprecedented burden on the health-care system.

Increased use of resources by an aging population puts a strain on the whole economic system.

The rest of the world also did well in the 1990s. Americans bought more imported goods and services. Likewise, the rest of the world, especially the Asian economies in four key communities (Taiwan, Hong Kong, Singapore, and Korea), bought increasingly larger quantities of American goods.

This rising tide of world trade not only raised living standards abroad but also created jobs and reduced unemployment at home. In the process, the increased globalization has made the United States more dependent on world trade. For example, the total monetary value of exports by American businesses in 1970 was 5.5 percent of the GDP. By 1998, it had grown to 11.3 percent.

THE ASIAN CRISIS

Although the U.S. economy continued to grow in the late 1990s, Asia suddenly slid into a recession, beginning with a pair of currency crises in Thailand and Malaysia. As the financial difficulties spread from one Asian country to another, their economies weakened and they cut back purchases of American goods, including medical supplies and pharmaceuticals. They also stepped up their efforts to export more to the United States by cutting prices. Meanwhile, the Japanese economy continued to be mired in a long period of stagnation. Its manufacturing sector continued to suffer from severe excess capacities, and its banking system from huge sums of insolvent loans.

The economic turmoil in Asia has slowed American exports and affected the earnings of many businesses that rely on selling goods and services throughout the world. The temporary setbacks encountered by these American export-oriented businesses are creating ripple effects throughout the domestic economy. The slowing of business activities in one segment of the national economy will eventually affect jobs and earnings of workers in other industries, including health care.

Countries around the world are becoming increasingly more interdependent. No country is immune to the economic events that happen in other countries.

 ## DEVELOPING A GLOBAL PERSPECTIVE IN NURSING

Nursing education and professional organizations in the United States have traditionally focused on health-care issues affecting people and their communities. In the last 30 years, however, transportation and communication technologies have drastically shortened the distances between people living in different parts of the world. In response, national leaders in the nursing profession have been advocating a greater awareness of the global and cross-cultural perspective of nursing. Nursing leaders emphasize that it is essential for nurses to take a global view in order to thrive as a group in the 21st century.

In her presidential inaugural message to members of the National League for Nursing, Rhetaugh Dumas appealed to all professional nurses who want to succeed in the complex world of the 21st century to see themselves as part of the global society. The challenge ahead, according to Dumas (1998), is to "expand nurses' personal and organizational boundaries to include the ideas of people whose perspectives and experiences are different from ours, and to create (or re-create) meaningful connections to one another and to our institutions and organizations. Otherwise, we will find ourselves 'lost in familiar places'" (p. 104).

Since the days of Florence Nightingale and Lillian Wald, nurses have been active in international activities to some extent (Simms, Price, &

Ervin, 2000). However, the recent national and international economic changes have profoundly affected health care; nurses thus need to increase their international activities in practice, education, and research. Modern-day nurses should understand diverse cultures in the United States and other countries where they may practice. The sharing of nursing values across cultures has gained renewed importance.

Two major organizations can mobilize nursing's influence at the international level (Ohlson & Styles, 1994). The International Council of Nurses (ICN) and the World Health Organization (WHO) play significant roles in health care worldwide and in promoting the global goal of health for all. The ICN is a federation of worldwide nursing associations managed by nurses and financed primarily by nurses. Its members are national nursing associations and individual members who are qualified to participate in ICN activities. The WHO is an organization of many health disciplines; nursing has always had an active role. Members of WHO are affiliated by country. Many opportunities exist for individual health professionals to participate in working assignments in various parts of the world.

Other nursing organizations dedicated to the advancement of international activities are the American Academy of Nursing and Sigma Theta Tau International. Both have active links with ICN, as well as having many independent practice-related activities. Recently, the American Organization of Nurse Executives has developed collaborative partnerships between nurse executives in various countries as part of an ongoing effort to develop an international focus.

TRANSCULTURAL NURSING

Nursing researcher Madeleine Leininger (1991) developed a conceptual framework of nursing based on cultural caring called the Sunrise Model. This model is based on the central idea that caring "is the central, dominant, and unifying focus of nursing" (p. 35). It begins with the premise that nurses learn to understand caring behaviors within a culture from those living in that culture. Cultural caring includes some universal aspects as well as some unique or diverse aspects.

Delivering culturally congruent care requires a cultural perspective that links lay and professional concepts of care. Cultural nursing interventions may be of three types:

1. Preservation or maintenance. Respect for and promotion of lay traditions
2. Accommodation/negotiation. Incorporation of the lay traditions into the plan of care

3. <u>Repatterning or restructuring</u>. Working with a client in respectful ways to find alternative ways of caring

Leininger and others in the transcultural movement have fostered a strong tradition of research and inquiry in transcultural nursing. This approach to nursing has been incorporated in many settings in the United States and across the world, especially in the underdeveloped parts of the world such as the Indian subcontinent, most parts of Africa, and some parts of Central and South America. Transcultural perspectives are used both in caring for patients and in managing a diverse workforce.

Transcultural care *is nursing care delivered with an understanding of different cultures.*

NURSING EDUCATION

The globalization of the world economy is influencing nursing education and practice (Fenton, 1994). There is a tremendous need for students, nurses, and faculty who have multicultural experiences. Many of the foreign nursing students who came to American schools for graduate education have now returned to their countries to provide leadership and to provide contact points for developing exchange systems in education and practice. Regional nursing associations around the world are responding to changes in global markets and the resultant introduction of new products and services and related occupational hazards and concerns. The global economy has also increased the availability of electronic communication; nurses in less developed countries can now access new health information without traveling great distances at high cost.

For many years, American nursing schools, especially graduate programs, have attracted large numbers of nurses from foreign countries. For example, Colling and Liu (1995) reported a 10 percent increase in international students enrolled in American graduate nursing programs from 1985 to 1995. This continued growth in the number of international nursing students studying in the United States is a testimony to the high regard in which American nursing education is held by nurses from the rest of the world.

Tlou (1998) suggests that international partnerships can be advantageous in education and service settings. An *international partnership* is a collaboration in which two or more institutions or departments carry out professional activities aimed at improving and developing knowledge for nursing education. Such a partnership can take the form of teacher and student exchanges, research activities, consultancies, or sabbatical appointments. For a partnership to succeed, both partners must see it as beneficial, and the sharing of information, resources, time, and expertise must be mutual. International partnerships in nursing education are growing as economies are shrinking.

> *International partnership is a collaboration in which two or more educational or health-care institutions carry out professional activities aimed at improving and developing knowledge for nursing education and research.*

Models of international exchange should go beyond student and faculty educational programs: Serious attention needs to be given to clinical exchanges. Nurse executives could facilitate these activities in much the same way as medical fellowships are arranged. For example, it is not uncommon for foreign physicians to be granted fellowships for clinical study and practice in academic health centers. International health conferences and distance learning programs are also bringing health professionals together from all parts of the globe, and the cross-fertilization of ideas is yielding new and unique therapies and partnerships.

NURSING RESEARCH

Ketefian and Redman (1997) reported that of the 110 universities worldwide offering doctoral degrees in nursing, 62 were in the United States and 48 in all other countries combined. These authors also noted the contribution of nursing research to the growing reputation of American nursing education. American nursing scholars and researchers have been active in both basic and applied research. They have published in a large number of reputable nursing journals and built up a worldwide reputation for both the quantity and the substance of their scholarly accomplishments.

Many American nursing researchers and practitioners have also been active in cross-cultural and cross-national collaborations with nursing colleagues in other countries. A good example is a project in which nursing faculty from the State University of New York at Buffalo participated in research in Nordic countries such as Finland and Iceland. These faculty members, according to a recent report by Marjorie A. White (1997), focused on such cross-cultural research topics as child abuse and the dynamics of Nordic families during and after pregnancy. Recently, nurses have found more opportunities for undertaking multinational research. The accompanying economic analysis presents one such example.

⊠ ECONOMIC ANALYSIS
⊠ MULTINATIONAL COLLABORATIVE RESEARCH

With the economic impact of health care affecting all countries, nurse researchers are developing international projects on the quality and costs of health care. Sochalski and colleagues (1998) noted that cost-containment pressures are leading hospitals in Europe and North America to reorganize their services and restructure their care-delivery systems. These reforms have created a target of opportunity for researching nursing-sensitive outcomes.

A collaborative team of nurse researchers from five countries (the United States, Germany, England, Scotland, and Canada) is pioneering such a research agenda. Researchers initially met in Bellagio, Italy, in 1996 to begin forming the international study. The vehicle for this research design is patient-focused care. It is hoped that this study will result in new ways to organize patient care that will improve both quality and efficiency.

NURSING RESPONSE TO GLOBAL CRISES

American nurses have in recent years responded to environmental and health crises in faraway places. According to Possehl (1998), exchange of microbes across global borders requires a universal change in our perspective on health care. For example, cyclospora clusters traveling on fresh fruits and vegetables can be found in California and Washington, DC, far from their original home in Central America. Bubonic plague and cholera have been found in North America, Asia, and Africa, and new strains of influenza and pneumonia are transported daily. In the post–Cold War world of globalization of business and industrial activities, cross-border movements of people, and ethnic violence and border disputes, American nurses have been busy responding to at least three types of global crises: large numbers of refugees, natural disasters, and emerging infectious diseases.

Refugees and Victims of Natural Disasters

Worldwide catastrophic events such as civil wars and ethnic conflicts have forced untold number of people to flee their homes to become refugees or displaced persons (Proctor, 1995). Natural disasters have added to the number of people needing medical and emergency health-care assistance.

True to their core beliefs and professional callings, American nurses have responded magnificently to the needs of displaced people from far-flung areas of the world. They have helped international relief agencies build their capacities to serve the needs of refugees and disaster victims. They have also actively participated directly in the delivery of needed medical and other charitable services.

Emerging Infectious Diseases and Environmental Protection

Many leading public health agencies in the United States, such as the Centers for Disease Control and Prevention (CDC) and the Institute of Medicine, are concerned about numerous infectious diseases that are emerging or resurgent and undergoing redistribution across geographic and national boundaries (Lederberg, Shope, & Oaks, 1992; CDC, 1994). Epstein, Cohen, and Larson (1997) cited several examples of these infectious diseases and their probable causes, including the following:

- A significant increase in schistosomiasis and Rift Valley fever caused by the building of dams in Africa
- The rapid emergence of multiple-drug-resistant strains of microorganisms caused by increasing environmental and clinical use of antibiotics
- The emergence of Argentine hemorrhagic fever associated with changes in the flora (i.e., tall grasses) and fauna (i.e., proliferation of mice and killing off of cats)

Emerging infections diminish labor productivity and absorb scarce health-care resources; as a result, they can drain the economies of many developing countries.

In collaboration with major public health organizations such as the CDC and the Institute of Medicine, the American Academy of Nursing (AAN) has made specific recommendations regarding the control of emerging infections and promotion of environmental balance from the nursing perspective (CDC, 1994). Highlights of these recommendations include the following:

- Support, interpret, and disseminate to the nursing community recommendations made by other leading agencies, focusing on implications for nursing.
- Collaborate with other professions and policy-making groups in mutual support, endorsement, and evaluation of global strategies to prevent or reduce the threat of emerging microbial diseases.

- Communicate with other nursing groups, recommending that they develop and disseminate policies and standards to their own constituencies to prevent the spread of emerging infections.
- Take leadership in major initiatives to focus on preventive strategies.
- Take an active role in promoting the science literacy of students in grades K–12.
- Promote a population-based, epidemiological, system approach for nursing education, practice, and research.
- Serve as a clear voice advocating for support for public education, public health infrastructure, and policies that protect the environment and promote ecological balance.

SHARING NURSING VALUES AND PRACTICES

Knowledge of health statistics in other countries has made U.S. health professionals aware that the United States no longer ranks at the top for common health status data such as infant mortality rates and death rates (Fenton, 1994). It is imperative that nurses work with health professionals in other lands to learn about their health promotion and illness prevention practices.

According to Ketefian and Redman (1997), American nursing education, theory, and practice reflect a set of deep-rooted values that represent the unique characteristics of American people and society. These values can best be summarized in the *Code for Nurses* of the American Nurses Association (1985). The preamble of this document reads, in part:

> When making clinical judgements, nurses base their decisions on consideration of consequences and of universal moral principles, both of which prescribe and justify nursing actions. The most fundamental of these principles is respect for persons. Other principles stemming from this basic principle are autonomy (self-determination), beneficence (doing good), confidentiality (respecting privileged information), fidelity (keeping promises), and justice (treating people fairly). (p. i)

These important professional beliefs have over the years profoundly influenced the core values and the clinical behavior of nurses in the United States. They have also been incorporated explicitly or implicitly in the theories and conceptual frameworks of the research conducted by American nurse scholars. Indeed, in the words of Ketefian and Redman (1997), these value assumptions "permeate the nursing literature" (p. 13). As nursing education, research, and practice become more internationalized and American nursing educational institutions experience rising global dominance, these values will be disseminated broadly across cultures and national boundaries. In keeping with the principles of transcultural nursing, the values and practices of nurses in the United States must be translated to other geographic locations in ways that are consistent with local cultures.

Understanding local culture and sharing values involve building new partnerships within communities in various countries. American nurses can learn much from nurses in other countries about working with health professionals and laypeople with differing levels of preparation. According to Bisch (1998), new partnerships for health are a reality today, no longer a vision for the future. As common health-care needs are identified in different parts of the world, nurses are learning to work with the private sector, industry, universities, and various communities in new ways to accomplish changes in health care. Faculty sharing and student exchange initiatives foster the development of partnerships that can yield productive cross-cultural nursing research. People-to-People International has been instrumental in bringing nurses together in a variety of exchange experiences via nurse-led delegations to various parts of the world.

 ## GLOBAL CHALLENGES FACING NURSING

The globalization of nursing presents a set of challenges and opportunities for which nurses should be prepared. Trade agreements have an impact on the health-care economy and subsequently affect nursing. Understanding marketing and establishing markets for nursing services will become increasingly more important in the 21st century.

THE IMPACT OF GLOBAL TRADE

The American economy by the late 1990s had become more dependent on global trade. The increased significance of world trade was in part enhanced by the economic growth in many parts of the world and in part by the passage of trade agreements such as the General Agreement on Tariffs and Trade (GATT) and the North American Free Trade Agreement (NAFTA). GATT was an important international trade treaty among major world trading partners. Its main purpose was to reduce tariffs and quotas so as to promote world trade. GATT began in 1946 with 23 countries. In 1995, it was replaced by a new international trade body called the World Trade Organization (WTO), with 117 member countries.

NAFTA is a trade agreement between the United States, Canada, and Mexico that took effect on January 1, 1994. The main purpose of this important trade agreement is to promote trade and prosperity in North America by lowering tariffs and reducing trade restrictions among the three countries that signed the treaty. As the volume of trade increased, so did the exchange of workers. For years, many Canadian nurses populated the cities along the U.S.–Canadian border. Recently, the Southwest regions of the United States have seen an influx of nurses with Trade-NAFTA visas from both Canada and Mexico (Stewart, 1998).

Just as a large number of foreign-trained nurses are working in the United States, so have many American nurses found employment and career opportunities abroad. However, the reasons that American nurses work abroad are different from the reasons that foreign nurses work in the United States. With the exception of those who work abroad for personal reasons, most American expatriate nurses do so for research collaborations, data collection, teaching, and refugee and disaster relief.

JOB OPPORTUNITIES ACROSS BORDERS

The higher living standards and stable political environment of the United States have for years attracted talented individuals, including those with nursing competencies and skills, to work here. During times of nursing shortages in the past, American policy makers and health-care institutions encouraged the immigration of large numbers of foreign-trained nurses. Today, it is hard to find a hospital anywhere in the United States that does not employ foreign-trained nurses.

In the 1960s and 1970s, foreign-trained nurses filled the vacancies that remained open because of nursing shortages. They also helped to ease the pressures on wages and benefits. Without them, labor costs in health care would have increased even more. However, during periods of nursing surpluses, foreign-trained nurses compete with American nurses for limited available jobs. Currently, nurses in Canada and New Zealand cannot readily find employment in their own countries and seek to find nursing positions in the United States.

GLOBAL MARKETS FOR NURSING SERVICES

In addition to having a high level of global consciousness, nurses need to acquire a set of practical problem-solving tools in order to excel in the new global health-care environment. It is important for nurses to understand marketing concepts and practices that have been employed successfully by business managers for marketing their products. These business concepts and techniques, when used appropriately, can assist in delivering more efficient health care and furthering nurses' professional careers.

Although marketing is usually seen as a business concept used in the for-profit economy, it can be applied to a wide range of nonprofit and professional settings, including health-care delivery and the activities of health-care professional groups. Marketing is a necessary building block of a successful business plan. When professionally and ethically applied, it can help its users to better serve their customers or clients and accomplish their organizational or group objectives.

Marketing *is a social and managerial process by which individuals and groups obtain what they need and want through creating, offering, and exchanging products of value with others.*

ECONOMIC ANALYSIS
WOMEN'S HEALTH AND MARKETING

As the result of successful marketing, the field of women's health is growing in popularity around the world, providing a unique opportunity for nurse-managed centers and nursing businesses. Successful marketing has occurred by the efforts of the American Nurses Association, the International Council of Nurses, and Sigma Theta Tau International in concert with the World Health Organization and the Institute of Medicine.

MARKETING OPPORTUNITIES

Mireille Kingma (1998) presented good examples on how to incorporate marketing into nursing career choices and professional development. Kingma pointed out a set of international and domestic opportunities that have become available to nurses, including the following:

- *Nurses' careers.* The role of nurses has expanded in a competitive health environment. In addition to the traditional role of caring for patients at the bedside, nurses increasingly perform expanded clinical and managerial roles in both direct patient care and medical decision making.
- *Entrepreneurship.* More and more nurses have decided to be their own bosses by creating their own health-care organizations to deliver services needed by patients or consumers. Home health care is a fertile area for entrepreneurial ventures. Case management services, medical informa-

tion management, and staffing agencies are also good examples. (See Chapters 9 and 10 for more information regarding nursing roles.)

- *Direct reimbursement.* In the long term, having nurses' services reimbursed directly by government health-care programs and private insurance companies is a critical step in the struggle for more professionalism. How to market nurses' services and value to the purchasers of health-care services is a challenge facing the nursing profession.
- *Consumer-driven services.* In the United States as well as many western European countries, nurse-led health promotion and maintenance services such as wellness centers, weight control clinics, and nutrition consultancies are gaining consumer acceptance and recognition by third-party insurers.
- *Partnerships.* Working together as a group is far more effective than working in isolation. Nurses are increasingly forming partnerships among themselves and with other health-care providers to increase productivity through the multidisciplinary team approach. The competencies brought by each discipline are given greater value when they are considered integral parts of the whole.

MARKETING TOOLS

The increased commercialization and sophistication of health-care financing and delivery have heightened the need for nurses to become aware of the business aspects of health care. One such aspect involves the use of the marketing mix concept to inform patients and third-party payers of what nurses have to offer.

Marketing mix is a key building block of modern marketing theory. It is used by businesses and nonprofit entities to pursue marketing objectives in preselected target markets. It is based on four marketing elements called the *four Ps of marketing*: product, price, place, and promotion.

Product is what a firm offers to the market. This is the most basic tool in marketing. The term *product* refers to the many attractive attributes of what is offered by a business firm. These include quality, design, features, branding, and packaging. In the realm of health care, for-profit and nonprofit providers such as hospitals, nursing homes, and pharmaceutical companies offer tangible products to the market. Marketing is a familiar concept to them. Other providers do not offer tangible products; they offer services such as physician services, dental care, and nursing care. To these providers, marketing is a relatively new and foreign concept. As nurses raise their professional standards and broaden their service offerings, the question of how to connect their services to the market and consumers is becoming critically relevant.

Price is the amount of money that customers are asked to pay. This element also includes such business practices as discounting, credit terms, allowances, and other arrangements to facilitate transactions. In health care, prices are more complicated than they are in the regular markets for consumer products. Health-care prices include not only the out-of-pocket payments made by patients and their families but also a complex web of insurance provisions such as copayments and deductibles. Nurses who offer their services or products directly to the market must be aware of the role of price in health care. The concept of *pricing*—the use of price as a strategic tool to promote a product—can help nursing entrepreneurs accomplish their professional and business objectives.

Place, the third tool in the marketing mix, refers to the various things that a firm does to make the product more accessible to the market. Having a good product at a reasonable price is essential but not enough. A successful business must identify the various parties that will help it to bring the product to the market and connect the product to the consumers. It must also promote the product.

Promotion represents the various activities that a firm undertakes to communicate the value of the service or product to the target customers. Promotion is not vulgar business practices or peddling products. When prudently and ethically done, it is a practice of using communications skills to reach out to consumers to explain to them what you have to offer and why your products will meet their needs.

For many years, nurses have worked hard to advance their profession. Much has been done to advance nursing science and effective nursing practices that enhance the quality of health care to individuals and their communities. However, more progress can be made if nurses become more knowledgeable about the various business aspects of health-care financing and delivery. Marketing tools are especially important to those nurses who wish to become entrepreneurs.

Marketing tools can be useful to professional nurses who provide direct patient care or manage the care of many people because these business skills can help them establish a variety of nurse-owned businesses. Simms, Price, and Ervin (2000) provide several examples of businesses established and managed by nurses. These businesses range from home health care, hospice care, nursing consultation, client care coordination, and parish nursing to a telehealth service. All these businesses required excellent marketing skills.

The four Ps of marketing *are four essential elements that constitute a successful business plan for bringing a product to the market: product, price, place, and promotion.*

✺ ECONOMIC ANALYSIS
✺ NURSING BUSINESSES

Nursing businesses can range from an independent practitioner providing services in a clinic or client's home to an international chain of nursing service providers. The oldest forms of nurse-owned businesses are in the community—home health, hospice, private duty, and nurse staffing businesses.

According to the International Labor Organization (1968), marketing involves six major business and managerial activities:

1. <u>Marketing research.</u> Activities concerned with obtaining information on available products or services, prices, consumer needs, gaps, and so forth. It is necessary to collect facts about the market so that decisions can be based on reliable, objective information.
2. <u>Product or service planning</u>. Activities concerned with developing a product or service so that it satisfies the customers and enables the enterprise or individual to use productive capacities or competencies fully.
3. <u>Pricing.</u> Activities concerned with determining the price of the product or service on the basis of costs as well as market factors such as distribution channels, level of prices of competitors' products or services, and the ability or willingness of customers to pay.
4. <u>Advertising.</u> Activities concerned with making the product or service known to the customers and creating demand for it. Advertising brings the customer to the product or service.
5. <u>Sales promotion</u>. Activities covering all aids to sales other than advertising. Sales promotion stimulates demand and increases purchases or contracts for services. Usually sales promotion moves the product or service toward the customer.
6. <u>Distribution.</u> Activities concerned with delivering the product or service to the customer, making it available and easy to purchase.

SUMMARY

Since the days of Florence Nightingale and Lillian Wald, professional nursing has played a leadership role among health professionals in linking clinical practice, education, and research. Both Nightingale and Wald were excellent administrators with exceptional business skills. However, most nurses tend to focus on their traditional role as providers of direct patient care rather than on economics.

A greater awareness of the interconnections between health care and the larger economic environment at both national and international levels is increasingly a prerequisite for competency in the 21st century. To develop this perspective, nurses must envision themselves as members of the global society. Health care in the United States is increasingly influenced by health concerns in other countries, internationally diverse clinical practices and research, and new organizational and management practices.

This chapter advocates a global perspective for nursing that incorporates useful economic and marketing concepts that can be easily transferred to nursing to help individual practitioners and professional groups improve their services and competencies. The use of acceptable business practices both extends professionalism and enhances career opportunities for nurses who are willing and able to adapt to the changing world of health care.

DISCUSSION QUESTIONS

1. Why is it important for nurses to take a global view?
2. Explain the interconnections between health care and the external economic environment.
3. Provide a few examples to illustrate the relationship between your local health-care environment and the events happening in the rest of the world.
4. Explain the American nursing values.
5. What are the four Ps of marketing?
6. Relate the concept of marketing mix to you as a future professional nurse and to the nursing profession as a whole.
7. Sketch your expected career path and discuss your professional aspirations.

 REFERENCES

American Nurses Association. (1985). *Code for nurses with interpretive statements*. Kansas City, MO: Author.

Bisch, S. A. (1998). Sharing in practice: New partnerships for health. *International Nursing Review*, 45(2), 51–54, 60.

Centers for Disease Control and Prevention. (1994). *Addressing emerging infectious disease threats: A prevention strategy for the United States*. Atlanta, GA: Author.

Colling, J. C., & Liu, Y. C. (1995). International nurses' experiences seeking graduate education in the United States. *Journal of Nursing Education*, 34(4), 162–166.

Dumas, R. (1998). President's message: Nursing and health care. *Perspectives*, 19(3), 104.

Epstein, P. R., Cohen, F. L., & Larson, E. (1997). Emerging infectious diseases: Symptoms of global change. *The Proceedings of the American Academy of Nursing 1995 Annual Meeting and Conference: Health Care in Times of Transitions*, Washington, DC. (pp. 67–77).

Fenton, M. V. (1994). Development of models of international exchange to upgrade nursing education. In J. McCloskey & H. K. Grace (Eds.), *Current issues in nursing* (4th ed., pp. 202–211). St. Louis: Mosby.

International Labor Organization. (1968). *Creating a market*. Geneva, Switzerland: Author.

Ketefian, S., & Redman, R. W. (1997). Nursing science in the global community. *Image: Journal of Nursing Scholarship*, 29(1), 11–15.

Kingma, M. (1998). Marketing and nursing in a competitive environment. *International Nursing Review*, 45(2), 45–50.

Lederberg, J., Shope, R. E., & Oaks, S. C. (Eds). (1992). *Emerging infections: Microbial threats to health in the United States*. Washington, DC: Institute of Medicine, National Academy Press.

Leininger, M. (Ed.). (1991). *Culture care diversity and universality: A theory of nursing* (NLN Publication No. 15–2402). New York: National League for Nursing Press.

Ohlson, V. M., & Styles, M. M. (1994). International nursing. In J. McCloskey & H. K. Grace (Eds.), *Current issues in nursing* (4th ed., pp. 407–415). St. Louis: Mosby.

Possehl, S. (1998). The long reach of bugs without borders. *Hospitals and Health Networks*, 72(13), 28–30, 38, 40.

Proctor, C. G. (1995). Identifying and responding to the needs of refugees: A global nursing concern. *Holistic Nursing Practice*, 9(2), 9–17.

Simms, L. M, Price, S. A , & Ervin, N. E. (2000). *The professional practice of nursing administration*. Albany, NY: Delmar Publishers.

Sochalski, J., Aiken, L. H., Rafferty, A. M., Shamian, J., Muller-Mundt, G., Hunt, J., Giovannetti, P., & Clarke, H. (1998). Building multinational research. *Reflections*, 24(3), 20–23.

Stewart, M. (1998). Global trade's impact on nursing. *American Journal of Nursing*, 98(1), 65–68.

Tlou, S. D. (1998). International partnerships in nursing education. *International Nursing Review*, 45(2), 55–57.

White, M. A. (1997). Global nursing collaborations. *Reflections*, 23(2), 22–23.

White House. (1999). *The economic report of the President*. Washington, DC: U.S. Government Printing Office.

SUGGESTED READING

Giordano, B. P. (1996). No passport is required to incorporate cultural appreciation into perioperative nursing practice. AORN Journal, 64(5), 679–680.

Hyde-Price, C. (1997). Global voice now heard. Nursing Standard, 12(10), 26.

Johnstone, M. J. (1998). Advancing nursing ethics: Time to set a new global agenda? International Nursing Review, 45(2), 43.

Lee, J. H. (1997). Making a world of difference: Nurse practitioners—a global perspective. Journal of Pediatric Oncology Nursing, 14(2), 52.

Ryan, D., Markowski, K., Ura, D., & Liu, C. Y. (1998). International nursing education: Challenges and strategies for success. Journal of Professional Nursing, 14(2), 69–77.

Thorne, S. (1997). Global consciousness in nursing: An ethnographic study of nurses with an international perspective. Journal of Nursing Education, 36(9), 437–442.

Part IV

Critical Professional and Economic Issues Facing Nursing

The last section of this book presents a variety of cutting-edge and emerging issues that can potentially affect the future of the nursing profession. These topics include managed care, cost-benefit and cost-effectiveness analysis, information technology, and quality assurance and improvement.

The triple challenge is to maintain high-quality health care that is accessible to health consumers regardless of their ability to pay. Managed care is a major response to the high cost of health care and the fragmentation of the delivery process. All health-care professionals must understand the structures of managed care, its operation, and the dynamics of how major players in the managed care process respond to the ongoing changes. Similarly, nurses' watchful presence is necessary to examine the impact of health-care policies on the availability of and access to health care, especially to traditionally underserved individuals. This vigilance is both noble and necessary as long as a significant proportion of the population continues to be without insurance.

Finally, nursing professionals need to understand key clinical economic concepts. Nurses must have the tools to analyze and evaluate the economic value of the health care they deliver. Cost-benefit and cost-effectiveness analyses are major analytical tools that facilitate decision making. By combining the outcomes and the costs of health-care interventions, these tools provide decision makers with useful information that can be acted on to improve the efficiency of their work.

Information technology encompasses another family of tools that can enhance communication among the major participants of health-care delivery and facilitate the collection, storage, and analysis of value-added data. An important component of information technology in health care is electronic medical records. Issues related to the development, use, and appropriate privacy protection of such records are discussed in this section.

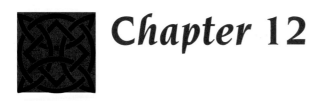

Chapter 12

The Impact of
Managed Care

Cyril F. Chang
Sylvia A. Price
Susan K. Pfoutz

LEARNING OBJECTIVES

- Define managed care and explain its significance.
- Review the history of managed care.
- Explain how managed care works.
- Give examples of managed care models.
- Compare how key developed countries manage their health-care systems.
- Explain how managed care has affected the health-care delivery system.
- Describe the effect of managed care on the hospital, home-care, and public health settings.
- Describe the impact of managed care on nursing.
- Explain the forces that seek to regulate the managed care industry.

WHAT IS MANAGED CARE?

More Americans are currently enrolled in managed care health plans than ever before. According to the National Center for Health Statistics (1998), about 66.8 million Americans (25.2 percent of the population) were enrolled in health maintenance organizations (HMOs) in 1997, an increase of 13 percent from 1996. Among Americans in government-sponsored health programs, 5.2 million were enrolled in a Medicare managed care plan of some form in 1997, and 15.3 million in Medicaid managed care plans (Health Care Financing Administration [HCFA], 1999a).

No single definition can adequately describe managed care because the term includes a complex range of organizational forms that are still evolving. Defined broadly, however, managed care is a health-care system willing to be held accountable both clinically and financially for the health outcomes of an enrolled population for a capitated (fixed) payment based on the covered services and enrollment size (Folland, Goodman, & Stano, 1997).

Managed care *is a health-care system willing to be held accountable both clinically and financially for the health outcomes of an enrolled population for a capitated (fixed) payment.*

Relative to traditional fee-for-service (FFS) health plans, managed care has two distinctive characteristics. First, it integrates the financing and delivery functions of health care into a single organized system. Second, it emphasizes the delivery of a coordinated continuum of services, from wellness care to acute care, with an emphasis on incentives to achieve cost efficiency.

Under traditional FFS reimbursement, insurance companies reimburse hospitals and physicians after the needed services are delivered. Providers earn more if they provide more. Under managed care, in contrast, keeping patients healthy means more profits for the managed care organization. Managers of managed care plans are therefore motivated to emphasize communication and coordination of care among physicians, nurses, and other health-care providers across different delivery settings. The essence of this delivery concept is that specific patient outcomes can be achieved by economizing resource use within a fixed budget.

A brief history of managed care, along with the system's financial implications, is provided in this chapter. Models of managed care are described. The discussion then shifts to the effects and implications of managed care on hospital, home-health, and long-term care. The chapter closes with an analysis of the impact of managed care on nursing.

 ## HISTORY OF MANAGED CARE

The precursor of managed care originated in 1932 when Ray Lyman Wilbur, MD, a former president of the American Medical Association, recommended prepayment to medical group practices that provided health services to groups of individuals such as farmers and teachers. The next two decades saw the establishment of early managed care organizations, some of which are still in operation to this day (Folland, Goodman, & Stano, 1997).

Key historic steps in the development of managed care included the following (Kongstvedt, 1997):

- In 1937, the Kaiser Construction Company sponsored the Kaiser Foundation Health Plans for workers and families who were building an aqueduct in the southern California desert to channel water from the Colorado River to Los Angeles. Similar programs were established later for workers who were constructing the Grand Coulee Dam in Washington State and at Kaiser shipbuilding plants in the San Francisco Bay Area.
- In 1944, the Health Insurance Plan of Greater New York was established as a nonprofit prepaid health plan in New York City to provide coverage for city employees.
- In 1947, 400 Seattle-area families organized the Group Health Cooperative of Puget Sound. It has served the Seattle area as a nonprofit consumer cooperative ever since, and has frequently been cited as a model of managed care organization.

Managed care health plans grew slowly in the early years of their history. A first impetus for growth came in the form of federal assistance authorized by Congress in 1973. That year, Congress passed the Health Maintenance Organization Act to provide federal funding for the expansion of HMOs. However, HMO enrollment did not grow as rapidly as expected in the next few years because the federal government was slow in issuing the necessary regulations. Another factor that impeded the growth of managed care was a host of costly and cumbersome rules and regulations regarding the comprehensiveness of the benefit package and the enrollment of individuals and groups without regard to their health status.

A second major event that stimulated the growth of managed care was the movement of corporate America in the 1980s from traditional FFS insurance to managed care plans for their employees. Employers realized that

no longer an insurer; it only provides management services (e.g., claims processing and case management) for a fee.

The members or *enrollees* of an MCO are the employees or association members who are insured. They receive the health services and, together with their employers or associations, pay for the covered services.

The last group of participants within a managed care system comprises the institutional and individual *health-care providers*, such as hospitals, physicians, and other health-care providers who are organized into a provider network to deliver services to members of an MCO. In many cities, providers are organized and represented by *management service organizations* (MSOs). MSOs are paid to provide contracting and administrative services for provider organizations. They specialize in the management of all business aspects of medical practice for the providers.

The health-care delivery system in the United States is now moving toward a payment system called the *capitation system*, under which MCOs are prospectively paid a per capita amount per month for a specified range of health services for a group of enrolled individuals. These services are either delivered directly by the MCO or through subcontracts between the MCO and independent providers such as hospitals, clinics, doctors, and other health-care practitioners. Capitation shifts the financial risk of providing services from insurance companies to MCOs and providers, forcing them to use health-care resources efficiently and effectively or suffer the financial consequences.

> **Capitation *is a prospective payment system that pays health plans or providers a fixed amount per enrollee per month to provide a defined set of health services based on enrollee needs.***

CAPITATION FEES

Under managed care, providers receive a fixed, prepaid fee, called the *capitation fee*, for each member assigned to their practices. These payments do not vary with the quantity of services consumed, and are paid on a per-member-per-month (PMPM) basis. Because some enrollees cost more than others to care for, capitation fees are usually adjusted by the age and gender of the enrolled population to reflect the cost differences in providing services.

A capitation fee can be calculated by dividing an MCO's projected total costs by the total number of member months (Grimaldi, 1995a). For example, if 3000 members are expected to be enrolled for a total of 12 months at a projected total cost of $4.5 million, the capitation rate would equal $125 per member per month. This is estimated by dividing $4.5 million by 36,000 "member months," which is equal to the number of enrollees multiplied by 12 months.

The MCO then divides its anticipated total costs into several categories, which include overhead and health expenses such as inpatient hospital care, emergency department use, and physician office visits. Each of the services has a projected utilization rate and a cost per unit of service that the MCO expects to pay.

Assume that an MCO expects a utilization rate of 120 days of hospitalization per 1000 enrollees per year, with each day of care costing $1200 on average. The enrolled members average 0.01 days PMPM of inpatient hospital care (120 days per 1000 enrollees divided by 12 months). The expected PMPM cost of inpatient hospital care would be $12 (0.01 × $1200). This calculation implies that the MCO can expect to pay $12 per member per month for inpatient care from the $125 capitation revenue. The PMPM costs of other services can be similarly estimated.

An MCO's overhead costs are fixed expenditures and are distributed over the total member months. The greater the amount of overhead costs, the greater the need for the MCO to sustain its market share in order to be financially viable. If enrollment decreases, the fixed cost per enrollee would increase, which would decrease the competitiveness of the MCO. The fixed payments imposed by the capitation system and the need to capture a sufficiently large patient base expose managed care plans to substantial financial risk. Grimaldi (1995b) stated: "Financial risk compels managed care organizations to track health costs and utilization closely, and systematically compare budgeted with actual performance" (p. 12). Inaccurate information may be costly because it results in avoidable losses and low quality of care. It may also impair an MCO's ability to remedy cost problems and calculate future capitation fees.

ECONOMIC ANALYSIS
CAPITATION VERSUS FEE-FOR-SERVICE REIMBURSEMENT

A patient who went in for cardiac bypass surgery in 1985 would have stayed about 13 days in the hospital. The hospital would have charged fees for the operating room, laboratory tests, X rays, pharmacy, and bed. Insurers would have paid for these expenses. In 1999, the patient would have stayed about 5 days and the hospital would be paid based on the diagnosis and not the actual medical expenses incurred, because the third-party payer has shifted from a cost-based reimbursement system to a prospective payment system.

MODELS OF MANAGED CARE

Managed care organizations can be for profit or nonprofit. They may be owned by for-profit insurance companies or nonprofit companies such as Blue Cross and Blue Shield Associations, physician groups, hospitals, or national health management firms. They can be organized in a variety of ways and are customarily classified into three major types: health maintenance organizations, preferred provider organizations, and point-of-service plans. (See Table 12–1 for a summary of major differences among these types of managed care.)

HEALTH MAINTENANCE ORGANIZATIONS

A health maintenance organization is a managed health plan that either administers health care or arranges for health care to be provided to its members for a capitated monthly fee (Fox, 1996). The philosophy of an HMO is to emphasize preventive health services that can avert costly treatments later, such as routine physical examinations, prenatal care, and proactive management of chronic conditions. In the United States, the number of people enrolled in HMOs increased from 33 million in 1990 to 66.8 million in 1997 (see Figure 12–2).

A health maintenance organization *is a managed care plan that orchestrates health services provided to its members for a fixed, prepaid fee. The plan usually shares financial risk with its providers.*

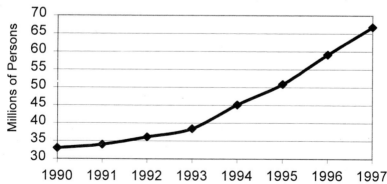

FIG. 12–2. Number of Americans enrolled in HMOs. (From National Center for Health Statistics. [1998]. *Health, United States, 1998.* **Hyattsville, MD: Public Health Service, Table 135.)**

TABLE 12–1. TYPES OF MANAGED CARE ORGANIZATIONS

Characteristics	Health Maintenance Organization (HMO)	Preferred Provider Organization (PPO)	Point-of-Service Plan (POS)
Definition	Managed care plan that provides, administers, or arranges for care to its members	Network of health-care providers, hospitals, and facilities that provides care to employee groups	Managed care plan that combines HMO features with choice at the point of specialty referral
Payment arrangement	Capitation: Pays providers a contracted fee per member per month	Negotiated fee for service	Capitation for within-plan providers and fee for service for out-of-plan referrals; consumers pay larger deductibles for out-of-plan services
Relationship with providers	Staff model pays providers a salary and owns facilities; group, IPA, and network models contract with one or more groups of providers and facilities	Plans contract with providers or provider groups as well as health-care facilities for discounted fee schedules	Combination of primary care HMO features with contract features of fee-for-service plans
Focus	Prevention and outpatient care		Flexibility in provider choice
Cost control	Discounted fee for service	Lowest fee Discounted fee through negotiation backed up by purchasing power	Lower costs for using services within plan; higher deductibles to prevent unnecessary out-of-plan utilization
Incentives	Keep enrollees well so as to prevent costly services	Providers can use volume to make up money lost in discounted fees	Keep enrollees satisfied with flexibility of choosing providers
Financial risk	Shares risk with providers	Health plan bears risk for covered services	Shares risk with providers and consumers
Choice of providers	Must choose within-plan care	Patients must use health-care providers within plan	Incentive to choose provider in the plan, although out-of-plan care is available

The relationship that an HMO maintains with its providers is paramount for its success. This is because the health services provided to patients must be procured from hospitals, physicians, nurse practitioners, and other health-care practitioners who participate in the plan. Without providers' co-operation, HMO enrollees will not receive cost-effective health services. It is therefore critical to develop a thorough understanding of the different ways that HMOs maintain relationships with their providers.

Depending on the financial arrangement and organizational relationships with providers, HMOs can be organized in a number of ways. The major HMO models are the staff model, the group model, the independent practice association (IPA) model, and the network model.

Staff Model

The staff model type of HMO employs its own physicians, advanced practice nurses, and ambulatory care nurses, who are salaried. These providers deliver health services only to plan members and usually practice at clinics owned and operated by the HMO. A major advantage of this model is that it exercises tight control over the providers' practice, thereby making it easier for the HMO to monitor utilization and costs. However, a major drawback is that the physicians in a staff model, who earn a fixed income and work a fixed number of hours to satisfy mandated encounter times, may provide patients with less attention than physicians working elsewhere.

Group Model

An HMO using the group model contracts exclusively with a group of physicians and, separately, with hospitals to provide services to its enrollees. The HMO usually pays the group practice a PMPM capitation fee for the provision of physician services. The major difference between a staff model and a group model is that in the staff model physicians are paid directly by the HMO, whereas in a group model physicians are paid by the physician group. Physicians in a group model can maintain greater autonomy and encounter less direct pressure from the HMO to cut costs than in a staff model because of this payment arrangement.

Independent Practice Association Model

The IPA, the fastest-growing HMO model, enters into a contractual relationship with solo or group practitioners to provide physician and nurse practitioner services to enrollees. In general, the IPA receives a PMPM capitation fee through a primary capitation arrangement with the health plan purchaser and reimburses IPA physicians through a subcapitation or a discounted fee-for-service subcontract. A *subcapitation* is a secondary capitation arrangement between the IPA and a group of physicians. This payment arrangement shifts the financial responsibilities of providing services for all or part of the enrollees of an HMO to the contracted physicians or physician group. A *discounted fee for service* is a payment arrangement whereby the physicians are still paid according to the services delivered, hence the term *fee for service*, but the fees are negotiated at a discount for assurance of a steady flow of patients from an HMO.

The major differences between the IPA model and the staff model are that the IPA provides an expanded choice of providers to enrollees and that physicians in an IPA can still see private paying patients. In a staff model, in contrast, enrollees do not have as much choice of providers because they must go to specific clinics staffed by the HMO physicians and may be seen by different physicians at each visit. Likewise, a staff physician can only see HMO enrollees.

Network Model

In this model, the HMO contracts with more than one physician group practice to provide services. Some HMOs contract with many small primary care practices (e.g., family practice, internal medicine, and pediatrics) under a subcapitation agreement. These physician groups can make referrals to specialists but are themselves financially responsible for reimbursing these referrals. Some network model HMOs contract with broad-based multispecialty groups that can provide a wide range of services from primary care to highly specialized services. The network model allows referrals to a wider range of physicians than either the staff model or group model described previously.

PREFERRED PROVIDER ORGANIZATIONS

A PPO comprises networks of hospitals, private practice physicians, and other health-care practitioners that provide comprehensive health services to employers and their employees for a negotiated fee. There are over 1000 PPOs in the United States. They serve over 20 percent of the insured population and account for half the total enrollment in managed care plans (Fox, 1996).

A preferred provider organization *is a health plan that contracts with a network of hospitals and physicians to provide health care to employers and their employees for a negotiated fee.*

A variety of entities, including insurance companies, professional organizations, hospitals, and physician groups, may sponsor PPOs. It is also common for a PPO to be jointly sponsored by a hospital and physicians. Unlike HMOs, PPOs do not assume the financial risk of arranging and providing health services; the sponsoring organizations do. PPOs also do not perform many of the functions customarily assumed by HMOs, such as utilization review, quality assurance, and insurance underwriting. They can be viewed as networks of physicians who agree to accept a discounted fee for service in exchange for a steady flow of patients.

Participating providers in a PPO usually are reimbursed at a rate about 15 to 20 percent lower than the local prevailing reimbursement rates. In return for lower fees, enrollees in a PPO agree to use health-care providers and facilities with whom the PPO has established a contractual relationship. PPOs can reduce costs by creating a network of health-care providers who provide services for prenegotiated fees.

POINT-OF-SERVICE PLANS

A point-of-service plan combines classic HMO characteristics such as capitation and coordination of service delivery with the PPO characteristic of enrollee choice of providers. Patients in a POS plan are required to select a primary care provider who manages and coordinates their health-care needs. Patients may choose a nonparticipating, out-of-plan provider at the point of receiving service, but they must receive a referral from the primary care provider who, in addition to providing primary care, serves as a gatekeeper. Enrollees must also pay a higher deductible or copayment, or both, for this privilege because these out-of-plan providers are usually paid on a fee-for-service rate. The POS plan appeals to enrollees who prefer the option of choosing providers outside the plan and are willing to pay extra for it.

A point-of-service plan *is a form of* **HMO** *in which participants must choose a primary care provider from a list of participating providers, who serves as a gatekeeper for referring specialty care. However, the consumer may choose a specialist who is not in the plan by paying a higher deductible or copayment, or both.*

✦ ECONOMIC ANALYSIS
✦ CHOOSING A HEALTH-CARE PLAN

A woman in her early 40s who works at an automotive plant must choose a health insurance plan during the open enrollment period offered by her company. A new union contract has just been approved, which offers three options for family coverage:

1. A traditional fee-for-service plan provides excellent illness care and choice of health-care providers. Participants do not need referral for specialty care. There is less preventive care provided, and all services require deductibles and copayments. There is a $10 copayment charge for all prescription drugs.
2. The health maintenance organization has specified providers for primary and specialty care. This plan provides excellent preventive care with a $5 fee per visit. Participants must have a referral for all specialty care and can only select providers from within the plan. There is a $5 deductible for prescription drugs, and providers must choose drugs from an approved list.
3. The point-of-service plan requires choice of a participating primary health-care provider as gatekeeper. If a referral is approved, the member may choose an in-plan physician at a $5 copayment or another physician at a 30 percent copayment. Prescription drugs are provided with a $5 copayment for approved medications, or a 30 percent copayment for out-of-plan medications.

This woman is a mother with three children aged 6 through 14. She carries the health insurance for the family because her husband is self-employed. As she prepares to make her choice, she identifies the following concerns and priorities for her family:

- Preventive services for the family are a priority, including well-child care, immunizations, regular women's health examinations (including mammography), and routine men's health care (including prostate screening).
- All family members are currently healthy.
- Both husband and wife are approaching the age when chronic illness is more prevalent. She has a family history of breast cancer. Both she and her husband work in jobs with environmental hazards. They both smoke one to two packs of cigarettes per day.

- She values choice in health-care providers. It is important for her to establish a relationship with a health-care provider who she can trust to coordinate each family member's care.
- Family members are not currently taking any prescription drugs.

This middle-aged woman's parents, both in their late 60s, are facing the same decision. Her father is retired from the same automobile plant. He must choose from the same three plans for his policy to augment Medicare. The older couple have the following concerns and priorities:

- Both parents have worsening chronic illnesses. Father has emphysema from smoking and exposure to occupational inhalants. He also has a history of myocardial infarction. Mother has osteoarthritis in the knees and hips. She is currently mobile but is approaching the time for joint replacement surgery.
- Both value the care provided by the specialists at a nearby academic medical center.
- Preventive services are important, but less than illness care.
- Both parents take prescription drugs, and they worry about future increases in those costs.

This extended family must match the needs of individual family members with the features of the three insurance options to make a choice that best serves the family members. This example illustrates the range of health plan choices and the health concerns and economic factors that affect consumer choice.

PAYMENT MECHANISMS AND FINANCIAL RISK

Methods of paying health-care providers have evolved to encourage everyone involved in the delivery of health services to become cost conscious. In its own way, each payment method provides incentives or imposes financial risk to affect the choices and decisions of both patients and their providers.

Financial risk in the delivery of health care is the likelihood of unforeseen monetary loss by a health plan because of lack of revenue, excess costs, or both in delivering obligated services. The traditional FFS payment mechanism places all the risk on the payer of health care. In other words, the insurer bears the burden of cost overruns. Newer payment methods, such as managed care and capitation, seek to share the financial risk with others who are involved in health care. Although there are many variations of payment systems, the basic three are described in the following sections.

Financial risk in the delivery of health care is the likelihood of unforeseen monetary loss by a health plan because of lack of revenue, excess costs, or both in delivering obligated services.

FEE-FOR-SERVICE PAYMENT

With a fee-for-service payment system, the provider is paid for each service rendered. Because income from medical practice increases as more services are delivered, providers have an incentive to provide more services, including some that might be inappropriate. This is the well-known problem of "moral hazard" in health care (Pauly, 1986). Under FFS payment, the financial risk is borne by the health plan that pays providers for all covered services.

A health plan under FFS may try to limit the amount paid for each service. An upper limit on reimbursement or a reasonable cost for each covered service may be established. These restrictions lower the payment for each service, but providers can make up for lost revenues by delivering a greater amount of services. Thus the health plan still bears the financial risk for covered services.

PPOs represent a variant of FFS payment. Under this fee arrangement, the health plan contracts with individual providers or provider groups for a discounted payment for each service. Enrollees are then required to select from a list of preferred providers who have agreed to accept the negotiated fees. This arrangement limits the amount of payment for each service, but does not eliminate the health plan's financial risk because providers can increase volume to maintain the same level of income. Many health plans thus resort to monitoring mechanisms such as peer review or utilization review to ensure the delivery of appropriate services.

PROSPECTIVE PAYMENT

Instead of reimbursing providers for each service delivered, health plans can pay a fixed amount that is predetermined for each procedure or episode of illness. In other words, the fee schedules are set ahead of time and providers adjust to them. Providers pocket the savings if they can deliver services at a cost below the predetermined rate. If the cost exceeds the payment rate, on the other hand, providers bear the loss. Under a prospective payment system (PPS), the incentive is to provide less care so as to keep costs within the reimbursement rate.

A good example of this system is the Diagnosis Related Groups (DRGs) system introduced by Medicare in 1983 to pay hospitals for inpatient services. Health plans shift part of the financial risk to hospitals by paying them a fixed amount based on the primary diagnosis of the admission. Because hospitals can only earn the specified amount for each episode of care, the incentive is to become cost conscious.

An undesirable aspect of DRGs is that providers may underprovide services because payments are fixed and predetermined. Inadequate services, such as premature discharge from the hospital, can result in inferior care and unacceptable outcomes. A quality assurance mechanism needs to be in place to monitor the appropriateness of care under PPS. Other shortcomings of DRGs include such provider practices as compensating for decreased earnings per episode of care by increasing the number of episodes of care or choosing a diagnosis that is reimbursed at a higher level. These abusive and inappropriate actions must also be closely watched and prevented.

CAPITATION PAYMENT

Capitation payment involves a fixed monthly payment called a capitation fee that is received by a health plan or provider for each enrollee. In exchange for this payment, the capitated party is then responsible for delivering a predetermined package of services to satisfy the health-care needs of the prepaid enrollees. Some health plans require their contracted providers to share the financial risk for maintaining the enrollees' health outcomes under a subcapitation contract. The expectation is that providers will develop a preventive focus and provide services in the most cost-effective manner. Providers under a capitated system have the incentive to provide fewer or smaller amounts of services because their income does not increase with the volume of care provided. There is some concern that this incentive might cause providers to withhold necessary care or not offer expensive treatments.

COST SHARING

All three methods of payment may include patient cost sharing using deductibles, copayments, or both. *Deductibles* are the costs of health-care services that the patient must pay before the health plan begins its share. *Copayments* are the amount of money, either a fixed dollar amount or a percentage of the cost, that must be paid by the consumer of health care.

The purpose of these out-of-pocket payments is to make consumers more cost conscious.

Cost sharing by consumers may be an access barrier for individuals with limited income because they may forgo needed services for financial reasons. Ongoing evaluation is necessary to examine the intended and unintended consequences of systems of payment that involve cost sharing and other financial incentives.

 ## MANAGED CARE IN THE PUBLIC SECTOR

The discussion of managed care so far has emphasized the pressures on private managed care plans to reduce costs and to remain competitive in attracting health insurance business. Although the public health-care system has the same pressures and concerns, it has unique characteristics and challenges that raise questions as to whether the principles of managed care are compatible with the goals of public programs that provide health care to elderly and poor people. At present, managed care organizations are gaining rapid inroads into the Medicare and Medicaid markets. The experiences of managed care in the public sector are of great interest to public officials, policy analysts, and nursing leaders alike.

MEDICARE

Medicare, the public system for health care for elderly people and for people with disabilities, is a critical political issue because the population is aging and the cost of health care to elderly people is rising rapidly. These health-care trends, in the words of health economist Victor Fuchs (1999), can "plunge the nation into a severe economic and social crisis within two decades" (p. 11).

Medicare began in 1965 as a traditional FFS program. Over the years, the Health Care Financing Agency (HCFA), the federal agency that administers Medicare, has tried to reduce costs and maintain quality with a variety of reform measures. In early 1983, for example, reimbursement for hospital services shifted to a prospective payment system using DRGs to pay hospitals for treating Medicare patients. Under this system, hospitals receive a set fee related to the primary diagnosis for hospitalization (see Chapter 4). There were some initial successes in slowing down the growth of Medicare inpatient costs. Over time, however, the costs of inpatient care to elderly people continued to rise (Zarabozo & LeMasurier, 1996).

Since its inception, Medicare has allowed HMOs to provide services to beneficiaries as private contractors. However, the complicated rules and regulations set by HCFA discouraged many managed care plans from partic-ipating. The regulations that became effective in 1995 under the Tax Equity and Fiscal Responsibility Act of 1992 made it easier and more attractive for HMOs to contract with HCFA. As a result, managed care enrollment of Medicare recipients rose rapidly, from 441,000 participants in 1985 to 5.2 million in 1997 (HCFA, 1998a).

> *Medicare-approved* **HMOs** *receive a monthly federal payment for each enrolled* **Medicare** *recipient. This payment varies from county to county depending on the local medical cost level.*

HCFA pays Medicare HMOs a monthly fee per enrollee based on the fol-lowing factors: age, sex, proportion of Medicaid-eligible subscribers, per-centage of subscribers residing in a health-care institution, percentage sub-scribing to a Medicare Part B (physician services) program, and the percentage of subscribers working and having other insurance. Together, these factors create many payment categories. The HMO establishes the fees owed it by estimating the number of subscribers in each payment cate-gory and calculating the average payment rate per person.

According to HCFA regulations, a participating HMO plan must meet the following requirements (Zarabozo & LeMasurier, 1996):

- Must contain a minimum of 5000 prepaid members in each organization (or 1500 in a rural plan)
- May not contain more than 50 percent of members eligible for Medicare and Medicaid (may be waived in poor areas)
- Must be able to provide or arrange for all Medicare services
- Must provide all Medicare A and B services available in the area
- Must have a 30-day open enrollment every year
- Must market the plan throughout the service area using HCFA-approved marketing materials
- Must be able to bear potential financial risk while the physician's risk is limited to 25 percent
- Must have sufficient administrative capacity to implement terms of the contract
- Must have quality assurance programs
- Must have records available for inspection
- Must ensure confidentiality of medical records

Is Medicare managed care working well? In terms of consumer choice, the situation has improved because more and more HMOs are entering the Medicare market to compete for subscribers. Between 1990 and 1997, for example, the number of Medicare HMOs more than tripled (HCFA, 1998a).

Statistics also show that 67 percent of Medicare beneficiaries resided in an area in which there was at least one HMO available; 58 percent of beneficiaries resided in an area with two or more HMO plans. The incentives for Medicare recipients to enroll in an HMO include low out-of-pocket costs and some additional services (e.g., vision care and preventive services) provided free or for a low copayment. HMO enrollees have been reported to be happier with their out-of-pocket costs than beneficiaries in traditional fee-for-service Medicare plans (HCFA, 1998a). In terms of perceived quality of care and ease of getting care, results are similar for FFS beneficiaries and HMO enrollees.

Medicare managed care is not without problems. For example, HMO enrollees express higher dissatisfaction with specialist care, provider concern for health, and the ability to get care by telephone (HCFA, 1998a). Another problem that might fundamentally affect the future of Medicare managed care is that there might not be a sufficient number of HMOs willing to participate in Medicare. HMOs participate in Medicare to retain enrollees in their plans after they become eligible for Medicare. However, as regulations tighten and reimbursement levels lag behind with inflation, HMOs may be reluctant to continue their participation.

Medicare remains a difficult political issue. Former HCFA administrator Bruce Vladek describes the positive impact of Medicare on increased access to health services for elderly people who previously could not afford them (Vladek, 1999). These services have contributed to increased quality of life, greater life expectancy, and decreased poverty. This transfer of resources to the aged and less fortunate remains in political dispute.

Many factors contribute to the rising costs of Medicare, and a variety of solutions are under consideration. Technology is viewed as a major source of cost increases both in the number of services provided and the cost per procedure (Fuchs, 1999). The financial impact of technological innovations, though modest at the beginning, grows as they spread through the health-care system. Although many innovations contribute to longer and higher-quality life for the persons benefiting from them, the question remains as to who shall pay for the costs. Either senior citizens must assume a higher proportion of the costs of their health care or taxpayers who work to support the Medicare program must pay more into the system.

Fuchs (1999) suggests that there are only three potential solutions to Medicare's financial dilemma:

1. Slow the growth of prices.
2. Produce more with the same or fewer resources by raising the level of efficiency in health-care delivery.
3. Slow the growth of services to clients.

A direct way to slow the prices of health care is to reduce reimbursements to providers. Fuchs (1999) argues that reimbursement cutbacks have been made and already achieved the biggest gains in reducing costs of which they are capable. Efforts to improve efficiency and eliminate waste and fraud should continue, but they cannot be counted on to solve all Medicare's problems. The major remaining way to limit the growth of costs is to limit the expansion of services, which most certainly will affect the care provided to Medicare beneficiaries. Because Medicare pays approximately one-half of health expenses incurred by elderly people, solutions must include measures to limit increases in health-care spending and improve the income of senior citizens so that they can pay a greater share of the cost (Fuchs, 1999).

MEDICAID

Medicaid is a program in which the states and the federal government partner to provide health services for the poor. Approximately 70 percent of Medicaid recipients are women and children (HCFA, 1999b). The remainder are elderly people or people with disabilities who are eligible for Medicare but cannot afford to pay premiums and deductibles.

Women and children on Medicaid have special problems accessing care because they frequently have intermittent eligibility and other barriers to receiving care (Hurley, Kirschner, & Bone, 1996). Another group of Medicaid recipients that has drawn public attention is low-income elderly and disabled beneficiaries who have dual eligibility for both Medicare and Medicaid. Medicaid pays the Medicare premiums, deductibles, and copayments for this group of disadvantaged persons. They represent about 29 percent of the total Medicaid population but account for approximately 73 percent of the services and expenses in 1996 (HCFA, 1998b). How to help the older and disabled poor without overburdening the system is a challenge that awaits a solution.

Medicaid has seen larger increases in managed care enrollment than Medicare has. Managed care options have been available to recipients from the inception of Medicaid, but both the insurance industry and Medicaid recipients showed limited interest in managed care for the first 15 years of Medicaid's history.

Three factors working together stimulated the growth of Medicaid managed care in the early 1980s. First, eligibility rule changes made the Medicaid population grow rapidly, putting an extra burden on the system. Second, total program outlays rose much faster than projected, making Medicaid the single largest social service program in many states. Third, managed care was perceived as an opportunity to limit expenditures just as it had in the private insurance market.

In 1981, the U.S. Congress passed legislation to encourage Medicaid to experiment with innovative ways of financing and delivering services (Hurley, Kirschner, & Bone, 1996). In 1982, Arizona became the first state to develop a statewide system using mandatory prepaid health plans to provide health care for the poor. Many states soon joined the reform movement to use managed care to expand services to the uninsured while controlling costs. The objectives of these state-initiated Medicaid reforms included the following (Hurley, Kirschner, & Bone, 1996):

- Competitive bidding for capitated contracts
- A primary care physician network for gatekeeping
- Copayments to decrease inappropriate service use
- Limited choice of providers after selection of the plan

Since the policy changes in the early 1980s, there have been dramatic increases in Medicaid managed care enrollment. In 1997, about 15.3 million people, or 48 percent of the total Medicaid population, were enrolled in Medicaid managed care (HCFA, 1999b). A wide range of Medicaid managed care plans and options have been implemented across the country with varying results (HCFA, 1999b).

Some plans were voluntary: Beneficiaries could choose to join managed care or stay in a fee-for-service system. Other plans were mandatory. Some states chose to consolidate all publicly funded programs for the poor and uninsured into a comprehensive managed care plan, whereas others opted to carve out certain specialty programs such as dental care and mental health and substance abuse services. Managed care *carve-outs* are subcontract arrangements that outsource or contract out certain specialized services to separate contractors who specialize in these services.

The effectiveness of these managed care programs is not clear because states evaluate their own programs and have not fully developed their evaluation procedures. They also tend to report positive outcomes and downplay unsatisfactory results for political reasons. Many states have reported decreased emergency department and hospital use—two main attractions of managed care. Others have reported improved consumer satisfaction. HCFA is closely monitoring the progress of the states that are experimenting with Medicaid managed care reform (HCFA, 1999b).

The future of Medicare and Medicaid remains a contentious topic for public debate and legislative actions. The major questions are who will receive services, what services will be provided, and how the services will be paid for. At the close of the 20th century, the United States was experiencing budget surpluses that allowed more options to be considered. However, national consensus on how best to serve older and vulnerable Americans remains elusive.

 ## INTERNATIONAL COMPARISONS OF MANAGED CARE

Like the United States, many developed countries are struggling with high health-care costs and confusion over whether market forces or government regulations can do a better job containing costs. Many of the countries have had years of experience with managed care of one form or another. A cross-country survey of health-care systems with a focus on health-care costs, health insurance coverage, and national health outcomes provides pertinent information for an international comparison of managed care.

Useful indicators for comparing health systems are the level of health spending, the percentage of population with health insurance coverage, and the health status of the general population. The Organization for Economic Cooperation and Development (OECD) collects and publishes both economic and health-care data for 29 developed countries around the world. It has recently reported that the United States has the highest level of health-care spending per capita as well as the highest percentage of the GDP spent on health care (Organization of Economic Cooperation and Development, 1998). Since 1960, the United States has increased the proportion of citizens with government health coverage from 6.9 percent to 33.3 percent of the population. However, most of the 29 OECD countries have universal health coverage.

The effectiveness of a health-care system can be evaluated by using economic factors such as the percentage of people with insurance coverage, national health-care spending per capita and as a percentage of gross domestic product, and the health status of the general population.

Another way to evaluate a country's health-care delivery is the health status of the population. Health-care utilization and distribution alone do not determine the health status of a population. Many other factors also affect health, such as the environment, heredity, and health behaviors. However, a comparison of health status among countries and across time can provide revealing information about the effectiveness of a country's health system.

The infant mortality and life expectancy rates are two basic health status indicators that are readily available. The median OECD infant mortality rate for 1996 was 5.8 infant deaths in the first year of life per 1000 live births. The

U.S. infant mortality rate for the same year was 7.8 (Anderson & Poullier, 1999). Life expectancy at birth for both males and females in the United States remains below the OECD median.

Life expectancy rates can be translated into "years of life lost," which measures the number of years a person died before the age of 70 that could have been prevented. The OECD median for 1995 was 3265 years of life lost per 100,000 life years for females, and 6281 years of life lost for males. The U.S. rate was estimated at 4591 years of life lost for females and 6281 for men (Anderson & Poullier, 1999). Taken together, these health outcomes do not suggest a high level of population health in the United States, notwithstanding the large amounts of health-care expenditures.

CANADA

Canada has maintained a publicly financed health-care system since 1957. A universal hospitalization scheme with first-dollar coverage (coverage with no deductible or copayment) was introduced first. Medical insurance for physician services was added in 1968. By 1971, all 10 Canadian provinces and 2 northern territories were participating fully in the combined medical and hospital insurance program based on five cornerstone conditions (Naylor, 1999, p. 11):

1. Universal coverage of all provincial residents on uniform terms and conditions
2. Public nonprofit administration
3. Portability of benefits among provinces
4. Comprehensive coverage of all necessary services provided by medical practitioners and hospitals
5. Maintenance of reasonable access to insured services, "unprecluded or unimpeded, either directly or indirect, by charges or other means"

The Canadian system has provided all residents necessary hospital, medical, and long-term care with no copayments for more than 40 years. Canadians have freedom of choice regarding physicians, who are private practitioners and not employees of the government or local health authorities. Prescription drug coverage is available to all, but requires cost sharing. The Canadian system is usually referred to as a *single-payer system* because there is no parallel private system in Canada: The government is the sole source of all payments for health care.

Over the years, large budget deficits have forced the federal government to reduce contributions to the 12 provincial and territorial health plans that compose the Canadian health-care system. The federal government has also limited fee increases for physician services and prevented additional charges for services beyond the health system reimbursement. Most physicians continue to be paid on the basis of a fee-for-service contract negotiated in each province between the provincial health authority and the medical association.

In recent years, better economic conditions have turned the chronic federal budgetary deficit into surplus. The federal and provincial governments as a result have engaged in active public posturing and private negotiations about the proper sharing of the costs between the federal and provincial governments. Another emerging issue is whether to expand the scope of services, such as offering better drug benefits and greater access to home care and other community-based services.

Still another issue facing Canadians is the question of whether integrated delivery systems (IDSs) can be adopted in the Canadian system. Shortell, Gillies, and Anderson (1994) define an IDS as "a network of organizations that provides or arranges to provide a coordinated continuum of services to a defined population and is willing to be held clinically and fiscally accountable for the outcomes and health status of the population served" (p. 47). The main advantages of an IDS are greater efficiency and better health outcomes. The coordinated delivery system combines acute care, long-term care, and community-based care under the management of a single health-care authority.

Health-care providers in Canada are still paid on a fee-for-service basis. How to integrate the various components of a health-care system within a largely fee-for-service scheme that resists integration remains largely unresolved. Yet Canadians support the single-payer system and are ambivalent about developing a separate system for those able to pay more. Incremental changes that promote integration, reform in primary care, a broadened scope of services, and continued improvement of quality are the current focus of the Canadian health system.

UNITED KINGDOM

The British National Health Service has existed since 1948, bringing together hospital, physician, and community health services under a national health-care system financed by general tax revenues. Over the years, this system has been hailed as a model of universal insurance coverage that yields outcomes comparable with those of other developed countries.

Because of fiscal pressures and complaints of long waiting lines and overcrowding in hospitals, England introduced quasi-market reforms under Prime Minister Thatcher of the Conservative Party in the 1980s. The goal was to gradually replace centralized control with market-based competition.

Taxation continues to fund the British National Health System. However, health-care providers have become more independent and now compete with other providers for service contracts with institutional health-care purchasers. These purchasers are either the district health authority or general practice fundholders, which are larger practice groups that are similar in many ways to American HMOs. Patients can choose physicians but can only change health authorities by moving.

To date, the limited evaluation data that exist seem to suggest that very little overall change has occurred in the British health-care system. For example, it was initially feared that providers might practice "cream skimming" by recruiting only healthy consumers to reduce the costs of care. However, there is no evidence that this has occurred. It was also expected that increased competition would expand consumer choice of providers. But there was little evidence to support this outcome either. The national government's control of the system is suspected of thwarting change and creativity.

The Labor government began to discontinue market reform in 1997. The reform introduced by the Labor government was described as a "third way" that was neither laissez faire nor central control. It created new organizational structures but at the same time retained some of the market reform provisions of the previous Conservative government.

The Labor reform has created two new national entities to address quality issues. The National Institute for Clinical Effectiveness sets quality standards, and the Council for Health Improvement enforces the standards (LeGrand, 1999). Dobson (1999) cites remaining challenges such as continuing inequalities, excessive waiting times, and geographic variations in quality. It is too early to tell whether the Labor government's reform will succeed.

JAPAN

Japan has a history of universal health coverage that achieves excellent health outcomes at a low cost. Citizens are free to select health-care providers, and providers have the flexibility to accept patients from a variety of health plans, which number over 5000. These independent health insurance plans fall into three major categories (Ikegami & Campbell, 1999):

1. Large-firm employees and their dependents are covered by Society-Managed Health Insurance; public-sector employees are covered by Mutual Aid Associations.
2. Small-firm employees are covered by Government-Managed Health Insurance in a single national pool operated by the Ministry of Health and Welfare.

3. Self-employed persons and pensioners are covered by Citizens' Health Insurance.

The three major health plans provide comparable benefits that include all approved medical and surgical procedures, pharmaceuticals, long-term care, dental care, and some preventive care. The federal government subsidizes the premiums for the poor. Funds for the elderly population are pooled from a combination of public and private sources. In short, the Japanese system of health-care financing is a hybrid of social insurance and voluntary contribution that thrives on the principle of public-sector and private-sector cooperation (Ikegami & Campbell, 1999).

The reasons for Japan's low health-care costs include lower rates of social problems associated with ill health (e.g., drug abuse), positive health habits and good nutrition, more equal income structure that limits poverty, and a health-care structure that promotes primary care with less invasive interventions. Price controls have effectively prevented aggressive growth in health-care spending. Medical fees have actually been reduced in recent years on services that were being used too heavily. Japan, in sum, remains committed to the principle of public and private cooperation in the financing and delivery of health care, with a heavy reliance on government for setting national standards and controlling costs.

This system continued with only minor changes for many years until new pressures in the 1990s forced Japan to reexamine its health system. New challenges include the growth of consumer consciousness, including ethical concerns; an aging population; and rapidly rising costs.

Rising costs have been a specific concern during the recession of the 1990s. Reform measures currently being debated include the following:

- Increasing patients' share of the costs
- Developing a separate plan for the elderly population
- Implementing a prospective payment system for hospital care similar to the DRG system in the United States
- Setting fees for prescription drugs that do not allow excessive provider profit

These proposals are predicted either to be difficult to implement or to have limited effect on costs and coverage. Most Japanese believe that their health-care system's problems are the result of the ongoing recession and will be relieved when the country overcomes its economic difficulties.

SUMMARY: INTERNATIONAL COMPARISON

Among all developed countries, the United States is the only one with no universal health coverage. The countries discussed here share common concerns over rising costs of health care, aging populations, and maintenance of quality of care. They have all recently modified their health-care systems to remain congruent with the values and priorities of the individual societies.

The United States leads in the adoption of market-oriented reform measures and remains firmly committed to the market approach to reform. But health outcomes in the United States are mediocre at best, and Americans have much to learn from other countries that have done better with less. Japan, in contrast, is the least committed to market reform and the most inclined to rely on the government to solve its health-care problems. It also has the best health outcomes, although its health care is not nearly as technologically advanced and expensive as that of the United States. No country seems to have found the "magic medicine," and no single model seems to be able to meet the needs of all countries, which differ vastly in cultural and ethnic backgrounds and economic conditions.

 ## THE EFFECT OF MANAGED CARE ON HEALTH-CARE SETTINGS

HOSPITALS

Available data from the National Center for Health Statistics show that managed care growth has significantly affected hospitals across the country. The shift from inpatient care to less expensive outpatient care has resulted in decreased inpatient admissions and a shorter average length of stay. Hospital profit margins are falling, and many hospitals are merging to find strength in size and market share.

Changes in hospital reimbursements have resulted in a trend of increased outpatient care and shorter hospital stays.

These changes have given rise to public and private efforts to restructure the organization and process of hospital care delivery to lower costs while maintaining quality. For example, redesign has resulted in slower growth of nursing positions in acute care settings (Buerhaus & Staiger, 1999). Meanwhile, new positions in a wide range of growing fields such as case management, information systems, and home health care have been created and made available to nurses with the proper training, credentials, and eagerness to learn and take risks (see Chapters 9 and 10).

HOME HEALTH CARE

Home-care agencies provide skilled professional care to patients in the home setting. Services include skilled nursing, home health aides, nutrition counseling, physical therapy, occupational therapy, speech therapy, and social work. With more Americans joining managed care, more patients are being discharged earlier from inpatient settings. Early discharge has increased the demand for home-care services.

The Balanced Budget Act of 1997 included several provisions that affect the delivery of home-care services. Home-care services were shifted from Medicare Part A, which covers hospital services, to Part B, which covers physician and ambulatory care services. Because Medicare Part B is optional and requires payment of a premium, this change could limit access to home-care services (National Association for Home Care, 1999).

Other provisions of the Balanced Budget Act established new reimbursement mechanisms. An interim payment system, which began on October 1, 1997, will be replaced by a prospective payment system in 2000. The interim system froze payments below allowable costs. This limitation has already resulted in the closing of at least 700 home-health agencies in 1998, leaving some communities without access to home-care services (National Association for Home Care, 1999).

ECONOMIC ANALYSIS
SURVIVAL STRATEGIES FOR HOME-HEALTH AGENCIES

Managed care practices are providing incentives for home-health agencies to develop cost-containment plans. Limitation of reimbursement has forced agencies to provide services at a lower cost or go out of business. Examples of ways that agencies are responding to this challenge include the following:

- Working within integrated systems to provide programs for patients who are discharged early
- Forming specialized services for patients who have received transplants or other high-technology care
- Developing mental health services in the home
- Developing preventive services
- Managing costs aggressively for each service component, such as travel, supplies, and employee processes

PUBLIC HEALTH

The line separating managed care and public health is getting increasingly blurred. Traditionally, public health agencies have been the primary organizations that promote community health through disease prevention, health assessment, and health-care delivery to the uninsured and underserved. The Institute of Medicine (1988) defines the mission of public health as "fulfilling society's interest in assuring conditions in which people can be healthy" (p. 7). The core functions of public health, according to the Institute of Medicine, are assessment, policy development, and assurance of access to adequate health care.

Managed care organizations pursue similar objectives of promoting healthful behaviors and utilization of preventive services. Under strong pressures from capitation and other financial restrictions, these managed health-care entities strive to improve the health of insured populations to avoid costly treatments as a consequence of ill health. They have relied on population-based data on health status and risk behaviors to help them prepare for the health-care needs of their enrollees. They have lately made impressive inroads into the public-sector insurance markets, taking responsibilities for the care of the aged, people with disabilities, and low-income children and adults. Because managed care organizations are increasingly engaged in many of the same functions as public health organizations, the question arises as to whether the two types of entities are on a collision course or whether they can cooperate and coexist in the increasingly more competitive health-care market.

At the state and local levels, health departments are in the process of refining missions and strategies. Public health agencies have sought new revenue sources to continue their services to the public. Many local health departments are negotiating managed care contracts to provide services that private managed care organizations have chosen not to provide. Some health departments have even begun to compete with private managed care organizations for the same services.

For health-care professionals on either the public health side or the managed care side of the health-care market, changes bring both threats and opportunities. For example, changes in funding mechanisms and mission present potential philosophical conflicts for public health professionals who sometimes wonder whether the needs of the entire community will continue to be met. Competition from the private sector poses a direct threat to the very existence of many local health agencies and the jobs of their employees.

Although the threats are real in public health, opportunities also exist. For example, public health workers, especially public health nurses, can use their skills in negotiation and organization to develop service contracts as private contractors for public health services. Examples of public health services that could be negotiated include school health, well-child services, lead screenings and follow-up, and senior services.

Opportunities also exist for developing partnerships or alliances with other public and private health-care agencies to develop joint ventures. An example is the development and maintenance of population-based health information systems. These data systems are expensive to set up and maintain. It is also inefficient to maintain separate systems for the public and private sectors. This is an excellent area of common interest in which the two sectors can join hands in developing a collaborative relationship for the benefit of the entire community.

These mutually beneficial relationships can be forged in a variety of ways, ranging from loosely formed alliances based on informal understandings to formal contractual agreements that spell out in detail the legal rights and obligations of all parties involved. Across the country, public health officials and private managed care managers are actively pursuing these opportunities (Halverson, Kaluzny, & McLaughlin, 1998).

Public health has unique concerns. Its missions and objectives may not always be congruent with those of managed care (Novic, Woltring, & Fox, 1997). However, under today's health-care climate of scarce resources and rising costs, the goal of achieving "health for all at an affordable cost" cannot be accomplished without cooperation between public health and private managed care.

 ## IMPACT OF MANAGED CARE ON NURSING

Managed care systems have wide-reaching effects on how and where health care is delivered. The growth of managed care and the emerging market-driven health-care system has radically changed the American health-care landscape, with resources increasingly being shifted from inpatient care to outpatient and community-based settings. Nursing must respond to the threats and opportunities that accompany these changes. Hospital administrators realize that they must compete not only on the basis of cost but also on quality. Cost cutting alone will not succeed in today's marketplace. As hospitals learn how to keep costs down and quality up, they will remain a major source of employment for nurses (see Chapter 9).

The demand for nurses in the outpatient and primary care settings, such as ambulatory surgical centers, primary care clinics, and public health facilities, will continue to rise. This shift of demand will be evident especially in nursing homes, home-health-care agencies, and a host of new managed care entities. Managed care, with its emphasis on cost effectiveness, may slow the growth of demand for nurses in the high-cost inpatient settings;

however, the demand for nurses in primary care, ambulatory centers, and long-term care settings will experience strong growth. If the strong growth in the expanding outpatient care settings more than offsets the slower growth in the inpatient care setting, compensation and employment levels for nurses will likely remain favorable. Concern over how nurses are coping with the unprecedented changes has led nursing leaders and major organizations to commission a number of major surveys.

As the location of patient care shifts away from the inpatient setting, opportunities and roles for nurses in outpatient settings will expand.

 ## ECONOMIC ANALYSIS
CHANGING ROLES FOR NURSES

A registered nurse (RN) who worked 8 years in critical care at a local community hospital recognized a shift in the ratio of nurses to patients in her unit from one RN to one patient to one RN to two patients. She liked to take care of one patient at a time, was confident in her clinical skills, and was looking for growth opportunities. She applied for a home-care position in the same hospital because the home-care department was expanding, although she had no home-care experience. She was accepted because of her strong acute care skills and enthusiastic attitude. The hospital provided continuing education for her to pursue this new role.

AMERICAN NURSES ASSOCIATION SURVEY

The American Nurses Association (ANA) commissioned a survey of registered nurses to measure the impact of managed care on professional nursing. This national sample of more than 7000 RNs included staff nurses, managers from all organizational levels, educators, clinical nurse specialists, nurse practitioners, and others who represent the broad spectrum of the nursing profession. Although 78 percent of respondents were hospital nurses, other settings were also represented (Shindul-Rothchild, Berry, & Long-Middleton, 1996).

There were geographic variations in the responses across the country, but many similar themes emerged from the survey results. Initial findings included reports of staffing reductions, increases in workload, and low morale, as well as a significant proportion (13 percent) of nurses who did not intend to remain within the profession. Another major finding was that 40 percent of the respondents claimed that they would not recommend the health-care facility where they worked to a family member or friend. Health care in those facilities was rated as excellent (9.9 percent), good (37.4 percent), average (38.8 percent), poor (12.2 percent), or very poor (1.7 percent) (Shindul-Rothchild, Berry, & Long-Middleton, 1996).

A follow-up analysis was conducted to identify factors that differentiated between facilities rated as poor or very poor and good or excellent (Shindul-Rothchild, Berry, & Long-Middleton, 1997). All 1016 respondents who earlier reported that their facility provided poor or very poor care were included in this analysis, along with a random sample from nurses who rated their facility as good or excellent. Ten factors—those relating to the structure, process, and outcomes of nursing care delivered in the facilities where the surveyed nurses worked—emerged as differentiating good facilities from poor ones. With each factor, a negative response was significantly associated with the facility being reported as poor or very poor. Many of the negative quality-related outcomes are those included in the American Nurses Association Report Card of Outcomes. The following are the 10 major factors that can cause quality to deteriorate at a facility (Shindul-Rothchild, Berry, & Long-Middleton, 1997):

Structure
1. Reduction of RN staff
2. Loss of the nursing executive without replacement

Process
3. Time to provide basic nursing care
4. Maintenance of professional standards

Outcomes
5. Patient or family complaints
6. Skin integrity
7. Patient injuries
8. Medication errors
9. Complications related to the admitting diagnosis
10. Likelihood of respondent to remain in nursing

ADVANCED PRACTICE NURSING SURVEY

Harrison (1999) conducted a survey to focus on the opinions of managed care held by clinical nurse specialists (CNSs) and nurse practitioners (NPs). The concern was that the ANA survey samples consisted primarily of staff nurses. Perhaps the threats and opportunities perceived by advanced prac-

TABLE 12–2. THREATS AND OPPORTUNITIES FOR NURSING IN MANAGED CARE

Threats Achieving 50% Group Agreement	Percent Agreement
Not alone, but managed care has contributed to:	
1. Increased paper chasing, hoop jumping	84.2
2. Tenuous job market for nurses, especially in inpatient settings	77.2
3. Encroachment on nursing practice by other disciplines, employers, and managed care personnel	77.2
4. Productivity demands limiting assessment activities	76.8
5. Workload demands allow professional collaboration	75.4
6. Rollbacks of gains in compensation, conditions, control	73.2
7. Diminished quality of care because of business focus	71.9
8. Band-Aid approach to complex needs	68.5
9. Limited ability of nurses to practice independently because they are restricted in managed care networks	68.4
10. Tension and friction between physicians and NPs/CNSs for control	63.1
11. Experienced nurses feeling useless without more training	61.4
12. Reduced self-esteem, exodus from profession	57.9
13. NPs/CNSs practicing more by the medical model	56.2
14. Erosion of confidentiality between client and nurse	52.6
15. Erosion of collective bargaining effectiveness	51.8

Opportunities Achieving 50% Group Agreement	Percent Agreement
Not alone, but managed care has contributed to:	
1. Exploration of new approaches to quality and cost-effective care	63.2
2. Expansion of nurse practitioner role in primary care setting	61.4
3. Professional nurses more effectively partnering with clients for health responsibility	56.1
4. Extension of NP role to emergency, urgent, acute care, and long-term care settings	54.4
5. Separation of the critical from not-so-critical thinkers in nursing, with prosperity for nurses who adapt	53.5
6. More focus on multidisciplinary clinical research outcomes	51.9
7. More involvement in health promotion and disease prevention	50.9
8. More practice opportunities in community outreach, primary care, ambulatory care, and home care	50.9
9. Professional nurses advocating for patients when potential for harm exists	50.8

Source: Harrison, J. K. (1999). Influence of managed care on professional nursing practice. *Image, 31*(2), 161–166.
CNS = clinical nurse specialist; NP = nurse practitioner.

tice nurses (APNs) would differ. A sample of 57 CNSs and NPs was recruited from California, a state with a high concentration of managed care. A three-round Delphi survey was used to determine the opinions of the participating subjects. Subjects initially responded to a question of how managed care affected professional nursing. Subsequent rounds provided the opportunity for subjects to agree or disagree with the proposed statements based on the responses from previous rounds of questioning.

For the second round of this Delphi survey, 36 statements were proposed to the subjects, including 16 opportunities and 20 threats. The criterion for deletion of a statement was that 50 percent of the sample must disagree or strongly disagree with the statement. No statements were deleted because none met that criterion. For a statement to be considered to demonstrate group agreement, 50 percent or more of the sample had to either agree or strongly agree with it. Group agreement was reached on statements regarding 9 opportunities and 15 threats (see Table 12–2).

The APNs surveyed saw opportunities in managed care for partnering with and advocating for clients, as well as expanding their practice in new directions and settings. The themes related to threats concerned decreased quality of client care and diminished professional identity and security. Client care was seen as threatened by productivity demands, insurance requirements, decreased time for thorough assessment, and decreased time to use assessment data. Professional identity and security were thought to be threatened by the declining number of positions in hospital settings, encroachment on the profession, limited opportunities for independent practice, and a more medical model of advanced practice nursing. Clinical nurse specialists rated the following threats at a higher level than nurse practitioners: decreased quality of care related to business focus, and the paperwork and hurdles required to achieve authorization for care or address denials. Nurse practitioners rated the opportunity of partnering with clients for health responsibility at a higher level than clinical nurse specialists.

SUMMARY

Managed care is one of the most significant developments in the recent history of American health care. The country's health-care system is currently being transformed by the concept of managed care, which relies on financial incentives and consumer choice to deliver quality services at a reasonable cost. It is likely to be the predominant model for health-care delivery and financing in the 21st century.

Most health-care experts now assume that the growth of managed care and a heightened level of competition will continue, easing the pressure on health-care costs. But the demographic trend of an aging population combined with emerging technological developments may offset the effects of managed care and competition. The net result is likely to be a slower growth of health-care prices and expenditures rather than an actual decline.

In this competitive environment, health-care organizations wishing to succeed will find that they have no choice but to continue to redesign and restructure their models of care delivery to meet the demand for high-quality, cost-effective health care. Nurses who work in this ever-changing environment, either for an employer or as owners of their businesses, face both an unpredictable future and many exciting opportunities. The ability to adapt, learn, and see opportunities in so-called threats is essential to nurses' personal satisfaction and professional success.

DISCUSSION QUESTIONS

1. Explain how managed care works and compare it with the traditional fee-for-service insurance plan.
2. Describe the roles of the major participants in managed care.
3. Explain the significance of the legislation regarding health maintenance organizations to the concept of managed care.
4. Why do nurses and other health-care practitioners need to be knowledgeable about the capitation mechanism for managed care organizations?
5. Differentiate among the managed care models in health maintenance organizations.
6. Discuss the major impact of managed care on Medicaid.
7. Discuss the major impact of managed care on Medicare.
8. What is the effect of managed care on the hospital, home-health-care, and public health settings?
9. Cite examples regarding how managed care has affected nursing.
10. How has managed care changed the health-care delivery system in the United States?

 REFERENCES

Anderson, G. F., & Poullier, J. P. (1999). Health spending, access, and outcomes: Trends in industrialized countries. *Health Affairs*, 18(3), 178–190.

Buerhaus, P. I., & Staiger, D. O. (1999). Trouble in the nurse labor market? Recent trends and future outlook. *Health Affairs*, 18(1), 214–222.

Cowan, C. A., Braden, B. R., McDonnell, P. A., & Sivarajan, L. (1996). Business, households, and government health spending, 1994. *Health Care Financial Review*, 17(4), 157–158.

Dobson, F. (1999). Modernizing Britain's National Health Service. *Health Affairs*, 18(3), 40–41.

Folland, S., Goodman, A. C., & Stano, M. (1997). *The economics of health and health care* (2nd ed.). Upper Saddle River, NJ: Prentice Hall.

Fox, P. D. (1996). An overview of managed care. In P. R. Kongsvedt (Ed.), *The managed health care handbook* (2nd ed., pp. 3–15). Gaithersburg, MD: Aspen Publishers.

Fuchs, V. R. (1999). Health care for the elderly: How much? Who will pay for it? *Health Affairs*, 18(1), 11–21.

Grimaldi, P. (1995a). Capitation savvy a must. *Nursing Management*, 26(2), 33–34.

Grimaldi, P. (1995b). Capitation's information imperative. *Nursing Management*, 26(4), 12–13.

Halverson, P. K., Kaluzny, A. D., & McLaughlin C. P. (1998). *Managed care and public health*. Gaithersburg, MD: Aspen Publishers.

Harrison, J. K. (1999). Influence of managed care on professional nursing practice. *Image: Journal of Nursing Scholarship*, 31(2), 161–166.

Health Care Financing Administration. (1998a). *The 1998 Medicare chart book*. Baltimore, MD: Author.

Health Care Financing Administration. (1998b). Medicaid vendor payments by eligibility group: FYs 1975–96. *Health Care Financing Review, Medicare and Medicaid Statistical Supplement*, 152–153.

Health Care Financing Administration (1999a). *Medicare and managed care*. Baltimore, MD: Author. Available: http://www.hcfa.gov/medicare/mgdcar.htm.

Health Care Financing Administration. (1999b). *National summary of state Medicaid managed care programs*. Baltimore, MD: Author. Available: http://www.hcfa.gov /medicaid/omc1998.htm.

Hurley, R. E., Kirschner, L., & Bone, T. W. (1996). Medicaid managed care. In P. R. Kongsvedt (Ed.), *The managed health care handbook* (2nd ed., pp. 761–778). Gaithersburg, MD: Aspen Publishers.

Ikegami, N., & Campbell, J. C. (1999). Health care reform in Japan: The virtues of muddling through. *Health Affairs*, 18(3), 56–75.

Institute of Medicine. (1988). *The future of public health*. Washington, DC: National Academy Press.

Knight, W. (1998). *Managed care*. Gaithersburg, MD: Aspen Publishers.

Kongstvedt, P. R. (Ed.). (1997). *Essentials of managed health care*. Gaithersburg, MD: Aspen Publishers.

LeGrand, J. (1999). Competition, cooperation, or control? Tales from the British National Health Service. *Health Affairs*, 18(3), 27–39.

National Association for Home Care. (1999). *Basic statistics about home care, 1999*. Washington, DC: Author. Available: http://www.nahc.org.consumer/hcstats.html.

National Center for Health Statistics. (1997). *Employer-sponsored health insurance*. Hyattsville, MD: Author.

National Center for Health Statistics. (1998). *Health, United States, 1998*. Hyattsville, MD: U.S. Public Health Service.

Naylor, C. D. (1999). Health care in Canada: Incrementalism under fiscal duress. *Health Affairs*, 18(3), 9–26.

Novic, L. F., Woltring, C. S., & Fox, D. M. (1997). *Public health leaders tell their stories*. Gaithersburg, MD: Aspen Publishers.

Organization for Economic Cooperation and Development. (1998). OECD *health data 98: A comparative analysis of twenty-nine countries*. Paris: Author.

Pauly, M. V. (1986). Taxation, health insurance, and market failure. *Journal of Economic Literature*, 24(2), 629–675.

Shindul-Rothchild, J., Berry, D., & Long-Middleton, E. (1996). Where have all the nurses gone? *American Journal of Nursing*, 96(11), 24–39.

Shindul-Rothchild, J., Berry, D., & Long-Middleton, E. (1997). 10 keys to quality care. *American Journal of Nursing*, 97(11), 35–43.

Shortell, S. M., Gillies, R. R., & Anderson, D. A. (1994). The new world of managed care: Creating organized delivery systems. *Health Affairs*, 13(5), 46–64.

Vladek, B. C. (1999). The political economy of Medicare. *Health Affairs*, 18(1), 22–36.

Zarabozo, C., & LeMasurier, J. D. (1996). Medicare and managed care. In P. R. Kongsvedt (Ed.), *The managed health care handbook* (2nd ed., pp. 715–740). Gaithersburg, MD: Aspen Publishers.

 ## SUGGESTED READING

Bonner, C., & Boyd, B. (1997). Managed care: Threat or opportunity for home health. *Online Journal of Issues in Nursing*. Available:
http://www.nursingworld.org/ojin/tpc2/tpc2_5.htm.

Buerhaus, P. I., & Staiger, D. O. (1996). Managed care and the nurse workforce. *Journal of the American Medical Association*, 276(18), 1487–1493.

Huntington, J. A. (1997) Glossary for managed care [On-line]. *Online Journal of Issues in Nursing*. Available: http://www.nursingworld.org/ojin/tpc2/tpc2_5.htm.

Shortell, S. M. (1996). *Remaking health care in America: Building organized delivery systems.* San Francisco: Jossey-Bass.

Turner, S. O. (1999). *The nurse's guide to managed care.* Gaithersburg, MD: Aspen Publishers.

Chapter 13

Access to Health Care

Cyril F. Chang

LEARNING OBJECTIVES

- ■ Explain the concept and importance of access to health care.
- ■ Illustrate the use of access objectives for national health promotion and disease prevention.
- ■ Review current statistics on access to health care.
- ■ Review the financial and nonfinancial barriers to health-care access.
- ■ Understand the racial, ethnic, and socioeconomic differences among Americans in access to health care.
- ■ Discuss access strategies and their relevance to nursing.

 ## THE SIGNIFICANCE OF ACCESS

Access to health care can be defined as the timely use of personal health services to achieve the best possible health outcomes (Millman, 1993). It is a critical goal of public health that has significant implications for both the American system of health-care delivery and the nursing profession.

Health-care access is the timely use of needed, affordable, convenient, acceptable, and effective personal health services.

Access is one of the key determinants of health status, along with environmental, lifestyle, and hereditary factors (Blum, 1974; Millman, 1993). Without access to adequate and high-quality health care, according to the World health Organization, the goal of health for all cannot be attained (WHO, 1978).

Access is frequently used as a performance measure in public health to gauge progress in health promotion and disease prevention. Health-care delivery in the United State is now moving to an outcome-based system that emphasizes, among other things, accountability for the health-care dollars spent (Kongstvedt, 1996; Sultz & Young, 1999). A reliable and well-designed mechanism to measure access to needed health services by the general population and its subgroups is essential for holding the health-care system accountable (Gold, 1998).

The U.S. health-care system is currently undergoing drastic and rapid changes. Both the government and the private sector are stepping up efforts to control excessive growth in health-care prices and expenditures. These important and sometimes painful measures raise the level of economic efficiency and eliminate waste in the health-care delivery system. However, the cost-cutting efforts have long-term effects on access that have not been carefully monitored and evaluated.

Nurses have a major responsibility for improving access. They have played a critical role and have been active in efforts to increase access at the local, regional, national, and international levels (Kalisch & Kalisch, 1982; Stevens, 1992). By calling attention to access issues through service, research, and active engagement in public debates, nurses can significantly influence public policies that affect the health of the general population.

In addition to its relevance to public health, acess to health care is also an economic problem. For most of the 40 million uninsured Americans (Swartz, 1997), unemployment or working at low-paying jobs that provide no or inadequate health insurance coverage is a major barrier to access to needed health care (Acs, 1995; Smith, 1997). Yet access is not a problem solely of the poor and uninsurable. Those who have the financial resources to acquire insurance coverage can have access problems too. Many people cannot get the type of care they need at a convenient time or place.

This chapter presents a systematic discussion of the issues and challenges involving access to health care. A major goal is to describe, explain, and analyze the various indicators of access and the conceptual differences in defining access. Another goal is to identify barriers to access and discuss ongoing public health efforts for improving access, especially those proposed for helping racial minority groups and other underserved population subgroups. A third goal is to explain the responsibility of nursing in improving access to health care for the American people and to identify available opportunities for nurses to participate in this important public health effort.

 ## THE CONCEPTUAL FRAMEWORK OF ACCESS

Over the years, the U.S. health-care system has experienced substantial changes in characteristics. The relatively simple, low-cost system of health care of the 1950s and 1960s has been forever replaced by a resource-intensive, high-tech, and high-cost system that routinely performs procedures that would be regarded as "miracles" by the standards of the earlier and simpler days. In the process, the concept of access to health care has also evolved from an earlier emphasis on utilization of health services in the 1960s and 1970s to a greater emphasis on efficiency, effectiveness, and health outcomes in the 1980s and 1990s. This evolution of the conceptual framework of access is reviewed in this section.

VICTOR FUCHS'S CONCEPTUALIZATION OF ACCESS

In an influential book on health policy choices entitled *Who Shall Live?*, health economist Victor Fuchs (1975) makes an important distinction between two types of problems involving access. The first type, labeled "special problems of access," are those that are faced by particular population subgroups in society, such as the uninsured and rural residents.

The problems facing the uninsured are mostly the result of poverty, according to Fuchs (1975). Medicaid and other health-care programs for the poor have to some extent eased the problems facing this group of individuals. But for those who have fallen through the cracks of the safety-net health-care system, access remains a serious problem. Even those who earn an income that is above the poverty level can lack health insurance because they are self-employed or work for employers that do not offer health insurance.

The special problems facing rural residents are not solely the result of poverty, although many rural residents are poor. Many rural residents have insurance coverage or substantial purchasing power to purchase health care. However, they do not have the same level of access to physicians, particularly specialists, and to health facilities as do those living in urban areas because physicians are reluctant to practice in rural areas and most rural areas do not have the population density to warrant a full-service medical facility.

> *Special problems of access are the problems facing the uninsured or the poor.*

For individuals or families who have insurance coverage or sufficient income to purchase health care, access can still be difficult. The problems such people face, called the "general problems of access" by Victor Fuchs, involve the inability of a health-care system to match demand with available supply. An example is an oversupply of surgeons and an undersupply of primary care physicians as more people come under managed care. Managed health plans need more primary care physicians than do traditional fee-for-service plans because these physicians play the role of gatekeepers while de-emphasizing inpatient care. Another example is a shortage of qualified critical care nurses in the inpatient setting when hospital critical care units are understaffed because many qualified nurses are withdrawing from the nursing labor market or practicing in other specialties. This may result in fewer staffed beds being available to patients in need. In both instances, insured patients cannot get the care they need because of the delivery system's failure to adjust to the changes in the marketplace.

The general problems of access are those faced by individuals who have insurance coverage in getting the care that their doctors have ordered.

The general problems of access and the special ones have different causes and require different solutions. General access problems mostly require an improvement in the functioning of the health-care and labor markets so that the imbalances in supply and demand can be quickly and smoothly eliminated. The special problems, in contrast, are more complex and multifaceted. They force us to re-examine such fundamental issues as whether the poor need access to health care more than they need other essential things in life such as food, housing, safety, and jobs; what the best way to help the poor is; and how much help to provide.

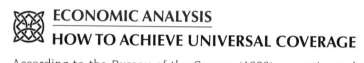

ECONOMIC ANALYSIS
HOW TO ACHIEVE UNIVERSAL COVERAGE

According to the Bureau of the Census (1998), an estimated 44.3 million Americans, or 16.3 percent of the total population, were without health insurance coverage during the entire 1998 calendar year. The reasons for lack of insurance, although complex, can be grouped into three categories:

1. Working for an employer that does not provide insurance coverage as a fringe benefit
2. Inability to afford insurance
3. Unwillingness to pay the insurance premium

Accordingly, health economist Victor Fuchs (1998) suggests that universal coverage can be achieved if two necessary and sufficient conditions are met. First, those who are too poor to pay for insurance coverage must be subsidized. Second, those who can afford to pay but are unwilling to pay must be required to have insurance. Addressing both conditions is necessary for improving health insurance coverage; failure to address either could make the situation worse. According to Fuchs (1998), if people who can afford to pay for insurance are not required to pay, they will choose to remain uninsured and only come back for public subsidies when they are sick.

THE ADAY AND ANDERSEN ACCESS FRAMEWORK

A group of applied sociologists, including Aday, Andersen, and their colleagues at the University of Chicago, began work in the 1960s on a conceptual framework of access to health care. The original Aday and Andersen model (Aday & Andersen, 1981) focused on explaining and predicting the use of health services, and suggested that use of health care at the individual level was related to a host of structural and process indicators. Structure indicators are characteristics of the health-care delivery system that affect the availability of health-care services. Examples include the human and material resources available to a health-care delivery system, which determine the volume of available health-care services; and the organization size and type, which can influence the distribution of services.

Process indicators, on the other hand, include the following (Aday & Andersen, 1981):

- *Predisposition to use services.* People of certain racial, religious, or ethnic backgrounds may be predisposed to particular diseases or health problems.
- *Factors enabling or impeding use.* Individual demographic characteristics, such as age and gender, and other socioeconomic variables, such as income, insurance coverage, and religious beliefs, can either enable or impede the use of needed health care.
- *The need for care.* These factors refer to the reasons for seeking health care, such as illness and injuries. People seek health care as the result of an evaluation by a health-care professional or as the result of a perceived need by the individual.

Over time, the Aday and Andersen model has evolved to distinguish between two types of access: potential and realized (Aday, 1993). *Potential access* refers to the ability and willingness of health-care systems to make health-care services available to targeted populations. The ability and willingness to provide access are influenced by the characteristics of the health-care system and the enabling characteristics of the patient population. The former characteristics include the health-care resources available in the area, the capacity of the health-care system, and organizational characteristics such as the types and mix of hospital ownership and the penetration of managed care in the health-care market. Enabling characteristics refer to socioeconomic factors of the community that influence residents' ability to afford health care.

Realized access refers to the type, site, and purpose of health services actually delivered by a health-care system. The types of services are categories of health services used by patients, such as hospital care, physician services, nursing care, and home care. The service site is the place where the service is delivered, such as the hospital, physicians' offices, and nurse-led and nurse-staffed primary care clinics. The purpose of utilization refers to the reasons for seeking health services, such as sickness, prevention, and health maintenance.

Most recently, Andersen (1997) has refined the earlier Aday and Andersen (1981) definitions of access by adding two additional types of access to health care:

- *Effective access* reflects a use of health services that results in an improvement in individual health and satisfaction.
- *Efficient access*, on the other hand, refers to a higher rate of return in health outcomes with the use of a unit of health service.

THE INSTITUTE OF MEDICINE ACCESS FRAMEWORK

In recent years, the development of an access framework has shifted from an emphasis on use of health care to health outcomes. An example of this shift is the 1993 Institute of Medicine (IOM) study of access indicators, which defines access as the timely use of personal health services to achieve the best possible health outcome (Millman, 1993). Under this definition, the IOM has identified five population-focused and outcome-based health policy objectives:

1. Promoting successful birth outcomes
2. Reducing the incidence of vaccine-preventable childhood diseases
3. Encouraging early detection and diagnosis of treatable diseases
4. Reducing the effects of chronic disease and prolonging life
5. Reducing morbidity and pain through timely and appropriate treatment

> *Health outcomes are the expected health results of a medical treatment or intervention.*

Based on the premise that access makes a difference in achieving these objectives, the IOM access framework links structural, financial, and personal barriers to access with the utilization of needed health services. Utilization is then related to health outcomes by mediating processes, including appropriateness of care, quality of providers, and patient adherence to treatment. By linking outcomes and effectiveness to access, it becomes possible to evaluate performance of the health-care system in terms of a set of multifaceted public health objectives such as access, cost efficiency, quality, and consumer satisfaction (Aday et al., 1993).

HEALTHY PEOPLE 2000

Healthy People 2000 is the most comprehensive national health promotion and disease prevention initiative ever undertaken in the United States (U.S. Public Health Service, 1991). Under the auspices of the U.S. Department of Health and Human Services (DHHS) and supported by private organizations, the Healthy People 2000 initiative began in 1990 and defined health objectives for the next decade. Healthy People 2000 defined three broad goals:

1. Increase the span of healthy life for Americans
2. Reduce health status disparities among Americans
3. Achieve access to preventive services for all Americans

To facilitate the accomplishment of these public health goals by the year 2000, measurable and modifiable health promotion and disease prevention objectives were organized into 22 priority areas. For each of the priority areas, one or more U.S. public health agencies were designated to coordinate activities for attaining the objectives and to monitor progress. These priority areas encompassed three approaches to health promotion and disease prevention (health promotion, health protection, and preventive services) and health information systems (surveillance and data systems). Specific objectives referred to health status outcomes, health behaviors, preventive services, and data monitoring needs. The original 22 priority areas of Healthy People 2000 are presented in Table 13–1.

Healthy People 2000 is a comprehensive national initiative for health promotion and disease prevention that began in 1990.

ACCESS TO CLINICAL PREVENTIVE SERVICES

Provision of clinical preventive services is one of the 22 priority areas of the Healthy People 2000 initiative. To monitor and evaluate national progress in achieving access to a wide range of clinical preventive services for every American, critical preventive services were grouped into eight categories, each having its own specific objectives, measurement indicators, and implementation timetables. These are summarized in the following list to illustrate how national objectives can serve as benchmarks for evaluating and monitoring the progress of a national project for improving access to cost-effective clinical preventive services.

TABLE 13–1. HEALTHY PEOPLE 2000 PRIORITY AREAS

I. Health Promotion
1. Physical activity and fitness
2. Nutrition
3. Tobacco
4. Alcohol and other drugs
5. Family planning
6. Mental health and mental disorders
7. Violence and abusive behavior
8. Educational and community-based programs

II. Health Protection
9. Unintentional injuries
10. Occupational safety and health
11. Environmental health
12. Food and drug safety
13. Oral health

III. Preventive Services
14. Maternal and infant health
15. Heart disease and stroke
16. Cancer
17. Diabetes and chronic disabling conditions
18. HIV infection
19. Sexually transmitted diseases
20. Immunization and infectious diseases
21. Clinical preventive services

IV. Surveillance and Data Systems
22. Surveillance and data systems

Source: U.S. Public Health Service. (1991). *Healthy People 2000: National Health promotion and disease prevention objectives.* Washington, DC: Department of Health and Human Services.

The Healthy People 2000 objectives for the Clinical Preventive Services priority area are as follows (U.S. Public Health Service, 1991):

1. Increase years of healthy life to at least 65 years.
2. Increase to at least 50 percent the proportion of people who have received, as a minimum within the appropriate interval, all of the screening and immunization services and at least some of the counseling services appropriate for their age and gender as recommended by the U.S. Preventive Services Task Force (1989).
3. Increase to at least 95 percent the proportion of Hispanics who have a specific source of ongoing primary care for coordination of their preventive and episodic health care.

4. Improve financing and delivery of clinical preventive services so that virtually no American has a financial barrier to receiving, at a minimum, the screening, counseling, and immunization services recommended by the U.S. Preventive Services Task Force.
5. Ensure that at least 90 percent of people for whom primary care services are provided directly by publicly funded programs are offered, at a minimum, the screening, counseling, and immunization services recommended by the U.S. Preventive Services Task Force.
6. Increase to at least 50 percent the proportion of primary care providers who provide their patients with the screening, counseling, and immunization services recommended by the U.S. Preventive Services Task Force.
7. Increase to at least 90 percent the proportion of people who are served by a local health department that assesses and ensures access to essential clinical preventive services.
8. Increase the proportion of all degrees in the health professions and allied and associate health profession fields awarded to members of underrepresented racial and ethnic minority groups.

THE NEXT STEP: HEALTHY PEOPLE 2010

The original Healthy People 2000 initiative focused on the health status of the nation and on desired directions for maintaining and improving the health of all Americans. To date, 47 of the 50 states have created health plans to implement health objectives for their jurisdictions. Healthy People objectives have also been used to measure the success of individual federal health initiatives, such as the Indian Health Service, the Maternal and Child Block Grant, and the Preventive health and Health Services Block Grant. Now individuals and organizations involved in public health are meeting to develop the next step, Healthy People 2010.

Currently, a collaboration of 350 member organizations and 300 state health, mental health, and environmental health agencies have developed objectives for the next decade. The Healthy People Web site (http://www.cdc.gov/nchs/about/otheract/hp2000/hp2000.htm) provides a wide range of information on the development of Healthy People 2010, interim status reports on Healthy People 2000, and other related publications.

In 1998, the DHHS began an initiative to address the elimination of racial disparities in health status. A description of this initiative can be found at their Web site (http://www.raceandhealth.hhs.gov). The six initial areas of disparity targeted for improvement are infant mortality, cancer screening and management, cardiovascular disease, diabetes, human immunodeficiency virus (HIV) infection and aquired immunodeficiency syndrome

(AIDS), and immunization rates. Through this initiative, DHHS is promoting research and supporting new programs to provide health services to underserved racial minorities and to reduce poverty.

 ## CURRENT ACCESS TO HEALTH CARE

Do most American people have adequate and timely access to needed health care? If not, what are the major barriers to access? Do serious differences in access to health care still exist among racial and ethnic groups years after the initiation of the Healthy People 2000 project? These and other questions can be answered by a review of available data collected and compiled by the National Center for Health Statistics and other federal agencies (National Center for Health Statistics, 1997, 1998).

CHILDREN'S ACCESS

Access to health care is especially important to children because a healthy childhood is the foundation of success and health in an individual's later life. Early access to health care is also related to health-care use in later life. Among the health-care services needed for a healthy childhood are prenatal care during a mother's pregnancy, vaccinations against childhood diseases, regular physician contact, ambulatory services, and health insurance coverage.

Children's access to health care affects health-care use and outcomes in later years.

Prenatal Care and Vaccinations

A healthy childhood begins with the good health behavior of the mother and adequate prenatal care. Early and consistent prenatal care, together with good health behavior on the part of the mother, increases the likelihood of having a healthy baby. To improve infant health through adequate prenatal care, Healthy People 2000 has aimed at achieving a goal of 90 percent of pregnant women receiving first-trimester prenatal care (U.S. Public Health Service, 1991), a goal that has not been achieved by 2000.

Another critical preventive service that improves the health of children is immunization against life-threatening and disabling childhood diseases. The Healthy People 2000 goal for immunization is a 90 percent vaccination rate by the year 2000 (U.S. Public Health Service, 1991). The recent trends in access to prenatal care for pregnant women and vaccinations for children are summarized in Table 13–2 and highlighted in the following list (National Center for Health Statistics, 1998):

- During the 1990s, prenatal care utilization rates for the country as a whole rose slowly and steadily. For example, the percentage of pregnant women beginning to use prenatal care during the first trimester rose from 75.8 percent in 1990 to 81.9 percent in 1996. Expansions in Medicaid coverage for pregnant women have been a major factor contributing to this trend.
- Considerable differences in the utilization of prenatal care existed among racial and ethnic groups. In 1996, according to the National Center for Health Statistics, Japanese and Cuban American mothers were the most likely to obtain early prenatal care (89 percent), whereas Native American and Inuit mothers were the least likely (68 percent).
- Prenatal care utilization is closely associated with the mothers' educational level. Pregnant women who have more education are more likely to start prenatal care early and have more visits. This was true in every race and ethnic group.
- In 1996, over three-quarters (77 percent) of children aged 19 to 35 months received the combined series of recommended vaccines consisting of four doses of diphtheria, tetanus, and pertussis (DTP) vaccine, three doses of polio vaccine, one dose of measles-containing vaccine, and three doses of *Haemophilus influenzae* type b (Hib) vaccine.
- A low vaccination rate is no longer associated with children's race and ethnicity. It is, however, still associated with family income level: Children from families with incomes below the poverty level are less likely to receive the combined series of vaccination than children from families with incomes above the poverty level (69 percent vs. 80 percent).

The data in Table 13–2 suggest that major differences still exist in health-care access and utilization by American children of different racial and ethnic groups. The data also indicate that the observed disparities in access are closely related to the socioeconomic status of the child's family, especially income level and the mother's education.

Physician Contact and Ambulatory Care

Regular physician contacts to assess children's growth and development and to ensure that their vaccinations are up to date are important to their health and normal growth. Children should have at least one physician visit a year (U.S. Preventive Services Task Force, 1989). In the United States, as suggested by the data in Table 13–2, lack of physician contact by children is closely associated with two socioeconomic factors: income and insurance status. Specifically, according to the National Center for Health Statistics (1998):

TABLE 13–2. CHILDREN'S ACCESS TO HEALTH CARE, 1996

	All Races	White, Non-Hispanic	Black, Non-Hispanic	Hispanic	Native American or Alaska Native	Asian or Pacific Islander
Maternal education	Percentage of prenatal care use in the first trimester among mothers aged 20 years and older					
Less than 12 years	68.0	72.2	61.3	67.2	59.7	69.3
12 years	82.0	86.1	72.2	77.1	68.7	77.9
13–15 years	87.8	90.5	80.2	83.2	75.0	84.1
16 or more years	93.9	95.0	89.9	89.0	87.4	89.7
Poverty level	Percentage of fully vaccinated children aged 19–35 months					
Below poverty level	69.0	68.0	70.0	68.0		
Above poverty level	80.0	81.0	78.0	74.0		
Family income	Percentage of children younger than 6 years with no physician contact during the past year					
Poor	11.2	11.0	10.9	10.8		
Near poor	10.1	9.9	9.3	10.7		
Middle/high income	6.9	5.3	5.3	5.0		
High income	4.1					
Family income	Percentage of children younger than 19 years with no health insurance coverage					
Poor	22.0	22.2	14.6	29.5		
Near poor	22.8	21.0	18.5	32.7		
Middle income	8.6	7.8	8.4	13.4		
High income	4.2	3.8	5.7	7.2		

Source: National Center for Health Statistics. (1998). *Health, United States, 1998.* Hyattsville, MD: U.S. Public Health Services, Figures 19–22.

- The percentage of young children without a recent physician visit varies inversely with family income. Eleven percent of poor children and 10 percent of near-poor children lacked a physician visit within the past year, compared with 4 percent of high-income children.
- Lack of a physician visit is also closely associated with lack of insurance coverage. Poor children without health insurance coverage were 2.8 times as likely to lack a recent physician visit as poor children with health insurance.
- In contrast to physician visits, the use of ambulatory care in hospital settings (emergency departments and outpatient departments) was almost 50 percent higher for children living in the lowest-income areas than those in the highest-income areas (79 visits compared with 54 visits per 100 children).

The Healthy People 2000 goal is for every child in the United States to be covered by health insurance (U.S. Public Health Service, 1991). The data discussed above clearly indicate that the goal of universal coverage has yet to be accomplished. It has been well documented that children without health insurance are more likely to delay seeking care or to go without care when such care is needed (Simpson, Cohen, & Parsons, 1997; National Center for Health Statistics, 1998). To remove the financial barriers to access for all American children, the Clinton administration and Congress took a concrete step by initiating the State Children's Health Insurance Program (SCHIP) under the Balanced Budget Act of 1997.

Health Insurance and the State Children's Health Insurance Program

Lack of health insurance is a major barrier to access to adequate health care for children in the United States (Newacheck, Hughes, & Stoddard, 1996). Currently, about 10 million American children—one in seven nationally—do not have health insurance and therefore are at significantly increased risk for preventable health problems (*Statement on the State Children's Health Insurance Program*, 1998). Lack of insurance is primarily associated with family income: Twenty-two to 23 percent of poor and near-poor children are uninsured, compared with 8.6 and 4.2 percent of middle-income and high-income children, respectively (National Center for Health Statistics, 1998). Children whose parents rely on Medicaid for health insurance coverage may also have difficulties finding physicians who are willing to treat them because of Medicaid's low reimbursement rates (Cykert et al., 1995). Moreover, many of the cost-cutting measures in state programs, such as cost sharing and benefit limitations, are known to raise barriers to access.

To provide affordable health insurance coverage to American children without insurance, President Clinton in his 1997 State of the Union address called for a bipartisan effort to launch the largest children's health insurance expansion since the enactment of Medicaid over 30 years ago. In August 1997, Congress passed, and the president signed into law, the Balanced Budget Act of 1997, which created a new children's health insurance program under Title XXI of the Social Security Act. Titled the State Children's Health Insurance Program, this new national initiative provides $24 billion over 5 years to help states offer affordable health insurance to previously uninsured children, especially those in working families whose income exceeds the Medicaid eligibility level but is insufficient to afford private insurance (*Statement*, 1998).

SCHIP is administered by the participating states and funded jointly by the federal government and the states. The states have three options in the design of their SCHIP programs. They can expand their Medicaid programs to provide coverage to uninsured children, create a separate health insurance program for children, or both. To date, 25 participating states have opted to expand Medicaid eligibility, 13 states have created separate state health insurance programs, and 10 states have used a combination of Medicaid expansion and separate state programs (Halfon et al., 1999).

To receive federal matching funds for children's insurance, states must submit a detailed state plan to the federal Health Care Financing Administration (HCFA). To maximize the number of children covered, funds must be used to cover previously uninsured children and not to replace existing public or private insurance coverage. States must also provide cost-sharing protections to ensure that families are not burdened with out-of-pocket expenses that they cannot afford. States can set the broad outlines of the program's structure and are given flexibility in tailoring their own programs to meet their own circumstances. At of the end of 1998, 52 plans—including those from two U.S. territories and the District of Columbia—had been submitted, and 40 plans had been approved (*Statement*, 1998).

ADULTS' ACCESS

It is important to an individual's health to have a usual source of health care, such as a particular doctor's office, clinic, health center, or other place for needed health care. Persons with a usual source have been shown to be more likely to receive a variety of preventive health services (Caplan & Haynes, 1996; Martin, et al., 1996). In 1996, approximately 23 percent of persons aged 18 to 64 had no usual sources of health care according to the 1996 Medical Expenditure Panel Survey (MEPS) (Weinick, Zuvekas, & Drilea, 1997). Among persons aged 65 and over, 9.2 percent had no usual source. A major cause of this situation is the lack of health insurance coverage. Individuals with no health insurance have fewer physician contacts and are less likely to receive preventive services.

Adults without health insurance are more likely to use more expensive emergency department services for health care than are those with insurance coverage.

Health Insurance

Lack of health insurance is a major barrier to access to health care in the United States. (Makuc, Freid, & Parsons, 1994; Bloom et al., 1997). The Healthy People 2000 goal regarding health insurance is for all Americans to have coverage, a goal that has not been achieved as yet, as demonstrated by the data presented in Table 13–3 and summarized in the following points.

- In 1994–1995, 18 percent of adults aged 18 to 64 years had no insurance coverage. Of those adults with insurance coverage, a majority (73 percent) had private insurance coverage, 7 percent had Medicaid or public assistance coverage, and 2 percent had other coverage, such as Medicare and military coverage.
- Among elderly individuals, less than 1 percent have no insurance because almost all are covered under Medicare.
- Lack of insurance coverage is closely associated with family income: The lower the family income level, the more likely it is for individuals in the family to have no insurance coverage.
- Across all income levels, there exist racial and ethnic differences in terms of insurance coverage: Blacks and Hispanics are more likely to have no insurance coverage than whites irrespective of the level of family income.
- Men are more likely not to have insurance coverage than women. This is true across all income levels and racial and ethnic groups.

 ECONOMIC ANALYSIS
THE EMERGENCY DEPARTMENT AS THE PRIMARY SOURCE OF HEALTH CARE

Most community hospitals in the United States offer emergency services. Many emergency departments (EDs) are state-of-the-art trauma facilities staffed by highly trained and expensive medical personnel. However, these facilities are frequently used inappropriately; for example, by inexperienced mothers seeking ED care for treating their children's common colds or sore throats and by homeless individuals

TABLE 13–3. ADULTS' ACCESS TO HEALTH CARE, 1996

Family Income	All Races	White, Non-Hispanic	Black, Non-Hispanic	Hispanic
Health insurance coverage among adult men aged 18–64 years				
Poor	44.1	37.9	44.4	58.7
Near poor	35.3	32.7	33.5	47.1
Middle income	13.8	12.8	14.5	20.7
High income	6.1	5.7	7.8	9.6
Health insurance coverage among adult women aged 18–64 years				
Poor	33.3	31.9	25.9	44.9
Near poor	28.6	27.5	22.8	41.5
Middle income	10.2	9.4	8.6	17.5
High income	4.4	3.8	6.3	7.8
No physician contact within the past year among adult men aged 18–64 years with a health problem				
Poor	21.2	20.3	20.8	24.4
Near poor	19.1	18.7	18.0	22.6
Middle/high income	14.9	13.4	13.0	17.2
High income	11.4			
No physician contact within the past year among adult women aged 18–64 years with a health problem				
Poor	11.7	11.5	10.5	14.3
Near poor	10.3	9.9	9.2	12.9
Middle/high income	5.7	4.8	5.3	7.1
High income	4.0			
Mammography within the past 2 years among women aged 50 years and older				
Poor	44.7	37.5	60.0	49.3
Near poor	48.2	47.9	57.4	38.2
Middle/high income	67.2	70.4	72.2	64.7
High income	76.3			

Source: National Center for Health Statistics. (1998). *Health, United States, 1998.* Hyattsville, MD: U.S. Public Health Services, Figures 43–48.

using the ED as an entry point for other services. Another problem is that emergency care does not provide the continuity of care that is possible from a health-care provider who is familiar with the individual. Follow-up of health concerns may not occur.

Nurse researcher Ruth E. Malone recently reported that at least 70 percent of the heavy ED users at two inner city hospitals in the San Francisco Bay Area were homeless, poor, or disabled people (Malone, 1998). The reasons for many of their ED visits were not medical. Instead, they used hospital EDs as a way to gain access to other types of low-tech care, such as rest, shelter, safety, showers, food, clothing, and social interaction.

Physician Contact

Timely and periodic physician contact is essential to one's health. Those who do not have adequate ambulatory care may suffer serious health consequences when they are ill. The prevalence of adults who have a physician visit at least once a year is a good measure of access to health care. The following points highlight physician contact data for American adults available from the National Center for Health Statistics (1998):

- In 1994–1995, 12 percent of adults aged 18 to 64 who reported a health problem had not had a physician visit in the past year. Among adults who reported a health problem, the proportion who had not had a recent physician visit was 31 percent. The likelihood of not having a physician visit in the past year among adults who reported a health problem is inversely related to family income, regardless of race, ethnicity, or gender. Poor men and women are much more likely not to have had a physician visit within the past year than their higher-income counterparts.
- Across all income levels, men are more likely not to have had a physician visit in the past year than women.

Mammography Screening

Access problems can also be seen in the lack of women getting cost-effective mammography screening. Breast cancer is the most common type of cancer in American women and a second leading cause of their death, after lung cancer. The American Cancer Society predicted that there would be an estimated 180,200 new cases of breast cancer in women and 43,900 related deaths in 1997 (American Cancer Society, 1997).

Early detection of cancer improves patient outcomes and decreases treatment costs.

A key factor in reducing the mortality rate associated with breast cancer is early detection with regular mammography screening, according to *The Clinician's Handbook of Preventive Services*, published by the U.S. Office of Public Health and Science and the Office of Disease Prevention and Health Promotion (1998). Both the National Cancer Institute and the U.S. Preventive Services Task Force recommend that women over the age of 50 should receive a breast examination and mammography screening every 1 to 2 years until the age of 70 (U.S. Preventive Services Task Force, 1996; National Cancer Institute, 1997). The Healthy People 2000 goal is for 60 percent of women 50 years and older to have had a breast examination and mammography screening within the past 2 years. The level of access to breast examination and mammography screening is highlighted in the following list (National Center for Health Statistics, 1998):

- In 1993–1994, 60 percent of women over the age of 50 reported having a breast examination and mammogram in the last 2 years.
- The percentage of women having a recommended breast examination is closely associated with family income. Women with high incomes are about 60 to 70 percent more likely than women in the lower income brackets to have had a recent mammogram.
- When controlling for income, black women are as likely or more likely than white women to have had a recent mammogram.

A clear message from the preceding discussion of access indicators for American adults is that many people—especially low-income and minority individuals—do not have adequate access to health care. The federal Agency for Health Care Policy and Research estimated that in 1996, 13 million (11.6 percent) of the roughly 110 million families in the United States experienced difficulty or delays in obtaining medical care (Weinick, Zuvekas, & Drilea, 1997). In addition, 46 million Americans (18 percent of the general population) did not have a usual source of health care. These figures had remained relatively unchanged since 1987. What are the factors that prevent so many Americans from getting the health-care services that they need?

BARRIERS TO ACCESS

A key to adequate access to health care in the United States is having sufficient insurance coverage. In most developed countries, health care is either provided directly by the government or covered by a government-mandated health insurance plan paid by employers and employees. In the United States, health insurance is voluntary. Unless covered by private insurance or a government-sponsored program such as Medicare or Medicaid, uninsured Americans must pay for health care out of their pockets or delay treatments. No wonder that the main barrier to access is lack of insurance coverage (Zuvekas & Weinick, 1999).

Lack of insurance is a major barrier to access to health care.

Nationally, according to a recent MEPS report (Weinick, Zuvekas, & Drilea, 1997), a majority of the families (59.8 percent) that experienced barriers to care singled out inability to afford care as the main reason for family members' difficulty or delay in receiving needed health care. Another 19.5 percent reported insurance-related reasons as the main obstacle to receiving needed health care. These reasons included ineligibility for insurance because of pre-existing conditions, treatments not being approved by the insurance company, inability to pay deductibles and copayments, referrals to specialists being required but unobtainable, and doctors refusing to accept the family's insurance plan. The remaining 20.7 percent of families experienced a variety of other problems, such as transportation, physical barriers, communication problems, child-care limitations, lack of time or information, or refusal to seek services.

In addition to financial barriers to access, there are many nonfinancial barriers, such as race and language difficulties (Weissman & Epstein, 1994). For example, according to the 1996 Medical Expenditure Panel Survey, 15.1 percent of the Hispanic families surveyed reported barriers to receiving health care. In contrast, 9.9 percent of black families and 11.4 percent of white families and families of other race or ethnicity reported barriers (Weinick, Zuvekas, & Drilea, 1997).

Geographic location is another serious nonfinancial barrier (Simpson, Cohen, & Parsons, 1997). In inner cities, for example, access may be lacking because physicians and other health-care providers are reluctant to practice there (Konrad & Li, 1995). Similarly, rural areas have far fewer doctors, hospitals, and other health resources than urban areas even though one-fourth of the population of the United States lives in rural areas (Ricketts et al., 1996; National Center for Health Statistics, 1998).

Religion is still another potential barrier because some religions discourage or forbid their adherents to seek certain types of medical care. In addition to religion, other personal values, practices, and preferences may lead individuals and groups to perceive the health-care system as incompatible with their culture. These and other nonfinancial barriers to access continue to present formidable challenges to the American health-care system, which is currently seeking ways to overcome barriers to health care for everyone.

✸ ECONOMIC ANALYSIS
✸ RURAL ACCESS TO HEALTH CARE

Since the advent of Diagnosis Related Groups in the early 1980s and the rapid growth of managed care in the 1990s, many community hospitals have come under severe financial stress. Many hospitals have closed as a result, and others have discontinued services that they could no longer support. These changes in the hospital industry have disproportionately affected rural areas. Unlike urban areas served by multiple hospitals, many rural areas are left with no alternate source of care once their only hospital closes its door or discontinues a service (Alexander, D'Aunno, & Succi, 1996).

ACCESS STRATEGIES

American nurses have been active in the forefront of efforts to improve health-care access. In the 1960s, for example, the American Nurses Association (ANA) supported and lobbied for the establishment of Medicare and Medicaid (Stevens, 1992). In 1980, it reaffirmed its commitment to the health of American people and their access to health care by declaring that nursing was accountable for the accessibility of health care (American Nurses Association, 1980). In response to President Bill Clinton's health-care reform in the early 1990s, a consortium of nursing organizations presented their reform agenda and promoted it as nursing's answer to health-care reform.

In recent years, the changes in health-care financing and delivery have presented new challenges and opportunities for nurses to contribute to the improvement of access. New nursing roles and delivery models that contribute to increased access include nurse-managed centers, walk-in and minor emergency areas in hospital emergency departments, advanced practice nursing in rural settings, and flight nursing.

NURSE-MANAGED CENTERS

Nurse-managed centers (NMCs) are community-based primary care centers led and managed by nurses. They are staffed by registered nurses (RNs); advanced practice nurses (APNs), including nurse practitioners (NPs) and certified midwives; and other nonphysician providers. They are usually associated with either an academic medical center or a school of nursing (Phillips & Steel, 1994) and typically serve underserved areas where a shortage of primary care physicians exists (Walker, 1994). Collaboration with physicians provides consultation and referral for services not provided at the center. The variety of primary care services offered include the following (Olmested & DeMint, 1997):

- Treatment of common colds, infections, earaches, and sore throats
- Performance of physical examinations

- Prescription of medication for chronic or acute conditions
- Management of chronic health problems such as diabetes and high blood pressure
- Delivery of screening and preventive services

Numerous studies have confirmed the quality of care provided by NMCs (Branstetter & Holman, 1989; Aiken et al., 1993). These centers have also been shown to be cost effective; NPs and their interdisciplinary practice teams produce appropriate patient outcomes, cost savings, reduced hospital length of stay, and diminished emergency department use (Cintron et al., 1983; McGrath, 1990). However, for survival in the long term, these centers must resist the temptation of becoming low-cost substitutes for the more expensive physician care. Instead, in the words of nursing researchers D. L. Phillips and J. E. Steel (1994), "nursing practice in NMCs should be promoted as a new, complimentary, community-based alternative that is responsive to patient needs" (p. 88).

Expanding nursing roles can provide improved access to health care economically.

NURSE PRACTITIONER–STAFFED MINOR EMERGENCY AREAS

Many people use hospital emergency departments (EDs) for minor, non-emergency conditions (Eastaugh & Eastaugh, 1990; Glick & Thompson, 1997). This inappropriate use of scarce health-care resources has not disappeared completely despite repeated attempts by health reform efforts and managed care organizations to reduce it. In recent years, hospitals have learned that many of the patients seeking care at EDs can be cared for in a cost-effective setting staffed by RNs and NPs (Buchanan & Powers, 1997). For example, a study reported that a majority of the 56 surveyed hospitals (58 percent) had opened a "fast track" minor emergency area (MEA) in their EDs (Nollman & Colbert, 1994). Another 25 percent of the surveyed hospitals were considering opening a fast track, and only 17 percent had not considered such an option.

The MEA is an excellent educational site for nursing and medical students in addition to providing a viable alternative to the more expensive ED care (Glick & Thompson, 1997). The large volume of patients with varied complaints in an MEA provides opportunities for students to gain experience and fine-tune clinical skills. By providing cost-effective emergency medicine and reducing crowding at the trauma center in the local community hospital, an MEA is an effective approach to improving access to critical care.

NURSE PRACTITIONERS AND RURAL HEALTH

Rural residents face many barriers to access to health care. Compared with urban residents, rural residents have higher poverty rates and tend to be in poorer health, and a greater percentage are elderly. Their health-care needs have not been sufficiently met because of higher rates of uninsurance and a shortage of health-care resources (Mueller, Patil, & Ullrich, 1997). With relatively few residents scattered in a large area, the demand for health care is insufficient to draw enough physicians to practice in rural areas. Furthermore, rural physicians are geographically isolated and cannot easily obtain consultations and backup coverage (Shi & Singh, 1998). However, these difficulties that discourage physicians to practice in rural areas present opportunities for nurses who can provide primary care and treat chronic conditions and are willing to practice in a rural setting.

Nonphysician health-care providers such as APNs and certified nurse midwives can make valuable contributions to improving health-care access in rural areas (Conway-Welch, 1991). Studies have shown that an increasingly large number of rural hospitals are employing NPs to enhance their delivery of outpatient services (Strickland, Strickland, & Garretson, 1998). They employ nonphysician providers for at least four reasons (Krein, 1997):

1. To extend care, assist physicians, or increase access to primary care
2. Because physicians are unavailable or too difficult to recruit
3. Because NPs or physician assistants are considered cost effective or more economical for rural areas
4. To gain Rural Health Clinic certification to become eligible for Medicaid and Medicare reimbursements

The Rural Health Clinics program was initiated by Congress in 1977 under the Rural Health Clinic Services Act (Public Law 95-210). It was designed to improve access to health care in underserved areas by allowing Medicare and Medicaid reimbursements for the services of midlevel practitioners in rural health clinics. To be designated a rural health clinic, a public or private physician practice, clinic, or hospital must meet several criteria, including location in a medically underserved rural area. The Rural Health Clinics program has been a major incentive for rural hospitals to employ nurse practitioners and physician assistants (National Rural Health Association, 1989; Shi & Singh, 1998).

Another impetus for the growth of employment of APNs in rural areas has been the establishment of community and migrant health centers (C/MHCs). Most of the C/MHCs are located in rural areas. They typically serve the rural poor and migrant farm workers, with a heavy reliance on nonphysician providers for service delivery (John Snow, Inc., 1990; Lewin-

VHI, Inc., 1995). Nationally, there were almost 700 C/MHCs in 1996, serving over 7 million patients annually (Shi & Singh, 1998).

TELEMEDICINE

An adjunct to nurse-managed centers in rural and underserved areas is telemedicine. Chapter 16 describes the development of this practice. Use of technology to connect relatively isolated health-care providers with others enhances providers' ability to consult on problem cases and provide specialty services not available locally.

Computer technologies are also increasingly used by individuals and families in their homes for monitoring and support functions. Pesut (1998) describes how consumers have access to lay information as well as free Medline access through the National Library of Medicine. Through this network of resources, consumers can locate all manner of comprehensive health information. Today, health information is readily available to consumers through the Internet. One of the most popular health information resources is HealthWorld Online (http://www.healthy.net). Other popular Web sites include WebMD (http://www.webmd.com), Mayo Clinic Health Oasis (http://www.mayohealth.org), and drkoop.com (http://www.drkoop.com).

FLIGHT NURSES

Flight nurses are nurses who provide patient care during air transportation. Their mission is to provide "safe and efficient transfer of patients while maintaining or improving the level of care" (National Flight Nurses Association, 1992, p. 1). Founded in 1980, the National Flight Nurses Association now has more than 1700 members from throughout the United States and 16 foreign countries (Reiser, 1998).

Most flight nurses provide patient care in fixed-wing aircraft or helicopters during the transportation of patients to a trauma center. They improve access by raising the chances of patients' surviving major trauma such as heart attacks and severe traffic accidents (Semonin-Holleran, 1996). They also provide medical services to residents in remote areas where no regular medical care is available.

Some flight nurses have found market niches and developed health-care businesses that deliver comprehensive medical services to customers who experience medical emergencies in remote areas on air, sea, and land (Jezierski, 1998). By marketing these services to business clients who travel frequently on company business, these new health-care entrepreneurs can earn a handsome return for their efforts and ingenuity.

SUMMARY

In the United States, access to health care is closely related to an individual's socioeconomic status. National data have shown that the health status of both children and adults and their access to timely and adequate health care are inversely associated with lower socioeconomic status. Poorer adults and children are more likely to lack adequate insurance coverage. They also lack the necessary financial resources to pay out-of-pocket expenses, which frequently become another financial barrier to access even for those low-income individuals with government-sponsored insurance coverage. Individuals in poor health need regular and routine medical attention to avoid future medical problems.

The federal Healthy People 2000 program has served as a national guideline for health promotion and disease prevention since its initiation in the early 1990s. Over the last decade, noticeable progress has been made in improving access to health care, especially for low-income adults and children. Medicare, Medicaid, and other health-care programs, such as community and migrant health centers and the Rural Health Clinics program, which try to improve access to health services in federally designated underserved areas, have had an important and positive impact on improving access to health care. However, much more still needs to be done in health education, promotion, and disease prevention and in access to health insurance and clinical preventive services to improve the health of American people, especially those of lower socioeconomic status. The beginning of this arduous task is to have a good understanding of the concept of access, the barriers to needed access, and ways to improve access.

DISCUSSION QUESTIONS

1. What is access to health care? How has the concept evolved in the last 20 years?
2. What is the significance of adequate access to health care?
3. What are the financial and nonfinancial barriers to access?
4. What are the missions and purpose of the Healthy People 2000 program?
5. What percentage of American adults and children do not have insurance coverage? What are the major reasons for not having insurance coverage?

6. How much progress has been made in achieving the original Healthy People 2000 objectives? How would you go about researching information relating to the progress of the Healthy People 2000 program?

7. Why is nursing responsible for access to health care? Provide examples of new nursing practice models and roles that can improve access to health care.

 REFERENCES

Acs, G. (1995). Explaining trends in health insurance coverage between 1988 and 1991. *Inquiry* 32,(1), 102–110.

Aday, L. A. (1993). Indicators and predictors of health services utilization. In S. J. Williams & P. R. Torrens (Eds.), *Introduction to health services* (4th ed., pp. 46–70). Albany, NY: Delmar Publishers.

Aday, L. A., & Andersen, R. M. (1981). Equity to access to medical care: A conceptual and empirical overview. *Medical Care*, 19(Suppl.), 4–27.

Aday, L. A., Begley, C. E., Lairson, D. R., & Slater, C. H. (1993). *Evaluating the medical care system: Effectiveness, efficiency, and equity.* Chicago: Health Administration Press.

Aiken, L. H., Lake, E. T., Semann, S., Lehman, H. P., O'Hare, P. A., Cole, C. S., Dunbar, D., & Frank, I. (1993). Nurse practitioner managed care for persons with HIV infection. *Image: Journal of Nursing Scholarship*, 25(3), 172–177.

Alexander, J. A., D'Aunno, T. A., & Succi, M. J. (1996). Determinants of rural hospital conversion: A model of profound organizational change. *Medical Care*, 34(1), 29–43.

American Cancer Society. (1997). *Cancer facts and figures—1997.* Atlanta: Author.

American Nurses Association. (1980). *A social-policy statement.* Kansas City, MO: Author.

Andersen, R. (1997). *Too big, too small, too fat, too tall: Search for "just right" measures of access in the age of managed care.* Paper presented at the annual meeting of the Association for Health Services Research, Chicago, IL.

Bloom, B., Simpson, G., Cohen, R. A., Parsons, P. E. (1997). *Access to health care. Part 2: Working-age adults* (National Center for Health Statistics, Vital Health Statistics, Series 10, No. 197). Washington, DC: U.S. Government Printing Office.

Blum, H. L. (1974). *Planning for health: Development and application of social change theory.* New York: Human Sciences Press.

Branstetter, E., & Holman, E. (1989). A nursing model of health care: A 10-year trend analysis. In National League for Nursing, *Nursing centers: Meeting the demand for quality health care* (NLN Publication No. 21–2311, pp. 117–127). New York: Author.

Buchanan, L., & Powers, R. D. (1997). Establishing an NP-staffed minor emergency area. *The Nurse Practitioner*, 22(4), 175–187.

Bureau of the Census. (1998). *October 1998 current population reports* (P60–208). Washington, DC: U.S. Department of Commerce.

Caplan, L. S., & Haynes, S. G. (1996). Breast cancer screening in older women. *Public Health Review*, 24(2), 193–204.

Cintron, G., Bigas, C., Linares, E., Aranda, J. M., & Hernandez, E. (1983). Nurse practitioner role in a chronic congestive heart failure clinic: In-hospital time, costs and patient satisfaction. *Heart and Lung*, 12(3), 237–240.

Conway-Welch, C. (1991). Issues surrounding the distribution and utilization of nurse nonphysician providers in rural America. *Journal of Rural Health*, 7(4, Suppl.), 388–401.

Cykert, S., Kissling, G., Layson, R., & Hansen, C. (1995). Health insurance does not guarantee access to primary care: A national study of physicians' acceptance of publicly insured patients. *Journal of General Internal Medicine, 10*(6), 345–348.

Eastaugh, S., & Eastaugh, J. (1990). Putting the squeeze on emergency medicine: The many pressures on today's E.D. *Hospital Topics, 68*(4), 21–26.

Fuchs, V. (1975). *Who shall live? Health, economics and social choice.* New York: Basic Books.

Fuchs, V. (1998). *Who shall live? Health, economics and social choice* (Expanded ed.). River Edge, NJ: World Scientific.

Glick, D. F., & Thompson, K. M. (1997). Analysis of emergency room use for primary care needs. *Nursing Economics, 15*(1), 42–49.

Gold, M. (1998). Beyond coverage and supply: Measuring access to healthcare in today's market. *Health Services Research, 33*(3, pt. 2), 625–652.

Halfon, N., Inkelas, M., DuPlesis, H., & Paul, W. (1999). Challenges in securing access to care for children. *Health Affairs, 18*(2), 48–63.

Jezierski, M. (1998). MedAire: Peace of mind in the skies—a flight nurses' dream come true. *Journal of Emergency Nursing, 24*(1), 71–73.

John Snow, Inc. (1990). *Impact of case management on health status in community and migrant health centers.* Boston: Author.

Kalisch, B., & Kalisch, P. (1982). *Politics of nursing.* Philadelphia: JB Lippincott.

Kongstvedt, P. R. (1996). *The managed health care handbook* (3rd ed.). Gaithersburg, MD: Aspen Publishers.

Konrad, T. R., & Li, H. (1995). Migrating docs: Studying physician practice location. *Journal of the American Medical Association, 274*(24), 1914.

Krein, S. L. (1997). The employment and use of nurse practitioners and physician assistants by rural hospitals. *Journal of Rural Health, 13*(1), 45–58.

Lewin-VHI, Inc. (1995). *The performance of C/MHCs under managed care: Case studies of seven C/MHCs and their lessons learned.* Fairfax, VA: Author.

Makuc, D. M., Freid, V. M., & Parsons, P. E. (1994). *Health insurance and cancer screening among women* (Advance data from vital and health statistics No. 254). Hyattsville, MD: National Center for Health Statistics.

Malone, R. E. (1998). Whither the almshouse? Overutilization and the role of the emergency department. *Journal of Health Politics, Policy and Law, 23*(5), 795–832.

Martin, L. M., Calle, E., Wingo, A., & Heath, C. W., Jr. (1996). Comparison of mammography and Pap test use from the 1987 and 1992 National Health Interview Surveys: Are we closing the gaps? *American Journal of Preventive Medicine, 12*(2), 82–90.

McGrath, S. (1990). The cost-effectiveness of nurse practitioners. *Nurse Practitioners, 15*(7), 40–42.

Millman, M. (Ed). (1993). *Access to health care in America.* Washington, DC: National Academy Press.

Mueller, K. J., Patil, K., & Ullrich, F. (1997). Lengthening spells of uninsurance and their consequences. *Journal of Rural Health, 13*(1), 29–37.

National Cancer Institute. (1997). *Cancer facts: Questions and answers about mammography screening.* Bethesda, MD: National Institutes of Health.

National Center for Health Statistics. (1997). *Healthy People 2000 review, 1997.* Hyattsville, MD: Public Health Service.

National Center for Health Statistics. (1998). *Health, United States, 1998.* Hyattsville, MD: Public Health Service.

National Flight Nurses Association. (1992). *Position paper: Role of the registered nurse in basic life support air transport.* Park Ridge, IL: Author.

National Rural Health Association. (1989). *Rural Health Clinic Services Act: Public Law 95-210.* Kansas City, MO: Author.

Newacheck, P. W., Hughes, D. C., & Stoddard, J. J. (1996). Children's access to primary care: Differences by race, income, and insurance status. *Pediatrics, 97*(1), 26–32.

Nollman, J., & Colbert, K. (1994). Successful fast tracks: Data and advice. *Journal of Emergency Nursing*, 20(6), 483–486.

Olmested, K. L., & DeMint, S. (1997). Nurse practitioner center expands access to primary care. *Healthcare Financial Management*, 51(2), 30–32.

Pesut, D. J. (1998). Electronic commerce and Internet-based health care. *Nursing Outlook*, 46(5), 201.

Phillips, D. L., & Steel, J. E. (1994). Factors influencing scope of practice in nursing centers. *Journal of Professional Nursing*, 10(2), 84–90.

Reiser, J. T. (1998). The National Flight Nurses Association—past, present, and future. *Journal of Emergency Nursing*, 24(6), 571–473.

Ricketts, T. C., Tropman, S. E., Slifkin, R. T., & Konrad, T. R. (1996). Migration of obstetrician-gynecologists into and out of rural areas, 1985–1990. *Medical Care*, 34(5), 428–438.

Semonin-Holleran, R. (1996). These nurses take flight. *RN*, 59(9), 57, 59–60.

Shi, L., & Singh, D. A. (1998). *Delivering health care in America: A systems approach*. Gaithersburg, MD: Aspen Publishers.

Simpson, G., Cohen, B., & Parsons, P. E. (1997). *Access to health care, Part 1: Children* (National Center for Health Statistics, Vital Health Statistics, Series 10–196). Washington, DC: U.S. Government Printing Office.

Smith, B. M. (1997). Trends in health care coverage and financing and their implications for policy. *New England Journal of Medicine*, 337(14), 1000–1003.

Statement on the State Children's Health Insurance Program before the House Commerce Committee, Subcommittee on Health and Environment, 105 Cong. (1998, September) (testimony of Nancy-Ann Deparle, Administrator, Health Care Financing Administration, U.S. Department of Health and Human Services). Available: http:www.hcfa.gov/init/testm918.htm.

Stevens, P. E. (1992). Who gets care? Access to health care as an area for nursing action. *Scholarly Inquiry for Nursing Practice*, 6(3),185–200.

Strickland, W. J., Strickland, D. L., & Garretson, C. (1998). Rural and urban nonphysician providers in Georgia. *Journal of Rural Health*, 14(2), 109–120.

Sultz, H. A., & Young, K. M. (1999). *Health care USA*. Gaithersburg, MD: Aspen Publishers.

Swartz, K. (1997). Changes in the 1995 current population survey and estimates of health insurance coverage. *Inquiry*, 34(1), 70–79.

U.S. Office of Public Health and Science and Office of Disease Prevention and Health Promotion. (1998). *The clinician's handbook of preventive services* (2nd ed.). Hyattsville, MD: Public Health Services.

U.S. Preventive Services Task Force. (1989). *Guide to clinical preventive services: An assessment of the effectiveness of 169 interventions. Report to the U.S. Preventive Services Task Force*. Baltimore, MD: Williams and Wilkins.

U.S. Preventive Services Task Force. (1996). *Guide to clinical preventive services* (2nd ed.). Hyattsville, MD: Public Health Services.

U.S. Public Health Service. (1991). *Healthy People 2000: National health promotion and disease prevention objectives*. Washington, DC: Department of Health and Human Services.

Walker, P. H. (1994). Dollars and sense in health reform: Interdisciplinary practice and community nursing centers. *Nursing Administration Quarterly*, 19(1), 1–11.

Weinick, R. M., Zuvekas, S. H., & Drilea, S. K. (1997). *Access to health care—sources and barriers: 1996. MEPS research findings No. 3*. (AHCPR Publication No. 98–0001). Silver Spring, MD: Agency for Health Care Policy and Research.

Weissman, J. S., & Epstein, A. M. (1994). *Falling through the safety net: Insurance and access to health care*. Baltimore, MD: The Johns Hopkins University Press.

World Health Organization. (1978). *Primary health care. Report of the International Conference on Primary Health Care*. Geneva, Switzerland.

Zuvekas, S. H., & Weinick, R. M. (1999). Changes in access to care, 1977–1996: The role of health insurance. *Health Services Research*, 34(1, Pt. II), 271–279.

SUGGESTED READING

Aday, L. A., & Andersen, R. (1975). *Development of indices of access to medical care*. Ann Arbor, MI: Health Administration Press.

Earle-Richardson, G. B., & Earle-Richardson, A. F. (1998). Commentary from the front lines: Improving the National Health Service Corp's use of nonphysician medical providers. *Journal of Rural Health*, 14(2), 91–97.

Penchansky, R., & Thomas, J. W. (1981). The concept of access: definition and relationship to consumer satisfaction. *Medical Care*, 19(2), 127–140.

Reinhardt, U. E. (1994). Providing access to health care and controlling costs: The universal dilemma. In P. R. Lee & C. L. Estes (Eds.), *The nation's health* (4th ed., pp. 263–278). Boston: Jones and Bartlett.

Woodside, K. J. (1996). Nurse practitioner educators join effort to improve access to primary care in New York City. *NLN Update* 2(1), 4–5.

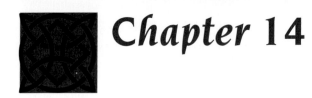

Chapter 14

The Relationship of Cost and Quality in Health Care

Robert W. Koch
Marylane Wade Koch

LEARNING OBJECTIVES

- Describe the economic and quality issues regarding health care that face the United States today.
- Describe the relevance of consumer surveys that address health-care concerns.
- Explain the relationship between quality and cost.
- Describe and analyze the role of the four national groups that are addressing cost and quality.
- Describe the nursing implications of cost and quality in health care.
- Describe implications for the future and give examples in which agencies or groups are making a difference in cost and quality improvement.

 ## ECONOMIC AND QUALITY ISSUES

A critical issue facing the United States is how to develop and implement a health-care delivery system that provides high-quality, affordable, and effective health care. Quality management leaders have for many years promoted quality improvement as the way to both improve quality and decrease costs in health care. Common sense supports the idea that improving quality can decrease costs; for example, emphasis on prevention minimizes expensive treatment of diseases. However, discussion continues as to whether the current applications of quality improvement are effectively used or are affecting rising health-care costs in the United States.

At the same time that health-care costs are increasing, many question the quality of care and services provided in this country. Although *quality* may be an ambiguous term, the goal of quality health care is to provide care in the appropriate setting at reasonable cost and with positive patient outcomes.

A *health-care delivery system that provides high-quality, affordable, and effective health care is needed.*

CONSUMER SURVEYS

Consumers are among those who question the quality of health care in the United States. Results of a national poll on how Americans perceive the health-care system demonstrated that Americans have lost confidence in the current health-care system. Eight of 10 Americans believed that there is something wrong with the U.S. health-care system. Seven of 10 stated they believe quality is compromised to "save money." Eight of 10 felt that quality health care is unaffordable for the average person. The most dissatisfied age group are those in their 30s and 40s (National Coalition on Health Care [NCHC], 1999a).

A national telephone survey entitled "Americans as Health Care Consumers: The Role of Quality Information," conducted by the Kaiser Family Foundation, the Agency for Health Care Policy and Research, and Princeton Survey Research Associates, found that 42 percent of Americans said their biggest concern in choosing a health plan is quality. Because consumers question both cost and quality in health-care services, the health-care industry is being challenged to take action to radically improve both (Agency for Health Care Policy and Research [AHCPR], 1996).

THE U.S. HEALTH-CARE SYSTEM

The current health-care delivery system is being investigated to evaluate the cost and quality of care. The largest alliance working to achieve necessary health-care reforms and improve health-care quality is the National Coalition on Healthcare, an organization of some 100 nonpartisan members who represent 100 million Americans in large and small businesses, large labor unions, the country's three largest religious faiths, large consumer organizations, primary health-care providers, and academic health-care centers. The Coalition commissioned a study to determine the condition of health-care quality in the United States. In a speech given to the national conference of state legislatures in December 1997, Dr. Henry Simmons, president of the National Coalition on Healthcare, summarized the state of the U.S. health-care system from his viewpoint (Simmons, 1997).

Dr. Simmons emphasized that in 1992, both presidential candidates agreed that our country's health-care system was in crisis. He told the group of legislators that the situation had only worsened: The problems our country faces with health care are more serious than before. Grave reforms are necessary to prevent the health-care problems of Americans from continuing to worsen. The Coalition released studies in 1997 that addressed three basic national concerns: cost control, health insurance coverage, and quality of care.

Cost Control

The first major problem is the rising cost of health care. Since the health-care reform debate began in the 1990s, costs have risen by 50 percent, or more than $500 billion (Simmons, 1997). Although there was a brief slow-down, health-care costs are rising at twice the inflation rate. Other countries provide health-care services for about half our cost and produce better health outcomes and patient satisfaction.

Despite major managed care initiatives, the Congressional Budget Office estimates that the existing costs of $1 trillion annually will increase by 50 percent over the next 5 years. Total health-care costs are thus projected to double to $2 trillion (see Chapter 4). Efforts such as managed care or bene-ficiary cost sharing have produced less results than desired. There is con-cern that these efforts will not result in sufficient cost containment over time to address the problem (see Chapter 12).

Health Insurance Coverage

The rising cost of health care contributes to the second problem: decreasing health insurance coverage. Daily, consumers hear news reports about the crisis of Medicare coverage for the country's senior population, a growing segment with increased health-care needs. Eighty million Americans are either uninsured or underinsured—10 million more than when the reform debate began. There are several reasons for this, but one key factor is that small businesses, representing a large part of the nation's economy, cannot afford adequate health-care coverage for workers. Many operate with contingent workers; thus, fewer employees are provided with health insurance.

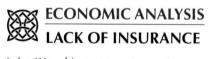

ECONOMIC ANALYSIS
LACK OF INSURANCE

John Wood is a computer systems analyst who worked for IBM for many years but now manages his own small business. When negotiating for health insurance coverage, the insurance agent tells him that compre-hensive coverage will be $450 per month for family coverage. However, if he hires the Web site specialist who has type 1 diabetes, insurance will cost $600 per month per family. John and his colleagues decide not to offer health coverage for the first year or so until the business is more established. This situation demonstrates the dilemma of small business owners regarding the provision of health insurance to a small number of employees.

Quality of Care

The third problem of the U.S. health-care system is quality of care. Although the focus remains on cost control, a critical concern is whether quality care is present, given the continued rise of costs. If the economic principle predicts that as quality improves, costs decrease, then what is happening in this country?

Major variations in care occur in the United States depending on geographical location; the amount of resources and practices in a given area can determine treatment. Major gaps in the medical knowledge base and in medical treatment exist across the country. Instead of one health-care system in the United States, there are many small systems operating in the various geographical areas.

Why is addressing variation of treatment and care important? Dr. Simmons (1997) asserts that "hundreds of billions of dollars of waste could be avoided and become available to provide necessary services to those currently served." He further contends that major quality issues such as treatment errors and deaths result from variance in health-care practices. Autopsy rates show a 35 to 40 percent rate of missed diagnoses (Simmons, 1997). In fact, an American Medical Association (AMA) poll suggests that more than 100 million Americans have experienced a medical mistake. Dr. Lucian Leape, physician board member of the AMA's National Patient Safety Foundation, states that the number of medical accidents in inpatient settings conservatively results in the deaths of some 300,000 people annually (Simmons, 1997). This is 7 times the rate of highway accidents in this country. The total number of inpatient medical accidents could be as high as 3 million, with a price tag of $200 billion each year (Simmons, 1997). The Harvard Medical Practice Study for the State of New York noted that if the New York medical accident rates apply across the United States, then about 180,000 people die annually as the result of negligence or medical injury. Half of these deaths are considered preventable. The Harvard team called this source of mortality the nation's "hidden epidemic" (NCHC, 1999b).

As public concern regarding costly health care with outcomes of less than desired quality grows, consumers must decide if they will accept this level of cost and quality or demand better. Simmons (1997) challenges each provider and consumer to take serious action to turn the tide of high health-care costs and poor-quality services. He reminds consumers that no other business in this country would be allowed to operate with such high expenses and quality problems. He questions, "Why do we continue to pay for and tolerate such poor care?" Groups such as the National Coalition on Health care advocate devising new approaches to deal with this costly problem. As more people become aware of the problems and believe they need a new look, consumer interests may force change.

THE COST OF QUALITY

Why is the cost of quality an important issue? Crosby (1979) states that the cost of quality is actually about the cost of "unquality," specifically in terms of waste. If there is a price for quality, how is it best understood and improved for saving resources and dollars? Two basic areas that affect the cost of quality are nonconformance and conformance.

The costs of *nonconformance* are the costs incurred by not having a quality product or service. Examples include the following:

- Rework (having to do work over because it was incorrect the first time)
- Scrap (having to discard the product because the work was substandard)
- Waiting (time wasted waiting for others to do work that affects one's own work)
- Downtime (incomplete product or service because of technology or machine breakdown)

Internal failures relate to the costs an organization incurs in scrap, rework, redesign, modification, overtime, corrective action, and downtime. External failures relate to the administrative cost of dealing with equipment failure and downtime and the subsequent loss of customer good will. When a product or service does not meet a standard and must be recalled or performed again, there can be increased costs in materials, human resource hours, or loss of customer loyalty. The product or service will actually cost more to rework than it would have cost to do it right the first time. This often means additional costs to the consumer as well as the provider, because costs are passed on. Crosby (1979) advocates doing things right the first time to save time, energy or effort, and money.

Nonconformance increases cost. When quality improves, cost is reduced.

The second cost of quality is *conformance*, or meeting requirements. The price tag for conformance is related to the following:

- Documentation, which includes producing paperwork and writing instructions
- Training
- Planning for prevention
- Inspection, which includes people, equipment, and other direct and indirect costs

Crosby (1979) advocates avoiding defects through planning, preparation, training, evaluation, and preventive maintenance. Conformance requires appraisal and measurement. These activities have their own cost.

Conformance is acting in accordance with a specified standard.

Some economic theorists believe that there is a minimum total quality cost that is the sum of costs for prevention, appraisal, and failure. Reducing any one of these elements will reduce the total cost. The key to achieving the minimum cost for quality is reaching a balance among the three elements. An example of balance is when reasonable prevention is employed, thereby reducing appraisal and failure. Unnecessary and excessive dollars spent on prevention measures alone can increase the total cost for the service or product provided above an acceptable level of cost or benefit. Such could happen if every American received immunizations for pneumonia when the disease primarily affects certain at-risk groups; the cost for this preventive measure in the total population would not be feasible compared to the benefit.

Godfrey (1999) states that for decades two ideas regarding quality have been under scrutiny. The first is the idea of *optimum quality*, or the point at which total quality costs are at a minimum. Much effort has been put into defining this elusive point. The second concept is that quality is a combination of prevention, appraisal, and internal and external failure. This concept became popular in the United States in the 1980s, when organizations began to realize savings by reducing the costs of each failure.

In the early 1990s, quality leaders questioned this approach, saying that minimizing quality costs can miss the point, which is minimizing the entire cost of production rather than any one subset of costs. This question arises when the organization moves to a focus on prevention costs, which soon becomes more accurately titled a focus on failure prevention and the total costs associated with it. Perhaps the best policy is to concentrate on the costs of failure, and justify the cost of preventive measures for one problem at a time (Godfrey, 1999).

 ## ECONOMIC ANALYSIS
PREVENTING MEDICATION ERRORS

Hospitals clearly want to minimize the impact of medication errors for patients. Elaborate automated medication delivery systems have been designed to provide the correct medications for patient use at the appropriate times. Some systems interface with charting systems to promote not only the accurate distribution of medications but also their correct charting. These elaborate systems for all units in the hospital have a very high initial cost for installation and training for use. In this situation economic analysis is critical because the monetary investment has to be examined relative to the large cost of major medication errors.

 ## AGENCIES ADDRESSING QUALITY AND COST IN HEALTH CARE

Addressing the concerns of cost and quality requires a multifaceted approach at both the local and national levels. Although most health-care providers or agencies have quality improvement processes in place to assist with this, certain groups have a more global charge. The agencies described in the following sections are well-defined, key groups that are currently monitoring and evaluating cost and quality in health care.

AGENCY FOR HEALTHCARE RESEARCH AND QUALITY (AHRQ)

Agency for Healthcare Research and Quality (AHRQ), formerly the Agency for Health Care Policy and Research (AHCPR), was established as the lead agency charged with supporting research to improve the quality of the US healthcare, reduce the cost, and improve access to needed services. The agency was established in December 1989 as part of the Omnibus Reconciliation Act of 1989 as part of the Department of Health and Human Services. There are 11 major divisions to achieve these objectives. Two key areas are the Center for Cost and Financing Studies and the Center for Quality Measurement and Improvement. The three strategic goals of the AHQR (1998) are as follows:

1. Support improvements in health outcomes
2. Strengthen quality measurement and improvement
3. Identify strategies to improve access, foster appropriate use, and reduce necessary expenditures

AHCPR (1995) issued an interim progress report to the National Advisory Council for Health Care Policy, Research, and Evaluation that addressed the impact on cost and quality of health-care services of research from the

AHCPR. The three main findings were that AHCPR products can and have reduced costs, that lower costs often mean higher quality, and that information can serve as a substitute for regulation.

ECONOMIC ANALYSIS
ADDRESSING COST AND QUALITY IN HEALTH CARE

The AHQR (1995) issued an interim progress report in 1995 to the National Advisory Council for Health Care Policy, Research, and Evaluation (10) that addressed the impact on cost and quality of health care services research from the AHQR. The three main findings were that AHQR products can (and have) reduced costs, that lower costs often mean higher quality, and that information can serve as a substitute for regulation.

Providers, payers, and health plans using AHQR recommendations reported cost savings and quality improvement. National cost savings from past research range up to $175 million per given condition. With cooperative providers, AHQR research can have a major effect of better and higher quality health care in the US. Assuming that specific findings only affected 1 in every 5 patients, cost and quality implications would include:

- Stroke prevention therapies could save $132 million dollars.
- Reduced use of acetaminophen could reduce kidney damage, saving $100-$140 million each year.
- Acute pain management protocols could shorten hospital length of stay, saving up to $81 million yearly with just hip replacement patients.

The Healthcare Research and Quality Act of 1999, signed by the President on December 6, 1999, reauthorized the AHCPR through the fiscal year 2005, or renewed the agency's original legislation. Changes include the renaming the agency and elimination of the requirement that this group continue to develop clinical guidelines. The agency is now charged with development of evidence-based reports and dissemination of these guidelines through the National Guideline Clearinghouse. More information about these changes is available on-line www.ahcpr.gov/news/ahrqfact.htm.

JOINT COMMISSION FOR ACCREDITATION OF HEALTHCARE ORGANIZATIONS

The Joint Commission for Accreditation of Healthcare Organizations (JCAHO) has developed its role to include new strategies for quality and performance improvement. JCAHO no longer mandates a specific model for accomplishing quality improvement. The expectation is that a model will include interdepartmental and interdisciplinary emphasis. JCAHO survey- ors assess both what the organization says it does and what it actually ac- complishes.

JCAHO has standards that address organizational performance in specific areas. The standards define maximum achievable expectations of perfor- mance relating to patient care and management. The components of the standard for improving organizational performance, for example, are plan- ning, designing, measuring, assessing, and improving. The definition of *per- formance* is doing things right and doing them well. The dimensions of per- formance that JCAHO addresses are efficacy, appropriateness, availability, timeliness, effectiveness, continuity, safety, efficiency, and respect and car- ing (Joint Commission for Accreditation of Healthcare Organizations, 1998).

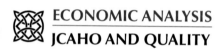

ECONOMIC ANALYSIS
JCAHO AND QUALITY

JCAHO strives to improve the quality of care for the public through ac- creditation and various related services that support performance im- provement in health-care organizations. One important part of perfor- mance improvement is making sure that quality data exist. If data quality is poor, health-care organizations risk making inadequate deci- sions based on inaccurate assumptions. This could result in inappro- priate, costly actions for the organization and the community at large. To be most useful, data should represent care and the outcomes of care in an accurate way. JCAHO expects data to be accurate, complete, and reported in a timely method.

JCAHO addresses principles for data quality control in the Joint Com- mission's Measurement Systems Attributes of Conformance. These attributes include validity and reliability, completeness, sampling method, outlier cases, data specification, internal and external stan- dards, auditability, monitoring process, documentation, feedback, edu- cation, and accountability. (For more information, see JCAHO's Web site, http://www.jcaho.org.)

NATIONAL COMMITTEE FOR QUALITY ASSURANCE

Another group active in evaluating health-care quality is the National Committee for Quality Assurance (NCQA). It is a private, nonprofit organization; the board of directors includes employers, health plans, quality experts, policy makers, consumers, labor representatives, and medical representatives. The mission of NCQA is to provide information on health-care quality in the marketplace, particularly to employers-purchasers and consumers. They strive to drive quality improvement and reward accountability in managed care (National Committee for Quality Assurance [NCQA], 1999).

NCQA encourages managed care health plans to focus on value and quality instead of pricing. The original activities of the organization were accreditation and performance improvement. They have recently expanded to accreditation of behavioral health-care organizations and physician organizations and verification of credentials.

NCQA studies confirm that public accountability, coupled with aggressive performance measurement, drives quality improvement.

NCQA offers an opportunity for standardized data comparison through the Health Plan Employer Data and Information Set (HEDIS). A national database called the Quality Compass is available through NCQA for HEDIS and accreditation information. It includes national and regional averages as well as benchmarks that set targets for quality improvement.

The NCQA released the third annual "State of Managed Care" report in 1999, documenting that healthcare plans who consistently practice public disclosure of quality indicators demonstrate steady improvement in these quality indicator measures. For example, the percentage of these health plans that used beta-blockers after a heart attack moved from 62.5 percent in 1996 to 79.9 percent in 1998 as a national average. Three-year public reports showed an even higher rate of use, 85 percent. It is believed that HEDIS has achieved these results by generating awareness of beta-blocker use as a proven way to save lives after a heart attack. The cost is relatively inexpensive compared with costs of treatment (NCQA, 1999).

In addition to clinical achievements, NCQA reported that a strong link exists between quality and customer satisfaction. Those plans with high scores in HEDIS Effectiveness of Care measures had consistently higher member satisfaction scores as well. Members remain with their plans when satisfied, which decreases administrative costs incurred in changing plans.

In summary, NCQA is a leader in managed care quality improvement, promoting accountability in health plans for quality, not just price.

OCCUPATIONAL SAFETY AND HEALTH ADMINISTRATION

The U.S. Department of Labor created the Occupational Safety and Health Administration (OSHA) to provide standards of safe practice in the workplace. OSHA is an important partner in risk and safety management, and likewise an important partner in quality improvement in health care. OSHA staff establish and enforce protective standards and provide consultation to 6.5 million employers with over 100 million workers. The vision of OSHA is "to be a world class leader in occupational safety and health, with a clear focus on protecting the safety and health of America's workers" (Occupational Safety and Health Administration [OSHA], 1999a). To achieve this vision, OSHA has three goals (OSHA, 1999b):

1. Improve workplace safety and health as evidenced by fewer hazards and reduced exposures, illnesses, and fatalities.
2. Change workplace culture to increase employer and worker awareness of, commitment to, and involvement with safety and health.
3. Secure public confidence through excellence in the development and delivery of OSHA's programs and services.

ECONOMIC ANALYSIS
OSHA REGULATION ON INDOOR AIR QUALITY AFFECTS HEALTH OF WORKERS

OSHA proposed a regulation in a 1994 *Federal Register* concerning poor-quality indoor air in the workplace. The OSHA document detailed the relevant effects of poor air quality in several categories, including irritation; pulmonary, reproductive, cardiovascular, and neurological effects; and cancer. Basically, breathing poor air can result in many health problems, including headaches, respiratory diseases, nausea, colds, influenza, Legionnaire's disease, and impaired judgment. Breathing tobacco smoke has been linked to heart disease, lung disease, low-birth-weight babies, cancer, and other illnesses (OSHA, 1999c). OSHA's role in investigating and monitoring indoor air quality in the workplace can save health-care dollars by preventing these adverse outcomes, can keep workers on the job with increased productivity when well, and can provide improved quality of work life.

NURSING FRAMEWORKS TO ASSESS QUALITY AND COST

Many individuals in the United States believe that high quality means high cost, or "you get what you pay for." Better products mean better crafting, which translates into more costly products. Although this stereotypical mindset is prevalent in our culture, health-care providers simply cannot afford the luxury of this delusion. One elementary economic principle that must constantly be remembered is that resources are limited and continuously shrinking.

Health-care providers are repeatedly challenged to examine the relationship between cost and quality. However, to do so these providers must become educated in the methodology used in assessing quality and its relationship to expense. This is critical for nurses as well.

Charles Hampden-Turner (1994) wrote extensively about the dilemma of cost versus quality. In his book *Charting the Corporate Mind*, he states that viewing quality versus cost as an either/or choice is disastrous for leaders today. Rather, as health-care providers, we must examine the phenomenon as quality *and* cost. Nursing must view cost and quality as one parallel entity rather than as two opposing entities.

Quality versus cost is not an either/or choice.

Because financial pressures have increased, attention to health-care costs and patient outcomes as the measures of the effectiveness of care delivery in health-care systems has increased. Determining nursing-specific outcomes by examining the impact of dependent and independent nursing interventions is essential.

Nursing researchers have attempted to determine the efficacy of nursing actions for a number of years. Aydelotte (1962) conducted a research study designed to demonstrate a causal relationship between nursing care and patient recovery as measured by "patient welfare." Eight years later, the Royal College of Nursing's study on nursing care attempted to develop a range of instruments and methods for studying the quality of nursing care (McFarlane, 1970). In the 1980s numerous studies were published that used outcome criteria. Nevertheless, the major difficulty has been in the establishment of valid and reliable outcome measures for determining the effectiveness of independent nursing actions.

However, some clinicians still function under the old belief that any consideration of cost is not ethical. Typically, it is argued that the clinician's responsibility is to provide the very best possible care for patients, ignoring the issue of the cost in clinical decisions. Yet health-care customers are no longer willing to accept this mode of practice and are requiring health-care providers to consider both quality and cost in rendering care.

As a profession, nursing is intimately involved with the financing and reimbursement issues associated with health care. Since the passing of the Balanced Budget Amendment in 1997, both nurse practitioners and clinical nurse specialists can receive direct reimbursement for services provided to Medicare beneficiaries. This reimbursement system is different from years past, when advanced practice nursing services could only be reimbursed through the billing of associated physicians. However, this reimbursement for nursing services is still governed by the regulations of individual states (see Chapter 1).

The Balanced Budget Amendment requires nurses to be more cognizant of their role in ensuring optimal quality at a reasonable cost. The challenge for nursing is to become more knowledgeable in this field as well as to develop a range of conceptual frameworks for practice that incorporate cost, quality, access, and outcomes. Nursing will continue to be under increased pressure to adopt more cost-effective treatment practices.

COST-EFFECTIVE NURSING CARE MODEL

The Nursing Role Effectiveness Model is one example that can be used to guide the assessment of the nurse's contribution to health care (Irvine, Sidani, & Hall, 1998). Based on the authoritative work of Donabedian (1980), this model focuses on the concepts of structure, process, and outcome related to quality (see Figure 14–1). Specifically, the model identifies four major areas that affect nursing's effectiveness: client health status, structure, nursing process, and outcome criteria.

Within each of the four domains are sets of variables that compose and define that domain. The first domain, client health status, addresses the characteristics and expectations of the client as he or she enters the health-care arena. Variables in this category include clinical and functional health status, expectation, and past cost. The client's clinical and functional health is described at the onset of care. Goals and expectations of care are then determined by the various reasons the individual pursues health care. Another variable in this domain is the past cost incurred by the individual for health care.

The second domain is structure, which addresses such variables as the characteristics of the nurse, the patient, and the organization. Nursing characteristics include nursing experience level, knowledge, and skill. Patient variables include the health-care recipient's age and physical functioning, the severity of the problem, and any comorbidities. Organizational vari-

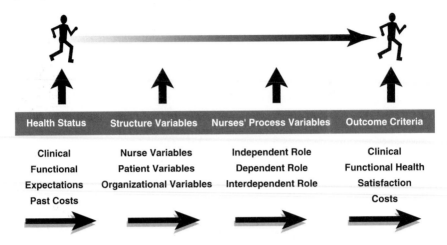

FIG. 14–1. The Nursing Role Effectiveness Model's application to quality improvement. (From Irvine, D., Sidani, S., & Hall, L. (1998). Finding value in nursing care: A framework for quality improvement and evaluation. *Nursing Economics, 16*(3), p. 112. Reprinted with permission of the publisher, Jannetti Publications, Inc.)

ables include staffing patterns, staff mix, nurse–patient ratios, and the type of nursing practice (team, primary, or modular nursing).

The nursing process category is the third domain and includes such factors as independent, dependent, and interdependent nursing roles. The creators of the model define the independent nursing role as performing those functions and responsibilities for which nurses (by profession and law) are accountable. The dependent role of the nurse concerns the execution of physician orders and treatments in a timely, accurate, and complete manner. Interdependent nursing roles involve activities that are partially or totally dependent on the actions and functions of other health providers. Examples of the interdependent nursing role include promoting and ensuring continuity of care and coordinated care.

The last domain is that of outcome criteria. The authors identified four variables associated with outcome: clinical outcomes, functional health, satisfaction, and cost. Six categories emerge from these variables:

1. Freedom from complications
2. Clinical outcomes, which include symptom relief
3. Functional health outcomes, such as self-care
4. Knowledge outcomes
5. Satisfaction
6. Cost outcomes

The model links patient and cost outcomes to the roles that nurses assume in health care. Specific nursing interventions, whether independent, interdependent, or dependent, can be examined for their impact on specific patient outcomes.The outcomes of independent nursing actions include symptom control, functional health status, knowledge, the self-care abilities of the patient and family, and the cost of providing care. The outcomes of dependent nursing actions relate to adverse events such as medication errors. The outcomes of interdependent nursing activities relate to team functioning and include outcomes such as effective interdisciplinary communication and coordination of care. Health-care team outcomes thus affect outcomes such as timely discharge, reduced length of stay, rehospitalization, and discharge costs.

Outcome criteria include four variables: clinical outcomes, functional health, satisfaction, and cost.

The application of this model for evaluating the effectiveness of nursing role performance and for guiding quality-improvement initiatives in various health-care settings is very promising. This conceptual model provides an efficient guide to selecting structure, process, and outcome indicators to consider in quality-improvement activities across many settings. The accompanying economic analysis gives an example of how the Nursing Role Effectiveness Model was used to guide quality improvement.

ECONOMIC ANALYSIS

 ## IMPLEMENTATION OF THE NURSING ROLE EFFECTIVENESS MODEL IN AN EMERGENCY DEPARTMENT

A team of nurses in the emergency department of a community hospital identified various problems related to lack of timely and complete assessment of febrile pediatric patients aged 2 years and younger. In their review of hospital records, they noted that no weight was recorded in the medical record for 30 percent of the patients. Obviously, this oversight could potentially lead to inappropriate antibiotic therapy because dosing is contingent on the child's age and weight.

The three outcomes identified by the nurses were as follows:

- Resolution of the fever, which was assessed within 48 hours of discharge from the emergency department through a telephone survey (clinical outcome)

- Patient or parent satisfaction with the care received in the emergency department (satisfaction outcome)
- Number of return visits to the emergency department for unresolved fever (cost outcome)

The emergency department staff closely examined the process flow from the time the patient registered in the emergency department until the time the child was seen and treated for the fever. The analysis revealed that the problem was organizational; that is, it originated in the coordination of care and communication between nursing professionals. In this analysis it became evident that the triage nurse conducted an initial assessment and then transferred the child with fever to a treatment room for further evaluation and treatment. The weight of the child was measured in the treatment room but was not consistently recorded.

The problem of delivering care was directly associated with the interdependent nursing role and could be resolved by refining the role responsibilities of the triage nurse. Once the roles of the staff registered nurse and triage nurse were clarified and changes in the triage and admission process were instituted to include having the child's weight measured and recorded in the triage area, the problem was quickly resolved. When clients' medical records were subsequently examined, the investigators found that the weight of the child was measured and documented for 100 percent of the patients examined. The remaining outcomes also met a satisfactory threshold when examined in the follow-up study (Irvine, Sidani, & Hall, 1998). The economic principles of balancing cost, quality, and effectiveness must be aggressively embraced by nursing when evaluating either new nursing interventions or existing nursing functions and activities.

COST-EFFECTIVE ANALYSIS

Another method used for evaluating the outcomes and costs of interventions designed to improve health is cost-effectiveness analysis (Stone, 1998). This methodology first appeared in the nursing literature in 1991 and has gained popularity for examining the cost outcomes of interventions and programs. The method includes such factors as the characteristics of the patient population, the decisions and possible alternatives, the degree of probabilities, the health benefits, and the estimated cost incurred by an intervention.

Cost-effectiveness analysis is the amount of benefit a treatment or intervention provides compared with alternatives. The concept of cost effectiveness assumes that resources for all services are limited and provides a measure of which service produces the highest benefit per dollar (Seigel, 1998).

For those grappling with increasing consumer demands and greater scarcity of resources, cost-effectiveness analysis is useful. Not only can this method of analysis aid in making decisions related to treatment and interventions, it can also aid policy makers to determine the allocation of resources and funding. Additionally, it allows better comparison between research studies that introduce various interventions for dealing with health-care issues (see Chapter 15).

Nurses need to become knowledgeable about cost analysis and to become experts in measuring and evaluating quality. Various professional organizations have been instrumental in establishing standards of care for their respective specialties. The purpose of such standards is to establish consumer safeguards and to direct nursing practice. Such standards are essential, and continued work in their development is ongoing. However, patient satisfaction is of equal importance as a measure of quality. Although consumers typically have marginal comprehension of professional standards, most have an opinion of what constitutes quality nursing care.

Patient satisfaction is an important indicator of quality care.

Evans, Martin, and Winslow (1998) report that patient satisfaction is a widely accepted indicator of quality care. A recent study completed by these researchers used a sample consisting of 1455 respondents from 2000 surveys collected over 9 months. Inpatient care surveys demonstrated that nursing care was the primary determinant of overall patient satisfaction. In the statistical analysis the beta coefficient was 0.61, whereas coefficients for other services were 0.09 or less. Nursing care in the outpatient setting was also seen as the major force in patient satisfaction. This result confirms studies done 15 years ago that reached the same conclusion: Nursing care is important to patient satisfaction as a dimension of quality care.

 ## VISION FOR THE FUTURE

In June 1998, the planning committee for the Forum for Health Care Quality Measurement and Reporting was initiated within the private sector to develop a comprehensive national plan for quality measurement, data collection, and reporting standards. The Department of Health and Human Services (DHHS, 1998) released a report entitled "The Challenge and Potential for Assuring Quality Health Care for the 21st Century." The report supports a national coordinated effort for quality improvement, such as the Forum.

The DHHS report points out that despite the many recent medical advances, 41 million Americans still remain uninsured. Also highlighted are the many quality problems of the current health-care system in the United States, including the following:

- Underuse of services, leading to additional complications and avoidable costs. Examples of underutilized services are screening processes such as Papanicolau tests and mammograms in women.
- Overuse of services, adding costs and sometimes leading to complications. An example is antibiotic treatment of the common cold, which leads to antibiotic-resistant microbes that could cost as much as $7.5 billion a year to expensive combat using more expensive drugs.
- Misuse of services, including missed diagnoses and unnecessary injury or death. One study showed that as many as 180,000 preventable deaths are caused by errors in hospital care.
- Variation of services across the United States, and even among regions and communities. For example, hospital discharge rates are 49 percent higher in the Northeast than in the West.

The DHHS report also highlights successful quality and cost improvement examples in the past decade (DHHS, 1998). For example, the New York State Department of Health released data that showed a reduction in cardiac bypass mortality by 50 percent over a 5-year period. A Michigan hospital reported an 80 percent reduction in drug reaction complications in a cardiac unit. A Boston asthma program decreased hospital visits by 86 percent and emergency department visits by 79 percent. In the United States in 1992, asthma brought some 468,000 people to the hospital, at an annual cost of $6.2 billion. The DHHS report concludes that poor-quality care results in sicker patients, increased disabilities, higher costs, and loss of trust from the public in the current health-care system.

U.S. PREVENTIVE SERVICES TASK FORCE

To decrease the costs of disease treatment and providers and to improve the quality of life, health promotion and disease prevention are of paramount importance. The Preventive Services Task Force was first initiated by the U.S. Public Health Service, but is now supported by the Agency for Health Care Policy and Research. It includes over 100 specialists from various disciplines and aspects of health care.

The U.S. Preventive Services Task Force released the second edition of its *Guide to Clinical Preventive Services* in 1995. The Task Force carefully reviewed over 6000 studies of 200 interventions for 70 diseases and conditions. In addition, the Task Force assessed 11 counseling topics (from prevention of household injuries to tobacco use), immunizations, and the use of aspirin and postmenopausal hormones to prevent disease.

The principal recommendations set forth in the *Guide* include encouraging physicians and nurses to provide frequent counseling on personal health habits, such as increasing physical activity and refraining from tobacco use. It recommends assessing individual risk factors and tailoring preventive care to the individual rather than just providing standardized counseling at annual check-ups. An important part of care provision is giving prevention information at every encounter, especially for high-risk populations who may not use clinicians on a regular basis. Another part is mutual goal setting and shared decision making between the health-care provider and the consumer in order to allow for personal preferences whenever possible.

The Task Force recommends counseling to prevent tobacco use in children, adolescents, and young adults, as well as offering guidance to those who desire to stop smoking. One in every five deaths in the United States is attributable to tobacco use, making it the most important preventable cause of premature deaths. Treatment for diseases associated with tobacco use is costly and preventable.

Another preventive measure is screening for colorectal cancer in persons older than 50, because colorectal cancer causes 55,000 deaths per year; colorectal cancer is the second most common form of cancer in the United States. Breast cancer is one of the leading causes of cancer in women; over 46,000 cases are reported annually. The Task Force recommends routine mammography and clinical breast examinations as a way to reduce these deaths. Health-care providers are also urged to encourage self-examination as a preventive measure.

The Task Force recommends screening for high cholesterol and other lipid abnormalities, especially in the older adult population and in young adults with coronary risk factors such as diabetes, high blood pressure, and family history. It also points out that screening for chlamydia infections in sexually active females could decrease the incidence of pelvic inflammatory disease by 50 percent. Other adverse and costly results of chlamydia infections include infertility and ectopic pregnancy.

These are just a few of the many recommendations concerning disease prevention and health promotion that have been made by the U.S. Preventive Services Task Force. The challenge is to implement these recommendations consistently in the practices of physicians and nurses across the United States and to motivate consumers to choose healthier lifestyles. These measures can prevent disease, disabilities, and death, thus resulting in improved quality of life and decreased associated health-care costs.

DISEASE MANAGEMENT

Disease management programs are touted as saving health-care dollars as well as improving the quality of life for health-care consumers. These programs are designed to provide proactive, integrated care and are targeted at those with risks, such as patients with chronic illnesses or those likely to experience a catastrophic outcome. These programs are of intense interest for managed care plans, which must provide costly care for high-risk, high-cost patients. Basically, disease management programs are aimed at health care's most costly patients. The goal is to keep patients well, or at least well managed, early in the disease process by preventive measures and by minimizing crises. This can be positive for patients and a good cost management strategy for providers (Marietti, 1999).

> *Disease management is established to coordinate care and maintain function for selected patients with costly diagnoses.*

Government agencies are taking a lead in developing disease management initiatives. An example of this is the Asthma Management Model, developed by an international panel of experts brought together in 1997 by the National Asthma Education and Prevention Program of the U.S. National Heart, Lung, and Blood Institute. An information system tool analyzes clinical problems and long-term effects associated with asthma. The system allows scientific-based decision making using evidence-based medicine in asthma management. The program has three components: research, education, and communication. The Asthma Management Model System has a Web site (*http://www.nhlbisupport.com/asthma/index.html*) that is continuously updated to provide clinicians with current information related to asthma treatment.

 ECONOMIC ANALYSIS
STROKE TREATMENT RESULTS IN COST SAVINGS

The National Institute of Neurological Disorders and Stroke (NINDS) is an institute that supports and conducts clinical investigations as part of the National Institutes of Health. It is a principal supporter of brain and nervous system research in this country, where about 700,000 people suffer strokes each year. Stroke is the third leading cause of death in the United States and the leading cause of adult disability, and carries a price tag of more than $40 billion each year.

Results from a study sponsored by NINDS demonstrate that treating patients with acute ischemic stroke with a clot-busting drug called tissue-type plasminogen activator (tPA) could result in substantial net cost savings to the U.S. health-care system (National Institute of Neurological Disorders and Stroke, 1998). For 1000 patients taking tPA, the estimated increase in hospital costs was $1.7 million. Treatment with the drug saves $4.8 million in nursing-home costs and $1.3 million in rehabilitation services, resulting in an overall net cost savings of $4 million for every 1000 patients. The potential cost savings for all stroke patients in the United States who are eligible for tPA treatment is estimated to be in excess of $100 million. This study is important because it not only addresses cost but also quality of life, which can be improved by decreased disability.

SUMMARY

In a recent interview, 94-year-old quality guru Joseph M. Juran was asked what industries could benefit most from adopting quality improvement principles. His response included "these enormous industries—government, health care, and academia" (Patton, 1999, p. 40). Health-care improvement in quality and cost management relates to all three areas. Juran further stated that certain major industries have "islands of excellence amid continents of mediocrity. . . . [T]hat's encouraging because the fact that there are islands of excellence means that it can be done" (Patton, 1999, p. 42).

As leaders look at the diverse data that support quality improvement in health care and reduction of health-care costs, there is encouraging evidence that these desired outcomes are possible. These outcomes can be actualized by concern and collaboration from the public and private sectors, from managed care health plans, from consumer groups, and from diverse provider disciplines.

Nurses have a major role in improving the quality of health care and in decreasing costs as practitioners, educators, researchers, and administrators. Numerous opportunities await the nursing profession as it understands the interconnected role of cost and quality and embraces measures to improve both.

DISCUSSION QUESTIONS

1. What are the current economic and quality concerns facing the U.S. health-care system today? Discuss consumer concerns as well as those raised by groups such as the National Coalition on Health Care.
2. Generally, it is believed that when quality improves, cost is reduced. Do you agree or disagree? Explain.
3. Discuss the basic factors that affect the cost of quality.
4. Name and discuss four national groups that are addressing cost and quality. Explain the role of each.
5. What are the nursing implications of cost and quality in health care? What are some recognized approaches?
6. Describe implications for addressing cost and quality for the future of health-care. Give examples where agencies or groups are making a difference in cost and quality improvement.

 REFERENCES

Agency for Health Care Policy and Research. (1995, September). *Better quality can cost less: The evolving role of* AHCPR. [online] Available: http://www.ahcpr.gov/about/quality.htm.

Agency for Health Care Policy and Research. (1996). *Americans as health care consumers: The role of quality information* [Highlights of a national survey]. Rockville, MD: Author. Available: http://www.ahcpr.gov/qual/kffhigh.htm.

Agency for Health Care Policy and Research. (1998, December). AHCPR *strategic plan.* Rockville, MD: Author. Available: http://www.ahcpr.gov/about/stratpln.htm.

Aydelotte, M. K. (1962). The use of patient welfare as a criterion measure. *Nursing Research,* 11(1), 10–14.

Crosby, P. B. (1979). *Quality is free: The art of making quality certain.* New York: McGraw-Hill.

Department of Health and Human Services. (1998). *The challenge and potential for assuring quality health care for the 21st century.* [online] Available: http://www.ahcpr.gov/qual/21stcena.htm.

Donabedian, A. (1980). *Exploration in quality assessment and monitoring: The definition of quality and approaches to assessment.* Ann Arbor, MI: Health Administration Press.

Evans, M. L., Martin, M. L., & Winslow, E. H. (1998). Nursing care and patient satisfaction. *American Journal of Nursing,* 98(12), 57–59.

Godfrey, A. B (1999). Quality management: Cost of quality revisited [On-line]. *Quality Digest.* Available: http://www.qualitydigest.com/apr/godfrey.html.

Hampden-Turner, C. (1994). *Charting the corporate mind: From dilemma to strategy.* Cambridge, MA: Blackwell.

Irvine, D., Sidani, S., & Hall, L. (1998). Finding value in nursing care: A framework for quality improvement and clinical evaluation. *Nursing Economics,* 16(3), 110–116.

Joint Commission on Accreditation of Healthcare Organizations. (1998). *Comprehensive accreditation manual for home care.* Chicago: Author.

Marietti, C. (1999). Seize the disease: Keep them well. *Health Informatics,* 16(3), 50.

McFarlane, J. K. (1970). Study of nursing—the first two years of a research project. *International Nursing Review,* 17(2), 101–109.

National Coalition on Health Care. (1999a). *Consumers lose confidence in health care system* [Press release]. [online] Available: http.//www.nchc.org/confidence.html.

National Coalition on Health Care. (1999b). *Key findings on quality of care in the United States.* [online] Available: http://www.nchc.org/emerge/keyquality.html.

National Committee for Quality Assurance. (1999). NCQA: *An overview.* [online] Available: http://www.ncqa/Pages/Main/overview3.htm.

National Institute of Neurological Disorders and Stroke. (1998, April 22). *New stroke treatment likely to decrease health care costs and increase quality of life.* [online] Available: http://www.aomc.org/NewsRelease/StrokeTreatment.

Occupational Safety and Health Administration. (1999a). *OSHA's mission: Over 100 million workers count on OSHA.* [online] Available: http://www.osha.gov/oshinfo/mission.html.

Occupational Safety and Health Administration. (1999b). A *high impact agency: Goals for the year 2000.* [online] Available: http://www.osha.gov/oshinfo/1pger1.html.

Occupational Safety and Health Administration. (1999c). *Indoor air quality.* [online] Available: http://www.osha-slc.gov/FedReg_osha_data/FED19940405.html.

Patton, S. C. (1999). A century of quality: An interview with quality legend Joseph M. Juran. *Quality Digest* 19(2), 40–42.

Seigel, J. E. (1998). Cost effectiveness analysis and nursing research—is there a fit? *Image: Journal of Nursing Scholarship,* 30(3), 221–222.

Simmons, H. (1997). *The state of our nation's health care system, a reality check.* Paper presented at the National Conference of State Legislatures annual meeting, Scottsdale, AZ. [online] Available: http://www.nchc.org/speech3.html.

Stone, P. (1998). Methods for conducting and reporting cost-effectiveness analysis in nursing. *Image: Journal of Nursing Scholarship,* 30(3), 229–234.

U.S. Preventive Services Task Force. (1995). *Guide to clinical preventive services* (2nd ed.) Washington, DC: U.S. Department of Health and Human Services, Office of Public Health and Science, Office of Disease Prevention and Health Promotion.

 ## SUGGESTED READING

Cherry, B., & Jacob, S. (1999). *Contemporary nursing: Issues, trends, and management.* St. Louis: Mosby.

Griffiths, P. (1995). Progress in measuring nursing outcomes. *Journal of Advanced Nursing,* 21(6), 1092–1100.

Koch, M., & Fairly, T. (1993). *Integrated quality management: The key to improving nursing care quality.* St. Louis: Mosby.

Nunnery, R. K. (1997). *Advancing your career: Concepts of professional nursing.* Philadelphia: FA Davis.

Price, S., Koch, M., & Bassett, S. (1998). *Health care resource management: Present and future challenges.* St. Louis: Mosby.

Tappen, R. M. (1995). *Nursing leadership and management: Concepts and practice.* Philadelphia: FA Davis.

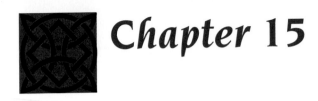

Chapter 15

Clinical Economic Analysis

Cyril F. Chang
William Robert Bartlett, Jr.

LEARNING OBJECTIVES

■ Introduce the concept of clinical economic analysis.
■ Discuss the importance of cost-identification analysis and provide nursing examples.
■ Examine the underlying theory of cost-benefit analysis and discuss the information needed for a successful cost-benefit analysis.
■ Define cost-effectiveness analysis and distinguish between cost-benefit analysis and cost-effectiveness analysis.
■ Discuss what costs and benefits should be included in health-care analyses and how to accurately measure them in evaluating health-care interventions.
■ Explore nursing examples of cost-identification, cost-benefit, and cost-effectiveness analyses.

Nurses and other health-care workers in the course of their work make decisions that affect the care of their patients. Many also participate in research and consulting projects in which they make decisions and recommendations on such clinical and public health questions as the following:

- Should scarce nursing personnel in a local public health department be set aside for home visits to deliver prenatal care to underserved pregnant women?
- Should nurse clinicians screen every patient who walks into a clinic for hypertension and elevated cholesterol levels?
- Should nurses spend time delivering smoking cessation messages to every cigarette smoker with whom they come into contact?

These and other decisions that nurses make can influence the health of a large number of people. But they also involve costs because the time spent performing these tasks cannot be dedicated to other useful purposes. Decisions must therefore be made in such a way as to use nurses' time and other health-care resources efficiently in order to deliver the best possible outcomes for the largest number of people.

THE SIGNIFICANCE OF ECONOMIC EVALUATION

In the past, health-care workers made medical decisions without paying much attention to economics. The primary concern when making decisions was whether the prescribed treatment or recommended course of action was prudent, beneficial, and necessary. Sometimes, providers took into consideration the wishes and preferences of patients and their families. But the overriding concern was always how well a procedure or treatment would work and whether the health benefits outweighed the inherent risks of treatment for an individual patient.

The persistent high cost of health care has made it clear that medical decisions cannot continue to be made solely on the basis of clinical considerations. Today, with health care being increasingly delivered on a fixed budget under managed care, health-care workers are being asked to make decisions that produce clinical benefits that are worth their cost. It is therefore essential that nurses and other health-care workers who share decision making with physicians recognize not only the health consequences but also the economic consequences of their actions.

Over the years, nurses have primarily been concerned with the health and welfare of their patients. In today's cost-conscious health-care environment, however, it is not enough to merely deliver health services that benefit patients. The services delivered must produce more benefits than costs than any alternative way of using the same resources. In other words, the services must be cost effective. This chapter introduces the concept of clinical economics and the three types of analyses useful for health-care decision making: cost-identification analysis, cost-benefit analysis, and cost-effectiveness analysis. These analyses will equip nurses with the necessary economic principles for making decisions that deliver the best health outcomes with limited resources.

 ## CLINICAL ECONOMICS

Clinical economics is a particular type of economic evaluation that assists in health-care decision making by assessing the relative merits of alternative courses of medical action or interventions. The underlying belief of clinical economics is that resources are scarce and should be allocated in such a way as to maximize the improvement in life and health for the general population. To achieve this goal, the following question is asked: Is this procedure, service, or program worth undertaking knowing that the resources involved will not be available for other things that are also beneficial?

Clinical economics involves economic evaluations of health interventions that assess the relative merit of alternative courses of action to assist in decision making.

Nurse clinicians, administrators, and researchers are routinely confronted with the need to choose among different ways of performing their tasks. Awareness of the concepts and principles for evaluating the available options and the tradeoffs involved is the key to delivering maximized health outcomes. In other words, concepts of clinical economics and their applications should be an integral part of the formal and informal decision-making processes in nursing research and practice (Chang and Henry, 1999).

A first issue to be settled in an economic evaluation is what analytical technique to use for evaluating a particular health-care intervention or program. Table 15–1 shows the three commonly used techniques in clinical economic evaluation: cost-identification analysis, cost-benefit analysis, and cost-effectiveness analysis.

Nurses who evaluate and communicate the value of their care will find that the three major methods of economic evaluation, though all useful in their own ways, have their strengths and weaknesses. Knowing what each of the three methods does, and its relative advantages and disadvantages, is critical for choosing the best analytical tool for the problem at hand.

 ## COST-IDENTIFICATION ANALYSIS

Cost-identification analysis tries to answer an important and straightforward question: How much does it cost? This question is answered by a thorough identification of the direct and indirect costs involved in a medical treatment or intervention.

Cost-identification analysis addresses the question of how much something costs.

For example, Eisenberg and Kitz (1986) used cost-identification analysis to document the cost savings from early hospital discharge of patients with osteomyelitis. They estimated that the total cost of care for conventional inpatient treatment was $2781. In comparison, the total cost of care using early discharge followed by outpatient antibiotic treatment was $2271. The potential total savings with an early discharge program were estimated to be $510 per patient based on this cost-identification study.

TABLE 15–1. THE THREE TYPES OF ANALYSIS IN CLINICAL ECONOMICS

	Cost-Identification Analysis	Cost-Benefit Analysis	Cost-Effectiveness Analysis
Definition	Determination and comparison of the dollar costs of different programs or procedures	Determination of whether the dollar value of benefits of a program or procedure outweighs its dollar costs	Determination of dollar cost per unit of outcome
Main use	To compare alternative options that produce the same or very similar outcomes with equal effectiveness	To evaluate programs that produce multiple outcomes (e.g., health outcomes plus quality-of-life improvement) or to compare programs that produce different types of outcomes (children's health vs. health benefits for older adults)	To compare alternative programs or procedures that produce the same or very similar type of outcomes but with unequal effectiveness and costs
Examples	Prenatal care delivered by nurse midwives and physicians who produce equal outcomes	A nurse-led intervention program for improving the quality of life and health outcomes for post-transplantation patients	The cost effectiveness of alternative smoking cessation programs, such as physician advice vs. advice plus pharmaceutical agents
Outcome measurement	No measurement necessary	Outcomes measured or valued in dollars	Outcomes measured in natural units such as number of lives saved or life-years gained
Results	Cost minimization	Maximum net benefits in excess of costs	Lowest cost per unit of outcome or greatest incremental benefits in excess of incremental costs
Formula	None	$NB = B - C$	C/E ratio
Type of projects	Clinical trials of new procedures or treatment options	A wide array of public projects, including health care, education, national defense, and public investment projects such as space exploration, highways, and dams	Clinical trials of new or experimental procedures or treatment options

Cost-identification analysis has also been used in determining the costs of health care and the financial burden of injuries and diseases. For example, Leigh and associates (1997) examined and estimated the annual incidence, mortality, and direct and indirect costs associated with occupational injuries and illnesses in the United States. They estimated that in the civilian American workforce, approximately 6500 job-related deaths from injury, 13.2 million nonfatal injuries, 60,300 deaths from job-related disease, and 862,200 illnesses occurred annually. In monetary terms, the total direct costs and indirect costs associated with occupational injuries and illnesses were estimated to be $65 billion and $106 billion, respectively.

ECONOMIC ANALYSIS
A NURSING APPLICATION OF COST-IDENTIFICATION ANALYSIS

Total parenteral nutrition (TPN) has traditionally been viewed as medical therapy that requires hospitalization, even in medically stable patients, because of the potential complications of infection, hyperglycemia, fluid and electrolyte imbalance, or air embolus. As managed care and capitated payment mechanisms force hospitals to operate in a more cost-effective manner, however, TPN and other therapies are being moved to the home environment for multidisciplinary management.

Curtas, Hariri, and Steiger (1996) used cost-identification analysis to study the cost of a nurse-led home TPN program. They reported the direct personnel costs of providing nutrition support in patients' homes to be $1982 per patient per year. However, when indirect personnel costs and the costs of furnishings and space were included, the service became more expensive, rising to $2070 per patient per year.

Currently, most of the costs of providing home TPN support are not reimbursable by third-party payers. By presenting reliable cost estimates and evidence supporting the value of services provided by a nurse-led home TPN team, this cost-identification analysis makes a compelling argument for third-party reimbursement for such services.

In addition to the systematic identification and estimation of costs, cost-identification analysis can be used to evaluate the relative merits of competing or alternative health interventions or procedures. For this purpose, however, cost identification should be undertaken only if there is reason to believe that the outcomes of the different procedures or interventions under consideration are the same. When the outcomes are the same, the intervention with the lowest total cost is the recommended one. Thus, cost-identification analysis is also referred to as *cost-minimization analysis*.

When outcomes are not similar, however, the intervention with the lowest cost may not be the most desirable choice. The lowest-cost option, although apparently saving money, may be so inefficient or ineffective that it is actually very expensive when the money spent is compared with the outcome achieved. In fact, the higher-cost alternative may be less expensive considering the greater quantity or better quality of health outcomes that it can deliver. In instances in which the outcomes of alternative courses of action are dissimilar, the decision should instead be based on the results of a cost-benefit analysis that takes into consideration both costs and outcomes.

 ## COST-BENEFIT ANALYSIS

Cost-benefit analysis is the most widely known form of economic and public policy evaluation. Developed over 50 years ago, it was used extensively in the 1930s during the Great Depression for public decision making in connection with flood control projects. Over time, cost-benefit analysis has been used with impressive results in a wide range of applications in such diverse fields as national defense, education, and health care.

> *Cost-benefit analysis provides information on the costs of resources used by a program compared with the benefits that the program creates.*

The term *cost-benefit analysis* has frequently been used incorrectly as a catchall term for cost-identification, cost-benefit, and cost-effectiveness analyses. It is more appropriate to use the name of the specific analysis method; for a comparison of the definitions, main uses, and other differences and similarities of these three methods, see Table 15–1.

Specifically, *cost-benefit analysis* refers to a form of economic evaluation that places monetary values on both the inputs and the outputs of a procedure, project, or program. *Inputs* are the resources and other factors used in carrying out a procedure or project, such as equipment and the providers' time. *Outputs* are the end results or outcomes. Economists use cost-benefit analysis to compare the dollar costs of the inputs used in delivering the service with the dollar value placed on the outcomes resulting from the service. This analysis is used mostly for comparing the relative merits of procedures or projects that are designed to achieve very different outcomes.

Inputs in economics are the manpower, materials, and equipment used in the production of outputs or delivery of services.

Outputs are the end products of a production process or the results of a procedure.

For example, public health officials are frequently presented with an array of projects to pursue. Some projects attempt to prevent childhood diseases through inoculation of infants, whereas others attempt to control pollution to improve the quality of air and water. The information generated from a cost-benefit analysis can assist both in choosing what projects to fund and in deciding how much to spend on each.

Another example of a situation in which cost-benefit analysis is useful is a nursing college facing a choice between funding an open house for high school seniors considering a career in nursing or funding training seminars for clinical specialists. The two projects serve different purposes, but the college has funds to support only one project. A cost-benefit analysis of the two competing projects can provide helpful information for this decision.

COST-BENEFIT FORMULAS

The basis of the cost-benefit analysis is simple: determining whether the benefits of a particular project outweigh its costs. If decision makers consistently choose only those projects that produce a surplus of benefits over costs, maximum investment returns can be achieved. To illustrate, consider the concept of net benefits to be defined as follows:

$$NB = B - C$$

In this formula, NB represents the expected net benefits of a project, B the expected total benefits from that project, and C the expected total costs.

Suppose three public health programs—a breast cancer screening program for adult women, a nutrition program for school-aged children, and an antismoking program for adolescents—are presented for funding. Suppose, too, that all three of the programs have been shown to be effective in achieving their intended objectives. A cost-benefit analysis can be applied to estimate the total benefits and costs of the three competing programs to determine the net benefits of each. An estimation of net benefits in terms of a common unit, dollars, makes it possible to discern whether a particular project generates greater net benefits for society than competing projects.

ECONOMIC ANALYSIS
A NURSING APPLICATION OF COST-BENEFIT ANALYSIS

Shared governance is one of the key strategies promoted by nursing scholars and executives for retention of professional nurses and enhancement of nursing autonomy and independence. In a case study of such a strategy, DeBaca, Jones, and Tornabeni (1993) applied cost-benefit analysis to a shared governance model at a short-term community hospital in San Diego over a 5-year period.

The shared governance program at the hospital began in 1988. The program's underlying philosophy was to support clinical practice using the principle of participatory management. A cost-benefit analysis was subsequently conducted by identifying and measuring both the direct and the indirect costs of the program and the direct benefits (cost savings) as well as the intangible, nonpecuniary benefits to the organization and the nursing staff. The total program costs over a 5-year period were $649,327. However, because of the elimination of administrative positions and other cost-saving measures made possible after nurses had gained greater autonomy and independence, the 5-year cumulative savings amounted to $5,837,126. The authors concluded that the hospital had more than recovered its financial investment by using the shared governance management strategy.

Frequently, the cost-benefit criterion is expressed as a ratio of total benefits to total costs (B/C) and not as net benefits (NB) in dollars. The main advantage of using the cost-benefit ratio to evaluate competing projects is that projects that are smaller in scale can be compared objectively with larger ones without being overwhelmed by the total dollar values that are typically associated with the latter projects.

A cost-benefit ratio is measured by dividing the total benefits of a project by its total costs.

This advantage can also be a disadvantage, however, because the ratio alone conveys some misleading information. For example, a small project in dollar terms may have an impressively high cost-benefit ratio. At first glance, it compares favorably with a larger project with a lower cost-benefit ratio. However, the larger project may be more attractive if funds are available because it brings about greater total net benefits than the small project. The ratio approach can also be misleading when its application involves a reduction of treatment or remedy costs that otherwise must be incurred in the absence of the project. The reduction in treatment costs can be treated either as an increase in program benefits (B) or a reduction in cost (C), but these approaches result in very different B/C ratios.

For example, an occupational injury prevention program may reduce the medical treatment costs associated with work-related incidents of injuries and illnesses by $100 million a year. The avoided treatment costs can be treated either as a part of the project's benefits (which increases the size of B) or as a reduction of the program's total costs (which increases the size of C). The former method raises the B/C ratio whereas the latter lowers the B/C ratio, resulting in very different conclusions regarding the worthiness of the project.

MEASURING COSTS AND BENEFITS

In carrying out a cost-benefit analysis, a series of three practical questions must be answered first: Which costs should be included in the cost-benefit calculation? Which benefits should be included? and How should future costs and benefits be treated?

Which Costs Should Be Included?

The answer to the first question depends in part on the perspective on which the cost-benefit analysis is based. The recommendation from the authoritative Panel on Cost-Effectiveness in Health and Medicine (a panel of experts on appropriate methods for standardizing the conduct of clinical economic evaluations convened by the U.S. Public Health Services in 1993) is to take the broadest perspective—namely, that of society as a whole (Russell et al., 1996). Accordingly, the three categories of costs that must be included are costs for health services, costs borne by patients and their families, and external costs borne by the rest of society (Robinson, 1993a).

Health-Service Costs. The first category of costs is payments for ambulatory services, hospital services, home-health-care visits, long-term care services, and medical supplies and drugs. In economic terms, these are the direct costs of providing health care.

These health-services costs can be divided into two types depending on whether the cost item has a tendency to vary with level of activity. The first type, *variable costs*, includes payments for most physician services, medical supplies, and drugs. Other examples of variable costs include the costs of hiring part-time nurses for the summer peak season and the costs of medical supplies that fluctuate with patient volume. The second type, *fixed costs*, includes most capital costs, such as maintenance and depreciation of buildings and equipment, and heating and lighting that must be used regardless of whether the hospital or clinic is fully occupied or not.

> *Variable costs are those that vary with the number of patients treated in a health-care facility.*

> *Fixed costs are those that do not change with patient volume.*

Costs Borne by Patients and Their Families. The third category of costs includes out-of-pocket expenses not covered by insurance and any costs in connection with caring activities that are borne by patients and their families, such as travel costs. These are all direct costs. In addition, there are indirect costs such as lost leisure time, foregone wages and salaries because of absence from work by the patients and family members who provide care, and psychological stress and suffering.

External Costs. Many public health programs, in addition to their direct costs of operation, impose costs on the rest of society. For example, public health and product safety regulations such as pollution control measures and food safety standards cost taxpayers money to enforce. They also increase the manufacturing costs and, eventually, the prices of consumer goods because it costs money to comply with the new rules and regulations and this cost is passed on to the consumer. These compliance costs are the indirect costs, which should be added to the direct costs to fully account for the resources involved in enforcing a public health or product safety program.

Which Benefits Should Be Included?

Let us now concentrate on the task of estimating the benefits associated with a given health-care decision. Health economists Santerre and Neun (2000) suggested that health-care benefits fall into four broad categories:

1. The medical costs diverted because an illness is prevented
2. The monetary value of the loss in production diverted because death is postponed
3. The monetary value of the potential loss in production saved because good health is restored
4. The monetary value of the loss in satisfaction or utility averted because of a continuation of life and better health

Of the four categories of benefits, the first is the most direct and easiest to estimate whereas the last is the most indirect and most difficult to quantify. The first benefit involves the identification of the direct medical costs that would have been incurred had the medical treatment or intervention not been implemented. The next two benefits involve an estimation of both the direct and would-be monetary losses in goods and services caused by an absence from work or lower productivity because of ill health. The last category of benefits is the monetary value of the pleasure and satisfaction derived from longer life and better health. In practice, this category is frequently ignored in cost-benefit analyses because verification of satisfaction is difficult. Most researchers simply estimate the first three types of benefits and use the results as a lower-bound estimate of total benefits.

How Should Future Benefits and Costs Be Treated?

Most health projects incur costs over a long period of time and yield benefits accruing many years in the future. For example, treatment for hypertension incurs costs regularly over many years. The benefits of such treatment, such as decreased likelihood of renal and heart diseases or stroke, also occur many years later in the form of avoidance of costly and invasive treatments.

In economics, it is generally accepted that a dollar today is more valuable than a dollar in the distant future. This is a reflection of the existence of time preference of money. Thus, the costs and benefits that will occur in the future must be *discounted* to their current values so that future benefits and costs will not be weighed as much as dollars spent or saved today.

Discounting is a method used to calculate the present values of a stream of future benefits or costs.

Discounting. Economists use the method of discounting to convert future benefits and costs to their present values. When future benefits and costs are discounted, the net benefits of a proposed project can be rewritten as follows:

$$NPB = \sum_{t=1}^{N} \frac{B_t - C_t}{(1 + r)}, \quad t = 1, 2, \ldots, N$$

In this formula, B_t and C_t are the expected benefits and costs in year t, r is the discount rate, and N is the total lifespan of the project in years. Expressed in present value terms, the net present benefits (NPB) of a project that is expected to generate benefits and costs for N years is defined as the sum of a stream of future net benefits discounted to their equivalent present values.

For example, a local health project that targets public housing residents has been estimated to generate $10,000 worth of benefits annually at a cost of $5000 in each of the 2 years the project has been in existence. The net benefits without discounting are $5000 per year, or $10,000 for the 2-year life of the project. But the net present value of the project using a discount rate of 5 percent is smaller:

$$NPB = \frac{(\$10,000 - \$5,000)}{(1 + 0.05)^1} + \frac{(\$10,000 - \$5,000)}{(1 + 0.05)^2} = \$9,297.05$$

This result means that the present value of the project's net benefits is $9297.05 rather than the cumulative amount of $10,000.

The Discount Rate. The previous formulas show that in addition to expected benefits and costs, a third variable, the discount rate, helps determine the relative merits of various health projects under consideration. Operationally, the lower the discount rate, the higher the expected net benefits are likely to be, and vice versa.

What is an appropriate discount rate for evaluating health projects? For cost-benefit analyses for government programs, the Office of Management and Budget (1994) recommended a discount rate of 7 percent because it is "a rate that approximates the pretax rate of return on an average investment in the private sector in recent years" (p. 9). For clinical cost-benefit analyses, the Panel on Cost-Effectiveness in Health and Medicine preferred a real annual rate of 3 percent (Gold et al., 1996). However, recognizing the widespread use of the traditional discount rate of 5 percent in health and medicine, the final recommendation of the Panel of Cost-Effectiveness in Health and Medicine was that future research should "conduct base-case analysis and critical sensitivity analyses using 5% as well as 3%" (Gold et al., 1996, p. 233).

Inflation. For projects that extend over many years, the effect of inflation must be taken into account in a cost-benefit analysis. Economic evaluation relies heavily on data drawn from financial statements and accounting records. These data on the revenues, expenses, assets, liabilities, and net incomes of a project are all measured in dollar terms. With inflation, however, a dollar may be worth substantially less 5 years from now than it is worth today. In other words, the purchasing power of dollars declines over time because of inflation. This presents a problem to cost-benefit analysis because a dollar of benefits or costs varies in worth at different points in time.

Inflation refers to substantial and sustained increases in the general price level that make goods and services everywhere in a country more expensive than before.

To control for the declining purchasing power of the dollar, economists convert the dollar amounts of expenditures and expenses originally recorded in accounting books and financial records into *real* or *constant* dollars. This is accomplished by dividing (deflating) the current dollar amounts by the consumer price index (CPI) compiled and published by the U.S. Bureau of the Census. For example, the CPI for 1996 is 157 for all urban consumers, and the CPI for the base period 1982–1984 is 100. Thus, $1 million worth of benefits or costs in 1996 is equivalent to $0.637 million (|$1 million/157|) 2100 in real or constant 1982–1984 dollars. When all costs and benefits from different years are expressed in terms of the dollars of the same base period, the effects of inflation no longer distort the true values of costs and benefits.

 ## COST-EFFECTIVENESS ANALYSIS

A major drawback of cost-benefit analysis is the difficulty involved in placing monetary values on the benefits of health-care interventions. This problem becomes obvious when quality-of-life issues and human lives are involved in the estimation because it is difficult, if not impossible, to put a dollar value on a human life. Cost-effectiveness analysis can avoid this problem.

Cost-effectiveness analysis evaluates competing programs that are designed to achieve the same or similar objective.

Cost-effectiveness analysis represents a more modest and manageable approach than cost-benefit analysis. It is used to evaluate competing programs that are designed to achieve the same or similar objectives. Because the program outputs are assumed to be the same, attention is focused on the identification and estimation of program costs, thus avoiding many of the difficulties of benefits estimation. For example, both physicians and nurse midwives can provide routine prenatal care, but the costs and effectiveness may be very different. Cost-effectiveness analysis can be used to evaluate the relative merits of the two types of health-care providers who can serve the needs of the same group of patients.

However, this very advantage is also the disadvantage of cost-effectiveness analysis. For example, cost-effectiveness analysis is unsuited for evaluating programs that produce multiple outcomes (e.g., a nurse-led intervention program that improves health outcomes as well as quality of life for post-transplantation patients). It is also inappropriate for comparing programs that produce different types of outcomes (e.g., home visits by public health nurses to pregnant women in low-income neighborhoods versus a community-based violence prevention program to improve quality of life and personal safety for community residents).

THE C/E RATIO

Central to a cost-effectiveness analysis is the construction of a cost-effectiveness (C/E) ratio. The numerator C of this ratio represents the costs of a program or intervention in dollars, and the denominator E represents the desirable outcome, such as years of life saved or number of people who have successfully stopped smoking. The ratio thus represents the dollar costs of a particular health-care intervention per unit of outcome. For example, school nurses are well suited for delivering antidrug messages to teenagers at risk of drug abuse. The cost effectiveness of this nursing role can be evaluated by calculating the costs of such intervention in a school environment per drug abuse case averted.

A systematic calculation of the C/E ratios of several competing intervention programs enables decision makers to answer a central question in cost-effectiveness analysis: "Given that some pre-specified object is to be attained, what are the costs associated with the various alternative means for reaching that objective?" (McGuigan, Moyer, & Harris, 1999, p. 749). For example, the nicotine transdermal patch has been clinically demonstrated as an effective aid in smoking cessation (Akehurst & Piercy, 1994; Orleans et al., 1994). But physicians and other health-care providers may be reluctant to recommend this treatment because of high treatment costs that include physician time and patch prescriptions. Cost-effectiveness analysis can assist in assessing the merit of nicotine patches compared with other effective smoking cessation methods.

In an analysis of nicotine replacement therapy, Wasley and coworkers (1997) found that the nicotine patch is not only clinically effective but also cost effective compared with other widely accepted antismoking treatments such as physician counseling and nicotine gum. Depending on age, for example, the average costs of nicotine patches per year of life saved range from $965 to $1585 for men and from $1634 to $2360 for women (in 1995 dollars). When the patch is added to a brief physician counseling session, the incremental costs per added year of life saved range from $1796 to

$2949 for men and from $3040 to $4391 for women. These figures compare favorably with the costs of the nicotine gum intervention, which range from $5792 to $8986 per year of life saved for men and from $9563 to $13,170 per year of life saved for women. The figures compare even more impressively with the C/E ratios of other pharmacological aids used in treating common, preventable conditions.

MEASURES OF EFFECTIVENESS

To express program costs per unit of output, a suitable measure of effectiveness that represents the treatment objective of a medical intervention must first be defined. Frequently, "life-years gained" are used as a measure of effectiveness in hypertension treatment and cancer screening programs. For example, Mandelblatt and Fahs (1988) reported that the early detection of cervical cancer through Papanicolaou tests saved 3.7 years of life per 100 tests performed and represented a cost of $2874 per life-year saved. Other commonly used measures of effectiveness include the following: lives saved, smokers who quit, cases treated appropriately, pain-free or symptom-free days maintained, cases successfully diagnosed, and complications avoided (Robinson, 1993b).

ECONOMIC ANALYSIS
A NURSING APPLICATION OF COST-EFFECTIVENESS ANALYSIS

Nursing scholars and administrators have both promoted case management as a model for improving the quality of health services while controlling costs (McKenzie, Torkelson, & Holt, 1989; Erkel, 1993). For example, nurse researcher Patricia H. Allred and her colleagues at the Medical College of South Carolina studied the administrative structure of nursing services and patient outcomes at a 517-bed academic health science center in the southeastern United States (Allred et al., 1995). They empirically tested the cost effectiveness of nursing case management in an inpatient acute care setting to explore the effect of practice environment on costs and outcomes. Central to the study was the concept of "practice environment," a term used to measure the degree of practice complexity and level of unpredictability of the work environment in a nursing unit.

The study found evidence supporting the theory that the interaction of case management and practice environment jointly determined the costs as well as the effectiveness of acute inpatient care. Specifically, after adjusting for quality differences, the average costs per patient were $7935, $12,078, and $14,527 for practice environments of moderate, high, and low levels of uncertainty, respectively. Clearly, case management achieved desired patient care outcomes in the moderately uncertain environment at a cost and quality level significantly better than that achieved in the practice environment characterized by either low or high environmental uncertainty. The authors attributed the better outcomes to the general practice environment of the hospital, the role differentiation of nursing managers, and the information coordination associated with case management.

 ## ADDITIONAL CONSIDERATIONS IN ECONOMIC EVALUATION

In addition to deciding whether to use cost-identification analysis, cost-benefit analysis, or cost-effectiveness analysis for an economic evaluation of a health-care intervention, two important decisions must be made: what perspective to take in the analysis, and what costs and benefits to include in the analysis.

PERSPECTIVES ON ECONOMIC EVALUATION

A health-care intervention can be evaluated from a number of perspectives, including that of the patient, payer, provider, or society. The choice of an evaluation perspective determines not only the types of costs and benefits to be considered in an economic evaluation but also the dollar amounts of them. Consequently, the conclusions drawn from the broadest perspective—that of society in general—can be very different from those drawn from the perspective of an insurer who reimburses providers for the care or a nurse clinician who provides the care.

Suppose, for example, that nurse educators from three hospitals wish to determine the financial impact of pooling critical care educators to conduct a citywide critical care education program. They expect that a coordinated program would be more cost efficient than the individual hospital-based critical care orientation that has dominated the local health-care system for quite some time. This issue is best assessed from the perspective of the health-care provider, because the benefits to society, the patient, and the third-party payer would be indirect and secondary.

On the other hand, the health-care provider's perspective would not be appropriate for a third-party payer wishing to determine if payments today for an outpatient nicotine withdrawal program will offset their future payments for treatment of smoking-related diseases. This question should be examined from the third-party payer's point of view, although some indication of societal benefits may potentially be extrapolated.

TYPES OF COSTS AND BENEFITS

Various costs and benefits can be included in an economic analysis of health-care decision making. These include direct medical costs, direct nonmedical costs, indirect morbidity and mortality costs, and intangible costs and benefits.

Direct medical costs are easily identified and include costs for hospitalization, drugs, physicians' fees, laboratory and diagnostic tests, rehabilitation, and durable medical equipment.

> **Direct medical costs are those costs related to the direct medical intervention, such as hospital charges and physicians' fees.**

Direct nonmedical costs are costs that significantly disrupt the lives of patients and caregivers. These may include the following:

- Loss of pay while either the patient or caregiver is unable to work
- Costs for special diets necessitated by the illness
- Changes of living arrangements or dwelling modifications to accommodate the needs of the patient
- Transportation to the physician or hospital

Indirect morbidity and mortality costs are costs that are borne by society as a result of the loss of productivity of an individual either by disability or premature death. When a patient dies or becomes incapacitated prematurely, society loses the values of his or her services or contributions. These losses are a cost to society and should be included in an economic evaluation that adopts the societal perspective. The following are examples of these indirect costs:

- The loss of future earnings and contributions to society because of the death of a female human resources director at a major consumer product company at the age of 35
- The reduction of earnings and contributions to society of a computer programmer who can only do part-time work after a major surgery

Finally, the costs that are most difficult to operationally define are the *intangible costs* associated with pain, suffering, or grief and other nonmonetary outcomes related to the disease or illness. These costs, though real and highly relevant to decision making, are notoriously difficult to measure. Examples of intangible costs include physical and psychological pain and distress associated with an illness or injury, and the inconvenience and disruption of lives caused by seeking treatment or adjusting to the disease.

> *Intangible costs are the emotional costs associated with pain, suffering, or grief and other nonmonetary outcomes related to the disease or illness.*

SENSITIVITY ANALYSIS

A criticism of economic evaluation is that regardless of how carefully the evaluation is designed and carried out, the results are subject to many uncertainties and bias. For example, the conclusion regarding the cost effectiveness of a particular antismoking program based on studying heavy smokers may or may not apply to those who smoke moderately. Similarly, the results based on a sample of men may or may not apply to women of similar characteristics. To deal with these uncertainties and biases, a sensitivity analysis is recommended (Russell et al., 1996; Weinstein et al.,1996).

Sensitivity analysis allows researchers to test the robustness of the results to see if variations in the values of important variables will significantly change the conclusions. For example, researchers may wish to change the underlying assumptions one at a time to see how sensitive the results are to such step-wise relaxation of estimation assumptions. This is referred to as *one-way sensitivity analysis*. An alternative to one-way sensitivity analysis is *multivariate* or *multiway sensitivity analysis*, in which more than one assumption is changed at the same time. By using either one-way or multiway sensitivity analysis, researchers can test whether results apply to a wide range of conditions or whether they are sensitive to the underlying assumptions and cannot be replicated when some of the basic conditions or assumptions are changed.

VALUE OF ECONOMIC EVALUATION TO NURSING

Nurses in both clinical and managerial roles can employ the economic evaluation methods presented in this chapter to communicate the value of nursing to different types of personnel within the health-care setting. Nurses have a unique vantage point from which to contribute to cost-analysis methods. The linkage between nursing and other disciplines is critical for demonstrating the value of nursing to patient outcomes. Once medical therapies are prescribed for patients, it is often the nurse who is responsible for aiding patients and families in attaining necessary medical resources.

Nurses also listen to concerns about the financial impact of goods and services that are not reimbursed by third-party payers. Additionally, the components defined as intangible costs, such as pain, suffering, and grief, provide a continual source of consternation and disagreement among health-service researchers. It is the nurse who attempts to relieve patients' pain and suffering and to moderate the grief experience of both patients and family members. Given this environment, nurses can apply state-of-the-art evaluation techniques to contribute to the delivery of health care that is both effective and cost effective.

Recognizing the significance of economic evaluation to nurses, the American Association of Colleges of Nursing (1996, 1997) has repeatedly recommended preparation at the baccalaureate and graduate levels for conducting and carrying out research on effectiveness, outcomes, and cost analysis. The analytical concepts and techniques explored in this chapter help nursing leaders and practitioners make rational, consistent, and effective decisions that maximize the beneficial outcomes for the health and well-being of a large number of people. They also help nurses to communicate the effectiveness of nursing interventions to patients, insurers, and other providers.

SUMMARY

This chapter presented three major approaches to the economic evaluation of clinical decisions from a nursing perspective. All three of the evaluation approaches can help nurses make rational decisions regarding cost effectiveness, but they differ in the questions addressed, the research design, and the types of cost and benefit data required.

The simplest and most modest evaluation method, cost-identification analysis, seeks to determine the costs of a treatment or intervention program. It applies to situations in which outcomes are the same or similar among options. Therefore, no outcome measurement is needed for this type of analysis.

Cost-benefit analysis measures both the benefits and the costs of an intervention in monetary terms. By a systematic calculation of how much the expected benefits exceed the expected costs of each of the available options, cost-benefit analysis provides a powerful tool for decision makers to make health-care choices that produce the most good for society.

> The third approach, cost-effectiveness analysis, is the preferred method of evaluation in medicine and health-services research. It measures outcome in natural units (e.g., years of life saved) and expresses evaluation results in terms of how much money a program costs per unit of outcome.

DISCUSSION QUESTIONS

1. What is clinical economics? Discuss the significance of clinical economic analysis to health care using nursing examples that you are familiar with.
2. What are the three different approaches to clinical economic analysis?
3. In your own words, describe the difference between cost-benefit and cost-effectiveness analysis.
4. Discuss the costs that should be included in a cost-benefit analysis.
5. Discuss the benefits that should be included in a cost-benefit analysis.
6. Discuss the concept of discounting. Why is discounting necessary in economic evaluation of medical interventions?
7. What is the sensitivity analysis? Discuss its purposes and significance.
8. Search the nursing literature and summarize the results of at least three articles based on, respectively, cost-identification analysis, cost-benefit analysis, and cost-effectiveness.

 REFERENCES

Akehurst, R. L., & Piercy, J. (1994). Cost-effectiveness of the use of transdermal Nicorette patches relative to GP counseling and nicotine gum in the prevention of smoking-related diseases. *British Journal of Medical Economics, 7*(2), 115–122.

Allred, C. A., Arford, P. H., Michel, Y., Dring, R., Carter, V., & Veitch, J. S. (1995). A cost-effectiveness analysis of acute care case management outcomes. *Nursing Economics, 13*(3), 129–136.

American Association of Colleges of Nursing. (1996). *The baccalaureate degree in nursing as minimal preparation for professional practice.* Washington, DC: Author.

American Association of Colleges of Nursing. (1997). *Joint position statement on education for nurses in administrative roles.* Washington, DC: Author.

Chang, W. Y., & Henry, B. M. (1999). Methodologic principles of cost analysis in the nursing, medical, and health services literature, 1990–1996. *Nursing Research, 48*(2), 94–104.

Curtas, S., Hariri, R., & Steiger, E. (1996). Case management in home total parenteral nutrition: A cost-identification analysis. *Journal of Parenteral and Enteral Nutrition*, 20(2), 113–119.

DeBaca, V., Jones, K., & Tornabeni, J. A. (1993). A cost-benefit analysis of shared governance. *Journal of Nursing Administration*, 23(7/8), 50–57.

Eisenberg, J. M., & Kitz, D. S. (1986). Savings from outpatient antibiotic therapy for osteomyelitis: Economic analysis of a therapeutic strategy. *Journal of the American Medical Association*, 255(12), 1584–1588.

Erkel, E. (1993). The impact of case management in preventive services. *Journal of Nursing Administration*, 23(1), 27–32.

Gold, M. R., Siegel, J. E., Russell, L. B., & Weinstein, M. S. (1996) *Cost-effectiveness in health and medicine*. New York: Oxford University Press.

Leigh, J. P., Markowitz, S. B., Fahs, M., Shin. C., & Landrigan, P. J. (1997). Occupational injury and illness in the United States: Estimates of costs, morbidity, and mortality. *Archives of Internal Medicine*, 157(14), 1557–1568.

Mandelblatt, J., & Fahs, M. (1988). Cost-effectiveness of cervical cancer screening for low income elderly women. *Journal of the American Medical Association*, 259(16), 2409–2413.

McGuigan, J. R., Moyer, R. C., & F. H. D. Harris (1999). *Managerial economics* (8th ed.). Minneapolis/St. Paul: West Publishing.

McKenzie, C., Torkelson, N., & Holt, M. (1989). Care and cost: Nursing case management improves both. *Nursing Management*, 20(10), 30–34.

Office of Management and Budget. (1994). *Guidelines and discount rates for benefit-cost analysis of federal programs* (Circular No. A-94 revised to include 1994 discount rates). Washington, DC: Author.

Orleans, C. T., Resch, N., Noll, E., Keintz, M. K., Rimer, B. K., Brown, T. V., & Snedden, T. M. (1994). Use of transdemal nicotine in a state-level prescription plan for the elderly: a first look at "real-world" patch users. *Journal of the American Medical Association*, 271(8), 601–607.

Robinson, R. (1993a). Costs and cost-minimization analysis. *British Medical Journal*, 307(6906), 726–728.

Robinson, R. (1993b). Cost-effectiveness analysis. *British Medical Journal*, 307(6907), 793–795.

Russell, L. B., Gold, M. R., Siegel, J. E., Daniels, N., & Weinstein, M. C. (1996). The role of cost-effectiveness analysis in health and medicine. *Journal of the American Medical Association*, 276(14), 1172–1177.

Santerre, R. E., & Neun, S. P. (2000). *Health economics* (Rev. ed.). Chicago: Irwin.

Wasley, M. A., McNagny, S. E., Phillips, V. L., & Ahulwalia, J. S. (1997). The cost-effectiveness of the nicotine transdermal patch for smoking cessation. *Preventive Medicine*, 26(2), 264–270.

Weinstein, M. C., Siegel, J. E., Gold, M. R., Kamlet, M. S., & Russell, L. B. (1996). Recommendation of the panel on Cost-Effectiveness in health and medicine. *Journal of the American Medical Association*, 276(15), 1253–1258.

 SUGGESTED READING

Boardman, A. E., Greenberg, D. H., Vining, A. R., & Weimer, D. L. (1996). *Cost-benefit analysis: Concepts and practice*. Upper Saddle River, NJ: Prentice Hall.

Gold, M. (1996). Panel on Cost-Effectiveness in Health and Medicine. *Medical Care*, 34(Suppl. 12), 197–199.

Siegel, J. E, Torrance, G. W., Russell, L. B., Luce, B. R., Weinstein, M. C., & Gold, M. R. (1997). Guidelines for pharmacoeconomic studies: Recommendations from the panel on Cost Effectiveness in Health and Medicine. *Pharmacoeconomics*, 11(2), 159–168.

Udvarhelyi, I. S., Colditz, G. A., Rai, A., & Epstein, A. M. (1992). Cost-effectiveness and cost-benefit analyses in the medical literature: Are the methods being used correctly? *Annals of Internal Medicine*, 116(3), 238–244.

Weisbrod, B. A. (1983). *Economics and medical research*. Washington, DC: American Enterprise Institute.

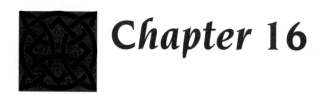

Chapter 16

Information Technology and the Economics of Health Care

Susan K. Pfoutz

LEARNING OBJECTIVES

- Describe the competing visions of computer technologies.
- Examine the information needs of nurses and other health-care providers.
- Describe the trends and developmental issues in the national information infrastructure.
- Discuss the history, trends, and issues in telehealth.
- Analyze the trends in distance learning that affect nurses and nursing education.
- Examine the computer skills required for nurses and the uses of computer information for nursing.
- Discuss the development of nursing information systems that incorporate data necessary for the evaluation of nursing care.
- Describe the use of computer technologies for dissemination and implementation of clinical practice guidelines.

 ## COMPETING VIEWS OF INFORMATION TECHNOLOGY FOR THE HEALTH-CARE INDUSTRY

It is imperative that health-care organizations achieve the desired goals of positive outcomes and efficiency in delivery of their services. Information technology provides tools that promise to assist in achieving these goals. This chapter discusses how these tools can be used to greatest advantage to advance the clinical and management components of health care. It also addresses the existing and potential economic contributions of technology applications to health care. An initial step is to examine ways in which information technology can be applied to solve existing problems. Selected applications of this technology are presented: telemedicine and telehealth, distance education in nursing, and practice guidelines for health-care delivery. This chapter focuses on the trends in information technologies affecting health economics; Chapter 17 addresses the specific use of computer information systems and standardized electronic medical records.

The organizations where nurses and other health-care providers work increasingly exist in an environment in which information must be available for provision of health services, documentation, administrative purposes, and evaluation of the cost and effectiveness of services provided. Information systems are used to evaluate economic data, staffing needs, and patient illness, as well as for budget projection and monitoring and analyzing changes in supply and demand. Computer technologies provide mechanisms to collect, manipulate, report, and transmit needed clinical and economic information in a timely fashion. The challenges for nursing are to envision the potential of evolving information technologies, use them to enhance the work of nursing, understand the trends and issues influencing the evolution of information systems, and use the data from these systems to support the economic basis for nursing and health care.

Although the term *information technology* makes one think of computers, it encompasses a wide range of mechanisms that interface or connect with each other. Information technologies include the following:

- Computers
- Telephones
- Static visual imaging by telephone or facsimile
- Moving visual imaging (video)
- Audio imaging

VISIONS FOR INFORMATION TECHNOLOGIES

Application of technology involves the ability to envision how that technology can make the current work easier, faster, more effective, and less costly. Technology can also transform the work being done by using new processes and mechanisms. In some cases technology applications lead to entirely new products or services not originally imagined. When examining technology, a beginning step is to examine the potential applications of technology.

Peter Drucker (1998) described the application of new technology by using the example of a previous information revolution: the invention of the printing press. This invention illustrates the progress of innovation, its economic impact on employment, and the development of new products. Soon after the development of the printing press, the monks who duplicated the Bible by hand were replaced by a much smaller number of technicians who operated the printing presses. For some time, the only product remained the same, the Bible. Publishers with the vision to identify potential uses of printing technology soon surpassed the technicians (printers) in importance to the publishing industry. Publishing expanded to include a wide variety of secular publications and other products.

This example also applies to the current information revolution: the computer. Drucker (1998) describes the purpose of any business as the creation of value and wealth. Up to this point most computer information systems have focused on the storage, manipulation, and retrieval of data for business operations. Information technology has less often been applied to management decision making and the identification of new concepts for businesses in the new era. New ideas require the capture of data from outside the organization to understand opportunities, changes, and threats. Application of computer technologies may actually transform the work to be done and the nature of the endeavor.

Two examples relevant to nursing and health care illustrate the transformation of work by computer and telecommunication technology (Drucker, 1998). Distance learning methods may challenge the existence of the free-standing university. Using distance education methods, education will likely shift from discrete programs of study to continuing professional education across people's work lives in convenient new locations such as the home, car, train, local school, or workplace. Similarly, health care is shifting from the fight against disease to the maintenance of mental and physical functioning. A focus on health maintenance and disease management requires access to information and communication between health-care providers and consumers, which is facilitated by information technologies and telemedicine or telehealth systems. Consumers have almost unlimited access to health promotion and illness information on the Internet and can communicate with health-care professionals through various telehealth mechanisms. The traditional education systems and health professions are being challenged to examine the new ideas defining the work to be done and to incorporate new technologies into health care.

An information system is an integrated set of computer applications designed to accomplish specific tasks.

Visions of the power of computer technologies vary from commercial uses to mechanisms that increase consumer access to information and link interested people together to participate in policy making. Although none of these diverse perspectives excludes the others, not all can be accommodated by the information infrastructure (Milio, 1996).

The first vision is a commercial one in which computers provide an expanding marketplace for products and services that create profits. Many businesses and health-care agencies view this technology as a means to increase the flexibility and efficiency of their work by bridging space and time.

Bill Gates (1999) has championed this view with his vision of "business at the speed of thought." In this perspective, information systems become a "digital nervous system" that can provide information for product design, customer feedback, production processes, marketing and distribution strategies, and inventory management. These systems provide immediate access to information for executives, managers, and line staff (Gates, 1999). The economic implications of such rapid information access include the following:

- Enhanced strategic planning that responds to market demand
- Enhanced consumer satisfaction related to this response to their needs
- Improved efficiency of operations by integrated use of information for purchasing, hiring, staffing, and production of services
- Enhanced evaluation of product and economic outcomes

In the health-care industry, these operational efficiencies would allow improved assessment and planning for needed health-care services, input to appropriate personnel decisions, and timely data for evaluation of outcomes compared with other facilities as well as with the cost of production.

> *Access to information facilitates economic efficiency by enhancing the organizational capacity to respond more rapidly to market supply and demand, consumer preferences, and need for changes in the processes of production.*

Milio (1996) describes computers as "engines of empowerment" that can be used to enhance the health of the public. This social perspective expands the number of individuals considered in infrastructure development to include the needs and desires of the consumers as well as the producers of health care. The federal government has advocated a public-service view of the information infrastructure in which all Americans have affordable access to technology regardless of their location or income. Others envision a populist function in which information facilitates participation in policy development. A similar but varying perspective is a public-interest one in which individuals and community organizations have access to a wide range of information that enables participation in discussion about public issues. These perspectives do not have as direct economic implications as the commercial perspective does. However, health care and human services will be used to the extent that they meet consumer needs and preferences.

To the extent that those needs and preferences are incorporated into initial program planning, providers of health care can get it right the first time.

ECONOMIC ANALYSIS
PUBLIC POLICY FAILURE: THE DEFEAT OF EXPANDED MEDICARE BENEFITS

In late 1988, Congress enacted the Medicare Catastrophic Coverage Act, which was designed to protect elderly people from the economic effects of catastrophic illness and to provide prescription drug coverage. Because the costs of extended illness and prescription medications can be financially devastating to the elderly population, changes were enacted to provide these benefits to Medicare recipients. Mechanisms to pay for these benefits included an increase in the Medicare premium. A vocal protest from some senior groups and other interested individuals resulted in the reconsideration of this legislation and the repeal of the act in 1989 (Gale & Stefl, 1992). Consensus had not been developed on the need for change nor on the specific mechanisms to remedy the problem. This resulted in constituent revolt against the enacted policy.

Information technology will greatly enhance the politics of health care because health-care decisions are made based on data collected and organized by computers. The following are selected examples of how access to information can influence political action (Milio, 1996):

- The U.S. Department of Justice developed the largest on-line legal database in the country, called JURIS. This system was accessed through a commercial network. When the contract was up for renewal, a public interest group called Taxpayer Assets Project lobbied for free public access. Individual and group pressure resulted in this service being made available to the public.
- The Environmental Protection Agency publishes the Toxic Release Inventory through paper reports, computer diskettes, CD-ROM discs, and electronic databases. This information enables local groups to pursue environmental action at the local level. The knowledge itself is not sufficient for change; however, along with the additional tools of organizational support, technical knowledge, and legal assistance, it can result in political change.

- Housing advocacy to prevent arson is enhanced by computer applications that can analyze data to predict the risk for arson. Again, this knowledge is not enough to prevent arson, but it provides an organizing tool to bring community people and organizations together. The computer-based information also provides a credible basis for discussion with community authorities.
- Information technology support groups, usually using volunteers, are a means to provide nonprofit groups in disadvantaged areas expertise in gaining funding and support to achieve access to information technologies. Support extends to customizing computer systems to the nonprofit agency, providing training, and assisting to resolve problems with systems because the staff in these agencies frequently turn over.
- Local, state, and federal government agencies have used information technologies to share information with constituents and to provide some services, including health-care services and education. Many localities use centralized computer locations that have easy-to-use interfaces for consumers.

Computer technologies provide enhanced access to information for health-care providers and consumers that facilitates improved decision making and participation in policy making.

A NURSING VISION FOR INFORMATION TECHNOLOGY

As individuals and groups throughout the health-care industry examine how information technology affects workers and the work to be done, so too are nursing leaders actively participating in the discussion of how information technology will be used in the health-care industry to facilitate the work of nurses. Nursing leaders and professional groups have participated in a variety of forums to identify the information needs of nurses; to ensure inclusion of nursing data in information systems; and to develop applications of these technologies for nursing practice, management, education, and research.

At the beginning of the 21st century, the discussion continues about what technologies and applications will best serve the nation's health. Nursing leaders who can use economic data from information systems can showcase the contributions of nursing to the health-care system and to the nation's health. Nursing leaders must also communicate nursing's economic contribution to public health care and participate in public policy.

A vision of health-care informatics in 2008 includes the following predictions (Collen, 1999):

- Few of the integrated managed care plans will survive the intense competition and expanding service needs of the aging population.
- Health care will be focused on both promoting health and treating illness.
- Large computer client databases will be standardized using standards imposed by the Health Care Financing Administration (HCFA).
- Although these standards will be difficult to achieve, they will facilitate improved management of care and use of data for research and evaluation.
- Clinical guidelines will direct much of patient care.
- Consumers will have smart cards that carry much of their health-care information, including genetic typing.

Health-care delivery will increasingly incorporate information technologies into clinical practice and management. Clinical practice guidelines and standardized formats for information will improve the evaluation of outcomes and cost of care. The demands of competition and an aging population will stimulate innovations in the use of technology for care delivery. The cost of these technologies will increase hospital expenses, but will be justified by the improved patient outcomes and decreased liability costs (Collen, 1999).

The National Advisory Council on Nurse Education and Practice (NAC-NEP) in the Department of Health and Human Services, Division of Nursing, has recommended directions for nursing and information technologies. This group recognized three significant federal technology initiatives that will continue to define the communication environment for health care into the 21st century: development of the national information infrastructure (NII), the Internet, and telemedicine or telehealth (Gassert, 1998).

THE NATIONAL INFORMATION INFRASTRUCTURE

The NII concerns the further development of the web of communication networks that facilitates the rapid transmission of information between distant points (Gassert, 1998). Which technologies will be used in the development of this infrastructure, particularly in remote areas, is unclear. However, it is clear that the volume, speed, and range of communication are rapidly expanding.

The national information infrastructure is composed of the electronic networks that are capable of communicating through a variety of media.

Several policy questions remain for the development of this communication network. Who will have access to this information? For whose interests will the infrastructure be developed? How will the important decisions be made? Consensus building is necessary to create standards that meet the needs of major users such as the government, businesses, and health professions. Currently, information technology in health care has emphasized administrative information rather than clinical or consumer information. Still, individuals and consumer groups are accessing information for their own purposes. If consumer needs are valued, additional design and access issues need to be addressed (Milio, 1996).

THE ROLE OF THE INTERNET IN INFORMATION DISSEMINATION

The Internet is a part of the communication system that links individuals and groups across the world. The Internet was originally developed by the U.S. Defense Department in 1969 as a mechanism for communicating data across time and space by linking vast numbers of computer networks together. This network has grown and become widely used by the general public. The development of the next-generation Internet will multiply the speed of communication, promote the use of new technological applications, and increase networking capacities that will enhance research (Nicholl, 1998).

> *Investment in the NII and Internet will affect the speed and breadth of access to electronic information as well as the scope of applications available.*

Nurses, other health-care professionals, and consumers can use Internet technology to access a wide variety of information for personal and professional use. The information available on the Internet includes both clinical and economic data important to health care and nursing. Telecommunication and computers will continue to enhance health care, public health, health-care provider and consumer education, research, and administration in the future.

Information Available on the Internet

Designated the *information superhighway*, the Internet uses both free roads and toll roads, the latter of which provide fee-based commercial services. Communication services are facilitated through electronic mail (e-mail) and bulletin boards. File transfer protocols allow the transmission of data from place to place. Other tools facilitate navigation through this vast network of information sites (Nicholl, 1998; Mascara, Czar, & Hedba, 1999).

ECONOMIC ANALYSIS
USE OF THE INTERNET FOR HEALTH-CARE INFORMATION

Breast cancer is an example of a condition that requires both consumers and health-care providers to have current information. The Internet provides multiple ways for both to access information.

Professionals and consumers can access scientific information regarding current research, therapies, and care management. A variety of locations also provide information on clinical practice guidelines for such related topics as pain management. These Internet sites may be created by individuals, U.S. federal government agencies, pharmaceutical companies, health-care organizations, or other organizations around the world. Access to medical literature searches at no cost can be attained through the National Library of Medicine Medline Service. An immense volume of information is available; both consumers and health professionals must sift through it to identify what is current, accurate, and appropriate for their particular use.

Consumers diagnosed with breast cancer may sign up for a chat group to talk with other patients with the same diagnosis for both support and information. In this forum, participants share their experiences concerning diagnosis and treatment, strategies for coping with this illness, and alternative therapies. Health-care professionals also have chat groups and other forums in which to discuss care and research issues. Professionals may also consult with experts in the field or other colleagues through e-mail.

These mechanisms provide access to a wide variety of information resources from the individual's home or workplace.

Types of Internet Resources

It is a challenge to sort out the vast amount of information on and features of the Internet. The following are types of commonly used Internet resources (Nicholl, 1998; Mascara, Czar, & Hebda, 1999):

- *Uniform Resource Locator* (URL). The address or unique identifier that locates the site or information of interest. Many sites also link to related information.
- *Bookmark*. A useful tool that stores the address for use another time without having to type the location each time.
- *Type of site*. Categories of locations on the Internet. Each type has its own address format and mechanisms for navigating the Internet.
  - *World Wide Web* (WWW). Developed by CERN (European Center of Particle Physics) in Switzerland, the Web uses a specialized language that allows linking from site to site.
  - *Gopher*. Software developed at the University of Minnesota.
  - *Telnet*. Facilitates connection with a remote computer to search databases, read text, and explore information, but not to transfer files.
- *Listserve*. A discussion group in which members communicate through e-mail. Discussion groups tend to provide a focus for either laypersons or professionals. Interested individuals join a listserve by sending an e-mail message to the host location of the group.
- *Usenet newsgroup*. A discussion group that is conducted by posting messages on a bulletin board. The user then decides how frequently to check or use the information.
- *Search engines*. Tools to locate multiple locations that reference a topic. There are many search engines. Users are encouraged to select a search engine appropriate to their needs. Search strategies can also be used to broaden or narrow the topic sought.
- *Government sites*. Location of government information. These sites are identified by the suffix .gov.
- *Association sites*. Location of nonprofit organizations. These sites have the suffix .org.
- *Corporate or private sites*. Location of corporations and for-profit sites. These sites have the suffix .com.
- *Education sites*. Locations for schools or organizations with a primarily educational focus. These sites have the suffix .edu.

Evaluation of On-line Information

Because technology enables anyone to place information on the Internet, it is important for nurses and their clients to evaluate the on-line information for correctness, timeliness, and bias. Although search engines can locate a vast amount of information, these tools do not examine the quality of information at the identified sites. Table 16–1 provides criteria for evaluating on-line information.

TABLE 16–1. CHECKLIST FOR EVALUATING ON-LINE INFORMATION

Credentials of author
- ☐ The author's preparation or background is given.
- ☐ The author's authority on the topic is provided.

Accuracy
- ☐ The author has provided references or resources for validation.

Date of creation
- ☐ The date when the material was written is provided.
- ☐ The date on which the material was posted is provided.

Bias
- ☐ The author and the sponsoring organization are identified.
- ☐ The purpose of the information is identified.

Completeness
- ☐ Sufficient information is available to address the topic adequately.
- ☐ Links to more information are provided.

Consistency
- ☐ The information is consistent with other sources the reader has examined.

Audience
- ☐ The audience for the information is identified.

Source: Adapted from Mascara, C., Czar, P., & Hebda, T. (1999). Internet resource guide for nurses and health care professionals. Menlo Park, CA: Addison Wesley.

The Internet provides a powerful communication technology to link health-care consumers, sellers, providers, educators, and researchers around the world. Potential users need to commit time to learn how to use this complex system, how to locate useful information in their area of interest, and how to evaluate that information for its reliability. Appendix B lists a variety of Web sites of interest to nursing and health care.

It is important to evaluate the quality of all information retrieved from the Internet. Although much information is available, there is no mechanism for screening the accuracy, currency, bias, and source of the information.

TELEHEALTH

Telemedicine is defined as "the use of telecommunications technology to send data, graphics, audio, and video images between participants who are physically separated" (Brecht & Barrett, 1998, p. 25). *Telehealth* is a broader approach that applies telecommunications to the health-care environment.

Because nursing is part of the larger health-care education and delivery system, the term *telehealth* will be used here. Telehealth technologies continue to evolve, providing new applications in education, prevention services, and therapeutic care. Nurses, as the largest number of health-care professionals, have a major role in the use of telehealth applications in a variety of health-care settings. Telehealth allows access to information and health services in areas where they do not currently exist. In addition, telehealth facilitates monitoring and disease management for patients while limiting costly home services.

Telehealth is an evolving delivery system for health care that uses telecommunications technology to provide health and illness services at a distance.

History of Telehealth

The history of telehealth dates back to 1876. Although telehealth techniques may be viewed as novel today, the telephone was the first distance health-care technology. Physicians and pharmacists were among the first professionals to see this invention as a valuable tool for their practices. Advances in technologies allowed the telephone to span ever-larger distances, including cross-continent communication. More recently, wireless technology has allowed penetration to remote areas (Viegas, 1998; Barrett & Brecht, 1998).

Modern telehealth began in 1948 with the sending of radiographic images over the telephone. By 1962 the University of Nebraska incorporated expanded technology for psychiatric consultations. Communication at longer distances led to clinical projects. In 1968 Massachusetts General Hospital conducted clinical consultations with Logan International Airport's clinical station, which was run by nurse clinicians (Barrett & Brecht, 1998; Strode, Gustke, & Allen, 1999). Since these first projects, many telehealth applications have been funded through the federal government to examine the feasibility of using telehealth to meet health-care and educational goals. By the 1990s teleconferencing had become much less expensive and used smaller, more accessible equipment. The focus of current projects is the evaluation of the cost, quality, and access provided by telehealth services (Viegas, 1998).

Access to qualified health-care providers is a primary concern in the development of telehealth. This focus has encouraged development of services in rural areas where there is often a shortage of health-care providers or of providers with specific expertise. Characteristics of health status in rural areas include younger mortality, increased chronic illness, increased infant mortality, and greater accidental injury. Geography in rural locations limits options for transportation, inhibiting the access to care. A 1997 survey conducted by the U.S. Office of Rural Health Policy reported that 30 percent of the 2472 rural hospitals use some form of telehealth technologies. The number of programs doubled from 40 to 82 in the period between 1995 and 1996. The monograph edited by Viegas and Dunn (1998) describes a wide range of telehealth applications by clinical specialty.

Telecommunication systems are frequently used by advanced practice nurses working in rural, public, private, and home settings. Communication with a licensed physician or other health-care professionals on the care team frequently occurs by telephone. Increasingly, home-health-care nurses monitor their clients' health status through telecommunication between scheduled visits. Applications include two-way video and diagnostic services such as heart and lung sounds, pulse oximetry, respiratory flow data, and blood glucose monitoring. Nurses in community settings and acute care settings frequently conduct follow-up contacts with clients by telephone. Telehealth technologies enhance the productivity of nurses by decreasing the number of home visits, particularly at a time when the costs of home-care services are being contained.

New technologies have the potential for increasing the use and possible applications of telehealth efforts. Telecommunication strategies for telehealth have usually used either interactive television or store-and-forward image and recording transmission using computers and remote monitoring. The development of higher-speed transmission as well as greater-bandwidth systems provides the capacity to transmit much larger quantities of data more quickly. Additional technology allows the transmission of images and other information in digital format. Although the cost of interactive video equipment is substantial, it is falling. A system that cost $100,000 in 1992 cost less than $20,000 in 1999. The volume of services remains a key in the cost of telehealth services (Viegas, 1998).

Facilitators and Barriers to Telehealth

Factors driving the expansion of telehealth include the following:

- Federal funding for projects
- Services becoming part of the telecommunication infrastructure
- Advancing technology
- Competition resulting from the deregulation of the telecommunication industry, which reduces costs
- Managed care
- State initiatives allowing reimbursement for services.

Although the advancements in technology and services are encouraging, many significant barriers remain. For example, the Health Care Financing

Administration and other insurance carriers require in-person contact for reimbursement for all services except radiology. HCFA is currently examining these reimbursement policies, and states are promoting reimbursement for distance services. The Federal Balanced Budget Act of 1997 requires HCFA to begin reimbursement for distance services in areas with a shortage of health professionals (Brecht & Barrett, 1998).

Provision of services to rural or distant areas requires the availability of a telecommunications infrastructure at a reasonable cost. The Universal Access Fund provision of the 1996 Telecommunications Deregulation Bill provides money to subsidize telecommunications services to rural nonprofit organizations, beginning in 1998. Although this provision will assist many areas to gain access to service, it will take time for these services to develop. Specific criteria for reimbursement of these services have also been developed (Brecht & Barrett, 1998; Strode, Gustke, & Allen, 1999).

Other barriers relate to the licensure of medical professionals. Because licensure occurs at the state level, telehealth services that cross state lines challenge current practice. Determination of liability and legal jurisdiction is related to the care provider of record and where that provider is located. These are thorny issues because states retain the right to regulate health-care practice. Dispute also exists regarding whether a local or national standard of practice should be applied to telehealth. Issues regarding the nature of the patient–provider relationship are affected and require definition of the roles of the consulting provider and the health-care provider or other personnel at the site where the consumer is located. Another legal and ethical issue is the maintenance of privacy related to information concerning the health-care consumer. Policies are needed for the audio, video, facsimile, and other transmission of data (Blair, Bambas, & Stone, 1998).

Organizational issues also challenge the practice of telehealth. The first issue is one of promoting and encouraging the organizational changes inherent in telehealth. Encouraging employees to adopt the new technology is a primary challenge. Next, there are many challenges involved in creating working relationships among organizations that have previously been competitive. Once working relationships are established, organizational structures and methods of operation must be integrated (Turner & Peterson, 1998).

Cost Feasibility of Telehealth

Cost is an important factor in evaluating any technology. A major concern is whether the cost of the technology is greater than the value of the service it provides. The earliest cost analyses examined the cost of sending electrocardiograms and phonocardiograms via the telephone compared with the cost of having equipment in each hospital. Cost analyses of telehealth have become more thorough over time.

Specific cost analyses of telehealth began in the 1970s. Some examples are the following (Moore, 1998):

- A telehealth project was established at the Sioux Lookout Zone in Ontario using three nursing stations equipped for distance consultations. The program did not justify the cost because the decreased cost of transport to emergency care did not balance the increased volume and utilization of services. Value could have been considered for increased access to care.
- A nursing-home telemedicine project in Boston in the late 1970s implemented the use of tone and voice paging systems, portable electrocardiogram machines, and telephone-coupled transmitters for the analysis of pacemakers. Results demonstrated that the group accessing the new technologies used more ambulatory care and significantly less hospital care than the comparison group.
- In the late 1970s the University of Washington Medical school began a satellite-based project serving several states in the region, reaching to Alaska. The cost of normal and emergency consultation was determined to be as cost effective as travel to the distant sites for either providers or patients.

Many of the early studies had conflicting results regarding the cost savings of telehealth services. The following variables remain relevant to evaluation of cost (Moore, 1998):

- *Equipment and technology.* Studies need to identify equipment costs.
- *Personnel.* Costs must include the salaries of those providing the actual services, technical skills, scheduling, and training and evaluation.
- *Transportation.* Transportation costs include the cost of those traveling (the provider or the client and family) and the nature of the travel (planned or emergency). Cost savings in telehealth include travel cost as well as the productive time that would have been lost during travel.
- *Time.* For telehealth costs to be cost effective the costs of travel and leisure time must be included.
- *Cost of local health care.* Studies have demonstrated that the cost of care at local or rural hospitals is less expensive than urban hospitals, another source of decreased health-care costs for people who are not transported. One Georgia study demonstrated that 80 percent of patients did not require transfer to higher-level care centers when using telehealth (Sanders, JH, Salter, PH, Stachura, ME, 1996).
- *Revenue generation.* Telehealth projects are in a favorable position when they can develop additional revenue through billing third-party payers.

Specific applications that have been shown to be cost effective include teleradiology, correctional health care, home care, and military care (Moore, 1998).

The cost feasibility of telehealth refers to the costs of the technology and services provided relative to the benefit gained. In telehealth this typically involves the cost of providing care relative to the anticipated reimbursement.

 ## ECONOMIC ANALYSIS
THE ARIZONA TELEHEALTH PROGRAM

A telehealth program was established in Arizona, the sixth largest state and one that has large geographic distances between populated locations. Much of the land contains large federal and Native American reservations. Approximately one-quarter of the population lives in rural areas with limited health-care resources that are designated as underserved areas.

In 1996 funding was sought from the federal government and the Arizona state legislature for the Arizona Telehealth Program. A system was chosen to handle the complex communications and limit the cost. Equipment for the entire network cost $192,000, compared with a typical cost of $155,000 per site. The entire network cost of equipment was $578,000 for video conferencing equipment and $400,000 for the store-and-forward equipment for multiple sites.

Three community sites and the Department of Corrections use the network for real-time interactive consultations as well as applications that store and forward data. Additional sites implement a dial-up system for radiology. By 1998, a total of 928 telehealth sessions had been completed, including 748 store-and-forward sessions and 65 cases of real-time video transmission. The teleradiology consultation system allows desktop review of the transmitted images. Expansion of services to provide urgent care consultations in the emergency department and cardiology consultations within the Heart Center are planned. Linkage to television facilities allows broadcast of continuing medical and nursing education (McNeill, Weinstein, & Holcomb, 1998).

DISTANCE EDUCATION IN NURSING

A specific application of telecommunications in health care is distance education. Nurses, along with other health-care professionals, have a need for continuing education to remain current in practice, as is demonstrated by state requirements for specified levels of continuing education for license renewal. Nurses in areas where universities are not located also need options for professional development through advanced degree programs. Nurses can use these same telecommunication technologies to provide health and disease management information to health-care consumers.

Many technologies can be used in distance learning, depending on the available equipment and the learning needs of students. One advantage of distance education is its flexibility in the delivery of educational programming, in both timing and format. With interactive television technology, one group of students and the teacher meet at the transmission site to broadcast to one or more groups of students at distance sites. In this format all students engage in learning at the same time (synchronous learning). This format allows students to interact with the teacher and students at other locations using video technology. With Internet courses, students access class information, participate in course discussion groups, and submit course requirements at the time of their choosing (asynchronous learning). Communication among students and the teacher occurs primarily through computer conferences and e-mail (Hartshorn, 1998). See Chapter 7 for more information on distance learning.

> *Distance learning provides opportunities for students to gain access to information for required continuing education or degree courses across long distances. Educational organizations can provide these learning experiences in a variety of formats.*

The economic evaluation of distance education is similar to that of any telehealth application. The cost of equipment and transmission must be compared with the cost of travel for faculty and students. In many instances, the distances between teacher and learners is so great that students could not participate in the learning experience without the technology.

 ## NURSING AND INFORMATION TECHNOLOGY

To apply the wide array of information technologies, nurses must learn to use these technologies, identify potential applications for nursing, and create information systems in all work settings.

INFORMATICS NEEDS FOR NURSING

Information technologies can enhance the development of qualified nurses and the provision of health services. Beliefs that form a foundation for the discussion of the informatics needs of nursing include the following (Gassert, 1998, p. 264):

- Learners are students, faculty, and clinicians.
- Nursing informatics is practiced within an interdisciplinary context that includes partnerships and collaboration.
- Efforts should target disadvantaged and underserved populations.
- Initiatives should be sensitive to other funding priorities.
- Collaboration is necessary for federal agencies and between federal and public agencies.

The strategic directions regarding informatics identified by the NACNEP advisory group include the following (Gassert, 1998):

- Education of students and practicing nurses in the core informatics competencies (use of word processing, e-mail, spreadsheets, databases, bibliographic retrieval, the Internet, the World Wide Web, and presentation graphics)
- Preparation of some nurses with specialized informatics skills
- Enhancement of nursing practice and education through informatics projects
- Preparation of nursing faculty in informatics
- Increased collaboration efforts among nurses, system developers, and health-care agencies in informatics

These strategic directions assist nursing as a profession to contribute to the information age in health care. By defining the general and advanced competencies within nursing, nurses with advanced skills can collaborate with others in developing information systems that meet the needs of nurses, health-care organizations, and consumers. Faculty members with informatics skills multiply their impact as they model those skills for students. The profession of nursing is then prepared to participate with other individuals and groups to achieve health goals, including the national health objectives of Healthy People 2000 and Healthy People 2010 (Gassert, 1998).

INFORMATICS, ECONOMICS, AND NURSING PRACTICE

The American Nurses Association (ANA) also regards computer technologies and information systems as being of vital interest to nursing and nursing economics. These information systems are crucial to the evaluation of health-care services. Because nursing data are critical to health policy development, information systems need to reflect nursing data for the evaluation of cost and outcomes. Therefore, the ANA is committed to having nursing problems or diagnoses, interventions, and nursing-sensitive outcomes included in information systems.

The Committee for Nursing Practice Information Infrastructure was created as an advisory group to the ANA to facilitate adequate representation of nursing data in information systems for the evaluation and support of quality nursing care. This committee collaborates with such organizations as the American Medical Informatics Association, the American Organization of Nurse Executives, and the Systematized Nomenclature of Medicine editorial board (another organization developing an interdisciplinary computerized system) to provide a nursing voice in decisions about informatics and the development of information systems (Gassert, 1998; Warren, 1999).

The ANA created the Nursing Information and Data Set Evelution Center to ensure that health-care information systems represent the work of nursing. This center has developed nursing standards by which to evaluate information systems. Creators of new information systems are aware that their systems will be evaluated according to how well they meet these nursing standards. Criteria include the following (Warren, 1999):

- Support of nursing practice by provision of clinically useful terminology
- A system that moves beyond currently recognized ANA vocabulary schemes or presents a rationale that builds on existing schemes
- Clear and unambiguous terms
- Documented testing of reliability, validity, and utility in practice
- A named entity responsible for a formal process of documenting evolving development and maintenance of the system, including tracking of deleted terms and version control
- A coding scheme that provides a unique identifier for each term

These efforts demonstrate involvement of the nursing profession in the ongoing dialogue on health-care informatics and the representation of nursing's information needs. The contribution of nursing care to patient outcome cannot be examined without having the elements of nursing care present in the information system being used. Chapter 17 describes the issue of nursing languages in information systems in more detail.

A nursing language (i.e., elements within information systems that represent nursing problems, interventions, and outcomes) is necessary to identify and evaluate the impact of nursing on patient outcomes.

The Nursing Minimum Data Set (NMDS) was designed at a 1985 conference at the University of Wisconsin–Milwaukee to standardize the core items necessary to represent nursing care. Nursing minimum data sets include nursing diagnoses, interventions, outcomes, intensity measures, and nurse identifiers. This concept was derived from the Uniform Minimum Health Data Set, which was designed to meet the core needs of multiple users. The most widely minimum data set is the Uniform Hospital Discharge Data Set, which is required for all hospitalized Medicare recipients. Since the development of the original NMDS, related nursing minimum data sets have been created to meet specific uses (Leske & Werely, 1992). The Nursing Management Minimum Data Set, for example, includes variables related to environmental resources, nursing resources, and financial resources (Huber & Delaney, 1998; Delaney, C. W., 1999).

Nursing minimum data sets include standard pieces of information recorded for each episode of care that provide comparable information for the evaluation of nursing care.

USE OF INFORMATION SYSTEMS TO ANALYZE PRODUCTIVITY

Central to the provision of cost-effective care is the concept of *productivity*, which is defined as the ratio of inputs to outputs (Productivity = Inputs/Outputs). Inputs reflect the materials, equipment, human resources, and time necessary to create a unit of a product. These inputs are then converted to dollars and referred to as *dollar costs*. The outputs reflect the amount of a product produced at a given quality (McHugh, 2000).

Productivity is the ratio of inputs to outputs for a given unit of service at a specified quality.

Frequently, health-care outputs have been quantified as units of service, such as patient-days or visits. Consumers and third-party payers seek prevention of illness or improved health and functional status as their desired outcome. The inputs to care are units of time, personnel, and equipment; health care reflects the actions of providers using these inputs to affect the outcomes of health and functional status.

Computer Simulations of Efficient Care Models

Computer simulations have been used to examine the processes of care to improve productivity. The following examples illustrate this concept.

- McHugh (1997) examined three nurse-floating patterns for their effect on wage costs and the resulting level of staffing (overstaffed compared with

understaffed shifts). The analysis demonstrated that the model that restricted floating nurses to units where they were competent to practice
was equally as cost effective as the model using unrestricted floating.
- Kalton and associates (1997) applied computer simulation modeling to
improve the process of providing multidisciplinary care to patients in a
cancer center. The computer simulation improved scheduling and decreased waiting times.
- Atkins (1995) examined staffing requirements in a psychiatric setting.
Two models were analyzed to determine the impact of managed care variables on staffing. Results demonstrated that as mean length of stay declined, reimbursement declined and the cost of care rose because of increased admissions and discharges.

These simulations demonstrate ways in which computer technology can be
used to design processes of care for testing in the clinical arena.

Efficiency and Productivity

Efficiency reflects the length of time required to accomplish a particular task.
Efficiency relates to productivity only indirectly. If small amounts of time
are saved per task, productivity is increased only when the time saved is applied to producing more units of service (McHugh, 2000). If a nurse saves 5
minutes using an intravenous pump instead of counting drops to determine the rate of the intravenous infusion, productivity is increased only if
the nurse accomplishes more productive work in the accumulated time
saved.

McHugh (2000) argues that managers' focus on encouraging staff to improve their work habits results in only small amounts of time saved. These
work habits often cannot be maintained and may not result in increased
productivity. Real and sustained gains in productivity are achieved by intro-
ducing new technologies and work processes. The scale of the work activity
affects potential changes in productivity. A 90 percent improvement in an
activity that consumes 1 percent of the nurse's time saves 4.3 minutes,
whereas a 20 percent improvement in an activity that takes 40 percent of the
nurse's time saves 38.4 minutes per shift. If there are 5 nurses on the unit,
the latter improvement would make 3.2 hours available for other activities
(McHugh, 2000). If the activity under scrutiny involves a large component of
time, such as medication administration or documentation, changes in process may achieve a productivity gain.

Technology may also provide a mechanism to improve productivity. In
the medication administration example, such technology could be computerized medication administration units. Technology analysis must focus on

currently available technology because potential technologies are not available for application (McHugh, 2000).

Efficiency reflects the speed with which a given task can be accomplished. Increased productivity results from efficiency only when the time saved can be applied to producing a higher quality or more units of a product or service.

Computer systems can assist nurses to increase productivity in the following ways (McHugh, 2000):

- Reducing the amount of time needed to complete tasks, particularly documentation and information transfer. Computer systems simplify data entry by using checklists or graphic representations. Entering the actual data is simplified by technologies such as light pens or trackballs. Computerized medication systems simplify administration of medications and immediately create charts for the nurse. This not only decreases the time required for the task but decreases medication errors.
- Expediting data transfer by directly entering data into the computer system from various machines, such as infusion pumps, monitoring systems, ventilators, and oximetry systems.
- Allowing for multiple uses or formats for data that are entered only once. Single entry of data prevents errors in transfer of data and saves time.
- Increasing the quality of outputs. Because data are already in the system, multiple report formats in specialized formats can be generated. Thus, data are available for quality monitoring.
- Providing reminders and other signals to support desired standards of care and reduce error. Quality is supported by the availability of clinical information that supports clinical decision making.

These examples demonstrate how information technologies can assist health-care professionals to model new processes of service delivery, improve efficiency, and evaluate both the technologies and processes of care delivery.

 ## CLINICAL PRACTICE GUIDELINES

Throughout this book the need to achieve positive health outcomes at the lowest possible cost has been emphasized. One mechanism for achieving these goals is the use of clinical practice guidelines, which are recommendations for practice developed by experts in the field based on available evidence (Cronenwett, 1999; Shanefelt, Mayo-Smith, & Rothwangl, 1999). The movement to establish clinical guidelines was stimulated by awareness of the limited use of research in practice, large variations in practice, the need to prevent significant rates of inappropriate care, and manage health-care costs (Brown, 1999; Shanefelt, Mayo-Smith, & Rothwangl, 1999).

DEVELOPMENT OF PRACTICE GUIDELINES

Health-care practice is based on a variety of information sources, such as tradition, rituals, experience, personal opinion, rules or procedures, local community customs, quality data, and research (Brown, 1999; Cronenwett, 1999).

Additional factors affect nursing practice and the willingness to implement changes in practice based on research. Nursing practice is affected by science, regulatory mechanisms, economic or insurance incentives, laws, regulations, and professional values and beliefs. To use research knowledge as the basis of practice several factors are necessary: a consistent knowledge base, awareness of the research and relevant practice recommendations, willingness, and resources to implement change (Brown, 1999; Cronenwett, 1999).

Even with a willingness to consider research-based practice, a review of existing literature is necessary to support the practice change. Despite the growth of research in nursing and health sciences, it is important to understand that evidence is not available to support or direct all areas of practice. Evidence for practice has been broadened to include not only research but also case studies and expert opinion (Cronenwett, 1999).

The Agency for Health Care Policy and Research (AHCPR) has developed the following grading systems to examine evidence for practice:

Levels of Evidence
Level I   = meta-analysis of multiple randomized clinical trials
Level II   = experimental studies (at least one)
Level III = well-designed quasi-experimental studies (at least one)
Level IV = well-designed nonexperimental studies
Level V   = case reports and clinical examples

Strength of Evidence
A = Level I evidence or consistent findings from levels II, III, or IV
B = Consistent finding from levels II, III, or IV
C = Inconsistent findings from levels II, III, or IV
D = Little or no evidence or level V evidence only
E = Opinion of expert panel

Much of the evidence available to nursing and other health professionals is at strengths C, D, or even E. The recognition that a high level of research support is not available for all areas of nursing practice has led to the examination of available evidence from all sources to determine the best practices at the present time.

> *Evidence-based practice is the use of the best available knowledge upon which to base nursing practice. Implementation of such practice should result in achievement of the best client outcomes.*

SOURCES OF PRACTICE GUIDELINES

One potential barrier to the use of single or multiple research findings in the form of practice guidelines is their availability to practitioners. Having practice guidelines on-line facilitates access to the best practice recommendations. Governmental and private information sources are available on the Internet. Some of these sources are freely available to anyone with Internet access; others require a subscription to access information.

> *The availability of clinical practice guidelines on the Internet provides access to current best-practice information developed by professionals in the field.*

Agency for Healthcare Quality and Research

This is a government agency that has convened interdisciplinary panels of experts to develop practice guidelines. In addition AHQR provides printed and Internet publications for the dissemination of these guidelines. A variety of practice information is available on the the new Web site for Agency for Healthcare Quality and Research (http://www.ahqr.gov).

The Cochrane Collaboration

The Cochrane Collaboration is an international nonprofit organization whose goal is to make current and accurate information about health-care practices available worldwide. Systematic literature reviews are conducted by the Collaborative Review Groups. The Cochrane Database of Systematic Reviews is available through subscription. Information is available at http://hiru.mcmaster.ca/COCHRANE?DEFAULT.htm or http://www.cochrane.de/cc/cochrane/crgs.htm.

Virginia Henderson Library

The Sigma Theta Tau International Honor Society for Nursing maintains the Virginia Henderson Library, which supports several initiatives to advance evidence-based practice. One mechanism is a database of nurse researchers with information about their research interests and publications. The *Online Journal of Knowledge Synthesis* publishes systematic reviews of the literature on nursing phenomena. Sigma Theta Tau also provides grant support to teams of nurse researchers to synthesize areas of nursing practice. These services are available on a subscription basis.

USE OF PRACTICE GUIDELINES

On-line practice guidelines assist the clinician to locate information, but are not sufficient for implementation of those guidelines. Zielstorff (1998) presents a model that elaborates the steps necessary to implement guidelines and points out related obstacles:

1. *Develop the guidelines.* Experts from the disciplines related to the area of knowledge review the existing knowledge and develop practice recommendations. Barriers to this process include an insufficient scientific base, conflicting evidence, and lack of evidence.
2. *Develop a protocol or algorithm with decision points to implement the guidelines.* This step is hampered by incomplete guidelines that may not address all clinical possibilities.
3. *Distribute the protocol within an organization.* This step includes education of clinicians and development of reminders to reinforce the protocol. Clinician use of guidelines is decreased by conflicting values and beliefs, ethical and legal issues, distrust in the protocol's validity, poor evidence for the impact of the practice, lack of clarity regarding its application to a specific case, and poor organizational support.
4. *Integrate the guidelines into the record system, with computerized reminders.* Computer support is limited by the available systems, the accuracy of data, and the effort and cost of implementing the guidelines.
5. *Examine the impact on processes and outcomes of care.* This step requires mechanisms for evaluation. Obstacles to evaluation relate to the systems for monitoring.

A systematic process can assist clinicians to implement current best practices. Guidance is also available to structure the use of practice guidelines (Henry et al., 1988).

ECONOMIC ANALYSIS
IMPLEMENTATION OF PRACTICE CHANGE FOR PAIN MANAGEMENT

A review of the literature has shown that pain management is limited in a wide variety of client populations. AHCPR has convened panels of experts to examine research knowledge of pain management and prepare guidelines to address both acute and chronic pain. The guidelines include a consumer guide, an abbreviated quick reference guide, and a longer publication that explains the development of the practice guidelines from existing research. Management of pain is placed into an algorithm to support practitioners' decision making.

One of the first aspects of pain management is accurate pain assessment. Guidelines have been established for the use of pain rating scales. This has become so common that pain assessment is frequently referred to as the "fifth vital sign." Nurses can access the pain management guidelines on the Internet in the abbreviated or full format. The research base with practice guidelines can be applied to the related client population in any health-care agency. The process of adopting the guidelines includes the following steps:

- Incorporation of a pain assessment tool into the clinical record.
- Implemention of a policy for the desired level of pain management, with specific procedures developed to achieve pain control.
- Incorporation of pain management into the quality improvement process, including pain management standards appropriate to the practice arena.
- Revision of procedures if desired standards are not met. Pain management could be included in routine competency testing.

This process demonstrates the ability of a health-care agency, no matter how small or remote, to access current best-practice information and to provide a high standard of pain management to their clients by using the synthesized research of experts in the field.

SUMMARY

This chapter has provided an overview of the issues and trends in information technologies that affect the economics of nursing and health care. New technologies are being created rapidly, and existing technologies are expanding their power and potential. Applications of information technologies are truly transforming the way health care is conceptualized, delivered, and financed. Nurses must be prepared to use these technologies in nursing practice, education, and management.

Economic health policy decisions will affect the direction of the national information infrastructure. These policies will affect access to the global network of information, the purposes it will serve, and the level of privacy that will be maintained. Nursing organizations and nurses with advanced informatics skills are participating in these policy debates.

Technologies for the delivery of health care and education across distances are rapidly expanding. Telehealth increases the access to health care for those without access to specialist care and provides support to health-care providers such as nurse practitioners. Distance education supports the continuing education of nursing professionals as well as formal education to assist the professional advancement of nurses.

Practice guidelines are designed to assist nurses and other health professionals to decrease practice variations, achieve desired outcomes, and reduce costs of care. The dissemination and use of these guidelines are facilitated by information technologies. Challenges remain in integrating available computer systems with patient data systems to enhance adherence to practice guidelines.

For all their advantages, computer technologies present a mixture of opportunities and threats. Cost provides a barrier to many health-care agencies, particularly smaller ones. Keeping current with new technologies and maintaining worker skills for using computer applications are constant challenges. Table 16–2 summarizes the benefits and limitations of computer technologies.

TABLE 16–2. COMPUTER TECHNOLOGY IN HEALTH CARE

Benefits	Limitations
Flexibility in manipulating data for multiple purposes	Specialized knowledge needed to use systems
Speed of retrieval and analysis	Lack of compatibility of formats and of interoperability
Accuracy in computations and manipulations of data	Usefulness depends on the quality of data entered
Instant communication across large distances	Privacy concerns (access of personal information by others)
Decreasing costs of hardware and software	High initial investment costs
Savings in time and travel	Lack of screening for accuracy, timeliness, or bias of information on the Internet
Potential for stimulating new applications	Rapid obsolescence

DISCUSSION QUESTIONS

1. What computer system applications would enhance the health-care work that you do?
2. How do you currently use the information superhighway? How could you better use this powerful tool in your practice?
3. What are your goals for enhancing your general or specialized nursing informatics skills?
4. How does your health-care agency use telehealth to extend services? If it doesn't use telehealth technologies, how could it expand into this area?
5. What distance learning opportunities are available to you?
6. How could you and your agency adopt clinical practice guidelines? How would you evaluate the economic consequences of the practice innovation?
7. What items would be needed to provide complete computer information systems in your setting? Estimate the costs.

 REFERENCES

Atkins, R. (1995). A computer based model for analyzing staffing needs of psychiatric treatment programs. *Psychiatric Services, 46*(12), 1272–1278.
Barrett, J. E., & Brecht, R. M. (1998). Historical context of telemedicine. In S. F. Viegas & K.

Dunn (Eds.), *Telemedicine: practicing in the information age* (pp. 9–16). Philadelphia: Lippincott-Raven.

Blair, P. D., Bambas, A., & Stone, T. H. (1998). Legal and ethical issues. In S. F. Viegas & K. Dunn (Eds.), *Telemedicine: practicing in the information age* (pp. 49–60). Philadelphia: Lippincott-Raven.

Brecht, R. M., & Barrett, J. E. (1998). Telemedicine in the United States. In S. F. Viegas & K. Dunn (Eds.), *Telemedicine: Practicing in the information age* (pp. 25–30). Philadelphia: Lippincott-Raven.

Brown, S. J. (1999). *Knowledge for health care practice*. Philadelphia: WB Saunders.

Collen, M. F. (1999). A vision of health care and informatics in 2008. *Journal of the American Medical Informatics Association*, 6(1), 1–5.

Cronenwett, L. (1999, March). *On the path to evidence-based practice*. Paper presented at the Conference on Evidence-Based Practice, Ann Arbor, MI.

Delaney, C. W. (1999, May). *Outcome visibility: The essential linkage of clinical and management data*. Paper presented at the Michigan Nurses Association Conference, Lansing, MI.

Drucker, P. F. (1998, August 24). The next information revolution. *Forbes*, 47–57.

Gale, B. J., & Steffl, B. M. (1992). The long-term care dilemma: What nurses need to know about Medicare. *Nursing and Health Care*, 13, 34–41.

Gassert, C. A. (1998). The challenge of meeting patients' needs with a national nursing informatics agenda. *Journal of the American Medical Informatics Association*, 5(3), 263–268.

Gates, B. (1999). *Business at the speed of thought: Using a digital nervous system*. New York: Warner Books.

Graves, J. R., & Corcoran, S. M. (1989). An overview of nursing informatics. *Image*, 21, 227–231.

Hartshorn, J. C. (1998). Distance education in nursing: Strategies, successes and challenges. In S. F. Viegas & K. Dunn (Eds.), *Telemedicine: Practicing in the information age* (pp. 167–173). Philadelphia: Lippincott-Raven.

Henry, S. B., Douglass, K., Galzagorry, G., Lahey, A., & Holzemer, W. L. (1988). A template-based approach to support utilization of clinical practice guidelines within an electronic health record. *Journal of the American Medical Informatics Association*, 5(3), 227–244.

Huber, D., & Delaney, C. (1998). Nursing management data for nursing information systems. In S. Moorhead & C. Delaney (Eds.), *Information systems innovations for nursing: New visions and ventures* (pp. 15–29). Thousand Oaks, CA: Sage Publications.

Kalton, A., Singh, M., August, D., Parin, C., & Othman, E. (1997). Using simulation to improve the operational efficiency of a multidisciplinary clinic. *Journal of Social Health Systems*, 5(3), 43–62.

Leske, J. S., & Werley, H. H. (1992). Use of the Nursing Minimum Data Set. *Computers in Nursing*, 10(6), 259–263.

Mascara, C., Czar, P., & Hebda, T. (1999). *Internet resource guide for nurses and health care professionals*. Menlo Park, CA: Addison Wesley.

McHugh, M. L. (1997). Cost effectiveness of clustered versus unclustered unit transfers of nursing staff. *Nursing Economics*, 15(6), 294–300.

McHugh, M. (2000). Computer information systems and productivity management. In L. Simms, S. Price, & N. Ervin, *The professional practice of nursing administration* (3rd ed.). Albany, NY: Delmar Publishers.

McNeill, K. M., Weinstein, R. S., & Holcomb, M. J. (1998). Arizona Telemedicine Program: Implementing a statewide health care network. *Journal of the American Medical Informatics Association*, 5(5), 441–447.

Milio, N. (1996). *Engines of empowerment*. Chicago: Health Administration Press.

Moore, M. (1998). Cost analysis of telemedicine consultations. In S. F. Viegas & K. Dunn (Eds.), *Telemedicine: Practicing in the information age* (pp. 229–244). Philadelphia: Lippincott-Raven.

Nicholl, L. H. (1998). *Nurses' guide to the Internet* (2nd ed.). Philadelphia: JB Lippincott.

Sanders, J. H., Salter, P. H., Stachura, M. E. (1996). The unique application of telemedicine to the managed health care system. Submitted to the American Journal of Managed Care HII

96. The emerging health information infrastructure: Enabling the vision, April 14–16, 1996. Washington: Georgetown University.

Shanefelt, T. M., Mayo-Smith, M. F., & Rothwangl, J. (1999). Are guidelines following guidelines? *Journal of the American Medical Association, 281*(20), 1900–1905.

Strode, S. W., Gustke, S., & Allen, A. (1999). Technical and clinical progress in telemedicine. *Journal of the American Medical Association, 281*(12), 1066–1068.

Turner, J. W., & Peterson, C. D. (1998). Organizational telecompetence: Creating the virtual organization. In S. F. Viegas & K. Dunn (Eds.), *Telemedicine: Practicing in the information age* (pp. 41–48). Philadelphia: Lippincott-Raven.

Viegas, S. F. (1998). Past as prologue. In S. F. Viegas & K. Dunn (Eds.), *Telemedicine: Practicing in the information age* (pp. 1–18). Philadelphia: Lippincott-Raven.

Warren, J. J. (1999, May). NANDA, NIC, & NOC: *Tools for the future.* Paper presented at the Michigan Nurses Association Conference, Lansing, MI.

Zielstorff, R. D. (1998). Online practice guidelines: Issues, obstacles, and future prospects. *Journal of the American Medical Informatics Association, 5*(3), 227–236.

 ## SUGGESTED READING

Dienemann, J. A. (Ed.). (1998). *Nursing administration: Managing patient care.* Stamford, CT: Appleton & Lange.

Duff, L., & Casey, A. (1998). Implementing clinical guidelines: How can informatics help? *Journal of the American Medical Informatics Association, 5*(2), 225–226.

Krous, M. (1999). Eight steps to successful hardware and software procurement. *Healthcare Financial Management, 53*(6), 60–64.

Majzun, R., & Clarke, K. (1999). Can information technology save health care quality? *Group Practice Journal, 48*(5), 11–18.

Moorhead, S., & Delaney, C. (1999). *Information systems innovations for nursing: New visions and ventures.* Thousand Oaks, CA: Sage.

Shi, L., & Singh, D. A. (1998). *Delivering health care in America: A systems approach.* Gaithersburg, MD: Aspen Publications.

Shomaker, D. (1993). A statewide instructional television program via satellite for RN-to-BSN students. *Journal of Professional Nursing, 9*(3), 153–158.

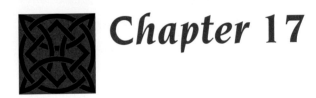

Chapter 17

Design and Evaluation
of Electronic
Medical Records

Marcelline Harris
Michael Bleich

LEARNING OBJECTIVES

- ■ Identify the difference between an electronic medical record and an information system.
- ■ Identify economic uses of electronic medical records.
- ■ Analyze the distinction between clinical data and clinical information.
- ■ Discuss the types of data and relationships among data that might be present in a conceptual data model for a hospital's nursing department.
- ■ Analyze how the model for nursing data is related to the examination of clinical and economic outcomes of care.
- ■ Examine challenges in representing and using nursing data and information in an electronic medical record.
- ■ Discuss strategies for evaluation of electronic medical records.
- ■ Examine the predictions for the future of electronic medical records.

ELECTRONIC MEDICAL RECORDS AND INTEGRATED INFORMATION SYSTEMS

Health care is an information-intensive industry, and the development of electronic medical records (EMRs) to support demands for data and information has become a national priority. A quote attributed to Simon Cohn of Kaiser Permanente reflects the financial and business imperative of EMRs: "Those with more detailed, reliable and comparable data for cost and outcome studies, identification of best practices, guidelines development, and management will be more successful in the marketplace" (Chute, 1997). Nursing, as the largest health profession, has a vital interest in the structure and format of the information systems used as tools to support the delivery of nursing care to patients and to demonstrate the contributions of nursing care to patient outcomes and cost effectiveness. The previous chapter described many aspects of information technology as they apply to nursing. This chapter specifically addresses the central role of the EMR in those information systems.

The many definitions and synonyms of the term *electronic medical record* reflect the evolving nature of our understanding of how electronic record formats can fully leverage technological advances. An electronic medical re-cord may also be referred to as a *computer-based patient record*, but the term EMR is used in this chapter. The Web site of the Computer-based Patient Record Institute (http://www.cpri.org) defines an EMR as "electronically stored information about an individual's lifetime health status and health care." Although comprehensive, this definition does not imply that *all* clinical data relating to an individual must be available in one record. The board of directors of the American Medical Informatics Association identifies four types of computer-based health records, not all of which are oriented to the care of individual patients (American Medical Informatics Association, 1997):

1. Records for institutions and delivery systems
2. Records for primary care and ambulatory care uses
3. Personal health records for individual use
4. Records for monitoring public health and the outcomes of care

The Institute of Medicine suggested three ways in which the EMR could affect the costs of health care. First, with more timely reporting of results, it is likely that redundant—and often expensive—testing will be eliminated. Second, administrative costs are likely to be reduced when claims can be submitted electronically, using a common form across payers. Third, clinician productivity is likely to increase when time is not lost waiting for patient records to be physically delivered to the point of care, when data can be entered once and used across applications as needed, and when the time needed for entering and reviewing records can be streamlined (Detmer, Steen, & Dick, 1997).

This chapter examines the components and design of EMRs as well as how they are useful for the evaluation of health-care delivery. The creation of an electronic record establishes a framework for recording health status, health services provided, and clinical outcomes. In connection with other components of the information system, it is possible to examine relationships among severity of illness, services rendered by various providers, outcomes of care, and the cost of those services. A particularly useful characteristic of EMRs is the efficiency of being able to enter data for the record one time with the potential of using that data for numerous purposes. Nurses have an important interest in this process for at least two reasons. First, a large proportion of the clinical data within patient records is collected and recorded by nurses. Second, the EMR offers promise as a mechanism to demonstrate the contribution of nursing to clinical outcomes and efficient care delivery.

Before discussing EMRs in some detail, it should be noted that the EMR is just one component of a health-care information system. The goal of *integrated information systems* is to link the EMR with other electronic data such as administrative data, enrollment files, and databases developed for specialized purposes (e.g., registries). Clinical, administrative, and information systems leaders must assess the organization's information needs and goals, particularly those related to the support of strategic planning and operational decision making. Table 17–1 summarizes the sources, uses, and limitations of selected databases common to many integrated information systems. Notice that *only* the EMR contains detailed clinical data in its original state. Much of the data in other databases has been abstracted, classified, and coded from the clinical record.

An electronic medical record is electronically stored clinical data that reflects an individual's health status and the health services received. Although the primary purpose of the EMR is to support the delivery of patient care, clinically derived data is also useful to support organizational processes such as strategic planning and operational decisions that consider both clinical outcomes and cost analysis.

The EMR is central to integrated information systems in health care because it represents both the health status and service data of health-care recipients. Given the centrality of the EMR to these data management systems, it is surprising that only recently has a national consensus begun to emerge over EMR content, data representation, and standards to support the interoperability of the EMR with other databases.

ELECTRONIC MEDICAL RECORD CONTENT

Although there is widespread agreement that the primary purpose of the EMR is to support the delivery of patient care, there is less agreement on the nature of the data required to accomplish this purpose. McDonald (1997) noted that the data embedded in the electronic data systems used to support hospital-based patient care could be clustered into 24 "islands," including the following:

- Admission, discharge, and transfer systems
- Anesthesia systems
- Cytology systems
- Diagnostic imaging
- Electrocardiograph carts with monitors
- Endoscopy
- Emergency room

TABLE 17-1. DATA WITHIN INTEGRATED INFORMATION SYSTEMS

Type	Source	Nature	Uses	Limitations
Administrative data (transaction systems)	Provider encounter	Data to support reimbursement activities, electronic formats *Example* Medicare UB-92: Patient and provider identifier specific to facility; patient name, address, birth date, gender, marital status, admission and discharge date, status, and insurance coverage; charge and billing data; diagnosis and procedure codes; payer; insurance group number; employer	*Primary Uses* Claims and reimbursement *Secondary Uses* Utilization studies, limited cost studies, and limited outcomes evaluations	• Different codes can be used to describe the same illness or procedure • Accuracy of coding varies across abstractors and facilities • No unique identifiers for patients, hospitals, providers • Inconsistent file formats across health plans • Limited or no detailed clinical data, or other data on sources of variability that affect outcomes
Enrollment files	Employers and individual subscribers	Employment and health plan data *Example* Name, address, and birth date of policy holder; type of coverage; employee identifier specific to employer; eligible beneficiaries; employers' name and address	*Primary Uses* Determine eligibility for coverage by health plan or government (e.g., HMO, Medicaid, Medicare) *Secondary Uses* Denominators and statistical adjustments when analyzing other data	• Variability in updating files across plans • Variability in data elements across plans • No unique identifiers for employers, employees, or beneficiaries • Limited or no clinical data

Specialized databases	Varies	Varies by purpose *Examples* Satisfaction surveys, disease registries, patient acuity systems, and quality indicator studies	*Primary Uses* Study special issues or populations of interest to specific constituents	• Expensive • Most are cross-sectional • Lack of unique identifiers to link records
Electronic medical record	Clinician notes; electronic data acquisition	Details of reason for visit, diagnosis, treatment, patient characteristics, follow-up plans, referrals, clinical outcomes *Examples* Clinical notes, laboratory data, imaging data, and pharmacy data	*Primary Uses* Describe what has occurred from the clinician's perspective *Secondary Uses* Cost and utilization studies, quality-of-care evaluation, and outcomes evaluation	• Record formats vary, and multiple records reside in each geographic location in which care was received • No uniformity (definitions and coding) for standardized data elements • Lack of unique identifiers to link records

- Home care
- Intensive care monitors
- Intravenous infusion control
- Laboratory system
- Nurse triage
- Order entry
- Outpatient pharmacy drug dispensers
- Pharmacy robot drug dispenser
- Pharmacy system
- Pulmonary function
- Radiology
- Risk management
- Scheduling and clinic charge system
- Surgery scheduling
- Transcription systems
- Unit dose dispensing machines
- Ventilator management

Clearly, the range of data and of systems in which the data are stored is diverse. The term *islands* is appropriate because of the freestanding nature of the data and systems employed in clinical settings today. For example, data embedded in an infusion pump may not be available for electronic transfer to an intake and output flow sheet.

Clinicians face distinct challenges when entering clinical data into any kind of record-keeping system. The concerns of brevity, ease of entry, and capturing the legal aspects of care are always present. Some clinical data can stand alone, whereas other data must be patterned in order to provide meaning. The transformation of pieces of data into an interpretable format results in the creation of *information*. For instance, a listing of vital signs (data) is not nearly as clinically compelling as a graphic portrayal of the vital signs over time (information). Rossi Morri, Consorti, and Galeazzi (1998) observed that in practice, the clinical data that professionals want recorded are embedded in a variety of record structures. Unfortunately, with the exception of data that are able to be presented in flow sheets, the synthesis of data into patterns or clusters to inform the clinician about the patient's clinical status has not been made explicit in most paper-based records or EMRs. Identification of relevant patterns is an important step in database design. These patterns can then be incorporated into applications that result in useful information.

Data must be processed and made available in ways that provide information that is useful to users.

ECONOMIC ANALYSIS
LACK OF DATA TRANSFER

Data about a patient requiring bypass surgery need to be shared among several departments to coordinate services, such as outpatient, radiology, admission, laboratory, operating room, critical care, cardiac rehabilitation, and home care. If the departments are not on a common network, or if they use different software applications, data cannot be readily transferred across the system to those who need the information, often called *end users*. For example, surgery scheduling may or may not be accessible to a nurse working in ambulatory cardiology. The discharge nurse may not have electronic access to scheduling information concerning follow-up medical appointments, home care, or cardiac rehabilitation. The home-care nurse is not likely to have access to hospital records. The ability to determine the clinical and cost outcomes across the entire episode of care is thus severely compromised.

Those who design EMRs realize that the task is far beyond moving the paper record to an electronic environment. Such an effort would merely serve to computerize the problems and limitations of the paper record. Rather, designers focus on the EMR as a component of an integrated information system and search for "reusable" or "exchangeable" data that can be used across computer applications. The goal is to select data elements that can be entered once and used for many purposes. This goal requires information system engineers to understand the data needs of end users by obtaining a vision of who the users will be and to what purpose the data will be put. This vision will drive the development of the EMR.

The strategic plan should provide direction in defining the data needs, including the nursing data needs, of the organization. Nurses at all points of the patient care delivery system need to participate in the process of creating conceptual models that diagram the nature and flow of the data and information that nurses require in EMRs. Building on this conceptual data model, software designers can employ additional data modeling strategies to represent real-world data in a computer-based model. This method allows a conceptual schema of clinical and business processes to drive specific data and information processing activities. An international multidisciplinary group, Health Level 7, is engaged in creating a reference model for all health-care data transactions, including the EMR. When completed, this model will provide designers with a model against which discipline-specific data requirements can be examined. The accompanying economic analysis describes how this process might work.

*For **EMR** data to provide information across multiple computer applications, requisite data elements for all uses must be identified. Relationships among data must then be described and the uses of the data specified so that a data model can be constructed.*

ECONOMIC ANALYSIS
IDENTIFYING DATA REQUIREMENTS

The health system for which you work has a stated goal of providing the highest-quality care in the region at competitive prices. As manager of the pediatric walk-in clinic, you begin to work with clinical and quality-improvement staff to identify relevant data by which you can benchmark your clinic's performance. A review of accrediting organizations such as the National Committee for Quality Assurance suggests the following data may be important to abstract from the EMR:

Illness Care
- Documentation that protocols representing best practices in the diagnosis and treatment of the presenting problem were followed
- Evidence that education of parents or family members was completed and was tailored to the child's condition and the family's readiness to learn
- Number of contacts required for the resolution of the problem
- Evidence of resolution of the presenting problem
- If hospitalization or other consultation was required, evidence that relevant clinical data were made available at the time of consultation
- Documentation of access and coordination of care across settings and providers

Well-Child Care
- Documentation of completion of age-appropriate history and physical examination
- Evidence that age-appropriate screening tests were performed (e.g., tuberculosis, vision and hearing, developmental assessment)
- Evidence that immunizations were reviewed and appropriate ones were administered

- Record of appropriate parental education and referrals being given
- Documentation that the child remains current with the appropriate level of care

Number and Cost of Services

- Clinical problems of children presenting in the clinic
- Services provided by the pediatric nurse practitioners and their compliance with agency standards
- Degree to which children meet the well-child care recommendations
- The quantity and cost of services provided, as well as supplies and equipment used
- Comparison of the providers in the walk-in clinic, such as variance among nurse practitioners or comparison of nurse and physician care

Analyzing the extent to which these recommendations have been met will require quality-improvement personnel to use automated tools to abstract clinical data from the EMR and then present it in some sort of aggregated and analyzed manner that conveys information about the quality and cost of care. This is not likely to be the same data display required by clinical users of the EMR. Therefore, when the design of the EMR is initiated, all end users of EMR data should be involved in the identification and conceptual mapping of data elements and data flow. The critical clinical and business functions that are to be supported by the EMR must be identified, and the relationships among EMR data and all users of that data must be described in a graphical manner. The software developers can then write code to support the desired data flows.

It is important to remember that many data elements needed in the EMR reflect patient conditions and situations; data are not "owned" by a single discipline. This presents a challenge for nursing. What, if any, discipline-specific data elements need to be designed into the EMR over and above those which are shared by all professional health-care disciplines? Are there clinical concepts unique to the nursing profession that nurses will want to record, store, and retrieve in order to provide effective patient care, demonstrate the contribution of nursing to outcomes, or aggregate for institutional and social policy considerations? Because the answer to this last question is a resounding yes, the details are being addressed with a sense of urgency by nursing leaders as the pace of information system development accelerates.

REPRESENTING NURSING CARE IN THE ELECTRONIC MEDICAL RECORD

In the current paper-driven world, it is a paradox that nursing data are absent from the coding and abstracting procedures that determine the intensity of care and services rendered to patients, given that nurses frequently have the most direct contact with patients across the continuum of care. Capturing nursing observations, interventions, and outcome descriptors in the electronic medical record is essential for representing the contribution of nursing to patient care. This information may influence bedside decision making, clinical research, and institutional and social policy setting in new and useful ways.

An international study conducted by Goossen, Epping, and Dassen (1997) investigated the purposes for creating nursing systems. The development, content, structure, and use of nursing information systems were of particular interest. The study concluded that a comprehensive nursing information system would:

- Support quality improvement
- Improve communication
- Support financial and other assessments of nursing's contribution to health care
- Stimulate research
- Improve effectiveness and efficiency of care
- Support complete, clear, and unified information in nursing records
- Support clinical decision making
- Support policy making
- Enable nurses and patients to plan, organize, coordinate, and control care
- Produce management summaries
- Enable and facilitate organizational change to improve care

In the same research, Goossen, Epping, and Dassen (1997) also reported consensus on the following characteristics of data in a nursing information reference model:

- Individual pieces of data, referred to as *atomic-level data*, should be present. The subsequent interpretations, decisions, and conclusions developed by the clinical nurse caring for the patient are also required and essential to the EMR.
- Data should be entered once and used many times.
- A nursing terminology and classification system should influence documentation, but free text should also be available to support documentation.

- A nursing minimum data set should be automatically retrievable from nursing information systems.

These characteristics are consistent with earlier initiatives in nursing information systems (Zielstorff, Hudgings, Grobe, 1993). If these characteristics are present in a nursing information system, the previously mentioned purposes for such a system can be attained.

Although the uses and criteria noted earlier provide a framework for nurses working in informatics to proceed with the development of information systems, they do not prescribe the specific atomic-level data elements, that is, the individual pieces of data that capture the domain of nursing. Traditionally, clinicians have recorded their clinical observations by entering numbers, terms, and phrases into the record. Much of the observational data is readily recorded in flow-sheet formats that accommodate both numbers and words. For example, we are all familiar with data represented by numeric symbols, such as weight and temperatures, and data represented by terms such as "good," "fair," and "poor" or "minimal assist," "moderate assist," and "maximal assist." In the EMR, data dictionaries provide references on acceptable reporting formats (e.g., pounds or kilograms) and the meaning of words (e.g., "minimal assist" means standby assistance only). Flow-sheet data are relatively easily stored and retrieved in an electronic medium provided clinicians use agreed-upon definitions and record the data in prescribed formats.

In addition to such clinical observations, nursing has a 25-year history of developing standardized languages that use specific *precoordinated phrases* to capture problem statements or diagnoses, interventions, and goals or outcomes. The nursing diagnoses put forth by the North American Nursing Diagnosis Association (NANDA) are an example of precoordinated phrases. Using such systems, individual nurses do not need to create statements to describe similar patient conditions. In some organizations, locally developed precoordinated phrases are used to describe phenomena of concern to nurses. To date, EMR initiatives concerning the use of precoordinated phrases have focused on *enumeration strategies* that assign codes to the precoordinated phrases and then essentially handle these enumerated phrases as nominal-level data. Hardiker and Rector (1998) note that such systems are important because they provide a way to formalize knowledge about nursing, have the potential to help determine the cost of nursing services, and contribute to making explicit the work of nursing.

Although the advantages of using precoordinated phrases are real, there is also a growing awareness that such vocabularies may not meet the criteria required of an EMR (Henry et al., 1998). Limitations include the following:

- Precoordinated terms and phrases represent a synthesis of the practice that may or may not reflect the phenomenon that the nurse desires to document. *Free text*, the use of the individual's own language or terms, is often required to support documentation at the level of clinical detail desired by clinicians caring for patients.
- The search to find a desired phrase within a list of all possible phrases often requires more user time than free-text data entry. Regardless of clinician or setting, productivity demands limit the time that staff can be expected to dedicate to structured data entry.
- Systems that use nursing-specific terminology are not user-friendly to disciplines unfamiliar with that terminology that may require the data in the nursing record for important secondary purposes. For example, a multidisciplinary team addressing pressure ulcers for a process-improvement effort would be remiss in excluding patient records coded with the nursing diagnosis of "altered tissue integrity." However, if the search was completed using "altered tissue integrity," an oversampling of records would be obtained because clinical records of other sources of tissue alteration (e.g., burns) would be retrieved.
- Standardization may actually present the danger of arresting progress if new insights into patient problems, responses, and effective interventions are not supported within existing structured-text systems. If language is the vehicle by which we communicate our knowledge of patients, then our systems must support unique clinician observations and insights.

The accompanying economic analysis describes how both standardized language and free text are necessary in EMRs.

Presently, a mix of standardized languages and free text is necessary to describe the work of nursing within the EMR.

 ECONOMIC ANALYSIS
DESCRIBING A PATIENT WITH A PRESSURE ULCER

Typically, the NANDA nursing diagnosis for a pressure ulcer is "impaired skin integrity." However, this label can also refer to other conditions, such as various types of burns and dermatitis. Although clinical tools within documentation systems, such as diagrams of the body, may guide notations about the clinical observations, documenting a nurse's synthesis of those observations as a problem statement in a clinically useful manner requires the nurse to use free text to enter a phrase such as "Patient admitted with stage II pressure ulcer, coccyx."

Retrieval of data on stage II pressure ulcers for analyses of best practices and costs of pressure ulcer care will be difficult if the only coded data entry is "impaired skin integrity." Individual records will need to be pulled and manually reviewed to correctly identify records related to pressure ulcers and eliminate from analysis those related to other skin integrity problems such as burns or dermatitis.

Newer methods to represent nursing work are under development. These methods are known as *compositional, concept-based terminologies*. The Systematized Nomenclature of Human Medicine Reference Terminology (SNOMED RT) is an example of this method. These systems do not require clinicians to select from predetermined lists of phrases; rather, clinicians document care narratively at the level of detail required, after which the narrative is electronically coded using natural-language processing techniques and, if desired, is mapped to standardized vocabularies, data sets, or any number of secondary applications. These terminologies have the advantage that clinical notes can be entered electronically at a level of detail and with the focus and emphasis desired by the clinician; the clinical data are then stored within a defined data model. Because the model is defined, data can be retrieved to support a variety of secondary uses within integrated information systems.

Whether the EMR documentation approach uses enumerated, precoordinated phrases such as standardized vocabularies and data sets or compositional, concept-based terminologies, there seems to be agreement that full coding of nursing practice in all its component parts is not possible at the present time. Likewise, it seems clear that a mixture of coded and free-text information will be needed to capture the essence of nursing. The question becomes, Which data are valuable enough to justify the mechanics of coding, and which can be left as free text? Capturing the essential data required to meet the *primary use* of EMRs—support of patient care—is a task that nursing leaders must address. The value of nursing's contribution to patient care is only supported when nursing data are included in the system and can be analyzed for patient and cost outcomes.

The coding systems that will ultimately drive the nursing component of the EMR are important beyond the primary need to describe the nursing care of patients. Important secondary uses of EMR data address changes in care delivery systems, demographics, and legislative and accreditation requirements. Managed care plans that emphasize integrated care across the continuum have stimulated a demand from purchasers of health care for data that reports the quality, costs, and outcomes of care. Contemporary approaches to health system management, billing, risk management, government reporting, and select clinical research all depend on the nature and type of data entered by clinicians. Obviously, a poorly designed clinical information system would severely strain the ability of an individual or organization to proceed with effective decision making because of such factors as the absence of essential data, the lack of uniform definitions, or the need to stretch existing data into venues beyond its rightful use.

The American Nurses Association (ANA), recognizing the need for data about and for nursing, has initiated a process to recognize vocabularies and data sets that reflect nursing. At the time of this publication, the ANA-recognized classification systems are the NANDA system, the Nursing Interventions Classification system (NIC), the Nursing Outcomes Classification system (NOC), the Nursing Management Minimum Data Set (NMMDS), the Home Health Care Classifications (HHCC), the Omaha System, the Patient Care Data Set, the Perioperative Nursing Dataset, and SNOMED RT. Links to Web sites that provide more information on each system are available at the ANA Web site (http://www.nursingworld.org/nidsec/classlst.htm).

UNRESOLVED DATA ISSUES

The challenge to identify essential data within the EMR is not unique to the domain of nursing. Davidoff (1997) summarized the questions EMRs raise for health care in general when he asked, "Can data serve as the agent for meaningful improvement in quality and cost? Is meaningful improvement possible without data? What data elements are necessary and sufficient?" (p. 770) The availability and decreasing costs of data acquisition and storage are seductive. We can find ourselves analyzing data "because it's there." Quality and cost evaluations are frequently driven by the available content and functionality of the database, rather than by knowledge of the data required to answer the relevant evaluation question. Evaluations should be conducted with a secure knowledge base and purposeful design. Only then will they be able to answer difficult questions, such as those associated with quality and cost.

A closely related issue concerns the overall accuracy of data within EMRs. The required level of accuracy associated with data collection and storage must be linked to its intended use: The higher the clinical and organizational stakes, the more accurate and timely the data need to be. The phenomenon of "the authority of black boxes" describes the blind readiness of stakeholders to accept conclusions associated with computer-generated reports. This phenomenon has been studied in paper-based records; limited work has been completed to evaluate the accuracy of data in EMRs and stakeholder response to reports based on that data.

Relevant clinical and cost data are necessary for meaningful analysis of nursing care. It is not sufficient to use data only because they are easily available.

The most immediate data concern centers on the interoperability of data elements within and across information systems. *Interoperability* refers to the ability to exchange data across computer systems and applications. Presently, even if EMRs were embraced and available in *all* clinical settings, disagreements over data elements and data architecture would likely exist. Simply put, different clinicians in different practice settings use different language to achieve documentation requirements. Similarly, different software developers and vendors use different approaches to technical components. For this reason, pervasive references are made to the health-care "Tower of Babel." To progress with the EMR, this tower must be eliminated so that systems can interpret the available information. Achieving interoperability is a noteworthy effort. Once accomplished, the limitation of paper-based records that exist in one geographic location and require clinicians to "go to the record" would be eliminated. Electronic data retrieval would replace the resource-intensive manual data collection that now occurs.

Congressional concern over the money spent on health-care administrative overhead resulted in passage of the Health Insurance Portability and Accountability Act (HIPPA) in August 1996. Areas addressed by this legislation include health insurance enrollment and eligibility; health insurance claims and information for encounters in managed care settings; identification numbers for providers, health plans, employers, and individuals; health data codes and classification systems; and security standards and safeguards. Clearly, all EMR content will be affected by interoperability standards resulting from this legislation. Various groups within the health-care industry are working intensively to develop and move toward national standards for health-care data. Table 17–2 lists the organizations addressing interoperability issues in the EMR. Readers are also encouraged to examine federal government Web sites (e.g., http://www.hcfa.gov and http://www.cdc.gov).

Moehr (1998) encapsulated the value of an integrated information system. His words reflect the depth and breadth of these systems' potential for enhancing nursing and patient care:

> If information systems would support high quality documentation of care processes with measures enforcing high data quality, it would be conceivable to automatically derive rules and other forms of knowledge representation. . . . [T]hese could feed the repositories of knowledge bases and guide access to patient records as well as treatment procedures, institutional management decisions, etc.[,] . . . [creating] a closed loop from care prac-

TABLE 17–2. SELECTED SOURCES OF INFORMATION ON EMR STANDARDS DEVELOPMENT

Organization	URL	EMR Standards Focus
American Medical Informatics Association (AMIA)	http://www.amia.org	Multidisciplinary association concerned with the development and application of informatics in support of patient care, teaching, research, and administration.
American National Standards Institute, Health Information Standards Board (ANSI-HISB)	http://www.ansi.org	Nonprofit organization that administers and coordinates U.S. private-sector voluntary standardization systems and serves as the official U.S. representative to the International Organization for Standardization (ISO). The Health Information Standards Board supports the voluntary coordination of health-care informatics standards among all U.S. standards-developing organizations.
American Nurses Association (ANA)	http://www.ana.org	Professional organization that represents registered nurses. Its Nursing Information Data Set Evaluation Center (NIDSEC) formally recognizes nursing data sets and classification systems. Contact information for developers is provided on the NIDSEC Web page.
American Society for Testing and Materials (ASTM)	http://www.astm.org	Developer and provider of voluntary consensus standards. ASTM Committee E31 on Healthcare Informatics develops standards related to the architecture, content, storage, security, confidentiality, functionality, and communication of information used within health care.
Computer-based Patient Record Institute (CPRI)	http://www.cpri.org	Serves as a forum for bringing diverse interests together to develop solutions for management of health information.

Organization	Website	Description
European Committee for Standardization, Technical Committee for Health Informatics (CEN TC251)	http://www.centc251.org	Develops standards that enable compatibility and interoperability between independent systems in health care.
Health Level 7 (HL7)	http://www.hl7.org	Models clinical and administrative data and EMR message protocols.
Institute of Electrical and Electronics Engineers (IEEE)	http://www.ieee.org	Not-for-profit international association that is a leading authority in technical areas, including computer engineering, biomedical technology, and telecommunications. The Medical Technology Policy Committee participates in the formulation of legislation, regulation, and policy in the United States.
International Council of Nurses (ICN)	http://www.icn.ch	An international organization of nurses, membership is through national nurses associations. The International Classification of Nursing Practice (ICNP) is a nomenclature and classification system designed to be integrated into multidisciplinary health information systems.
International Organization for Standardization (ISO)	http://www.iso.ch	A worldwide federation of national standards bodies from some 130 countries; its mission is to promote the development of standardization and related activities in the world.

tices to knowledge repositories and knowledge-based decision support . . . a feedback loop where scientific insights are augmented and refined as scientific evidence is used, where the use of evidence-based decision-making spawns more evidence in a fraction of the time and at a fraction of the cost involved at the present. (p. 168)

 EVALUATION OF ELECTRONIC MEDICAL RECORDS

Increasingly, developers and users are being asked to demonstrate the value of EMRs. This is a difficult task. As Paul Clayton, president of the American Medical Informatics Association, wrote in 1998, "In my opinion, the health care industry has yet to recognize the potential cost-effectiveness that our (information) systems can help achieve. We may have expedited the billing process but, except for a few notable examples, we have not yet had a significant impact on the decision-making process at the point of care" (p. 2). Clayton's approach suggests that evaluation activities are broader than financial applications.

Recent discussions concerning the evaluation of EMRs and information systems suggest that there is a professional obligation to evaluate these systems. Anderson and Aydin (1998) wrote: "[T]here is an ethical imperative for conducting (information) system evaluations. . . . [F]ailure to perform such evaluations becomes a shortcoming that is itself ethically blameworthy" (p. 57). Three issues are at the forefront when evaluating information systems: the capacity of the system to protect patient rights and confidentiality, the scope and efficacy of decision support, and the justification of financial and resource expenditures.

PROTECTION OF CONFIDENTIALITY

The ethical obligation to protect the confidentiality of information has long been recognized in nursing and is supported in documents such as the ANA's *Code for Nurses*. However the presence of integrated information systems raises new questions concerning medical record confidentiality. Most commonly, evaluation of EMR confidentiality rightly emphasizes system access and authorization validation. Access is typically restricted to those sections of the record for which one has authorization. Evaluation plans should also account for developments that tighten system access and authorization. These developments include encryption technologies that code data so that they are not usable to unauthorized personnel, password protection, and electronic trails that can be audited to demonstrate the paths of data transfer.

Specific organizational policies associated with electronic confidentiality are required and should be monitored for compliance. As an aside, the safeguards present in paper-based records are generally monitored through medical records departments if the record is inactive. However, when the record is active, there is wide agreement that access to the entire record is widely available to anyone with reason to access any portion of the record.

The current situation concerning the protection of confidentiality in EMRs is best described as dynamic. Clinicians and information technology personnel will be challenged to work together not only to stay abreast of and respond to changing laws, regulations, and standards, but also to proactively develop and influence organizational data security policies, procedures, and practices. The Computer-Based Patient Record Institute is an excellent resource for current information on EMR confidentiality (as well as other EMR issues). The National Research Council (1997) recommended that an assessment of security risks in protecting health information include the value of the assets being protected, the vulnerabilities of the system, potential threats to security, the costs of failure and recovery, and the organization's degree of risk aversion. Many other readily available resources on confidentiality in EMRs support these dimensions of evaluation. Clearly, evaluation of protection of confidentiality requires broad participation across different disciplines in organizations.

> ***Confidentiality of EMRs is maintained through technologies that provide controlled access and authorization to patient information.***

DECISION SUPPORT

Another focus of EMR evaluation concerns the magnitude and efficacy of decision support systems. Davidoff (1997) argued that when large databases are used to predict clinical states and influence treatment decisions, they become like clinical instruments. This use of the EMR has many pitfalls because the assumptions on which such decisions and predictions are based are largely unexplored. Expert panels of clinicians may be needed to judge the adequacy of the decision rules embedded within a software program. Evaluation can be expanded to include whether decision support was used or should have been used by clinicians, and the adequacy of the courses of treatment used. Evaluation should also examine the appropriateness of the use of electronic decision support in decision making.

Decisions derived from data within computer-based decisions are only as good as the knowledge base on which those decision support systems are founded.

FINANCIAL ANALYSIS

There are many ways to evaluate EMRs economically, such as calculating returns on investment (ROI) or performing cost-benefit analysis or cost-effectiveness analysis. A full discussion of these mechanisms is beyond the scope of this chapter, but each method will be discussed briefly.

ROI analysis is used by businesses to make decisions regarding capital investments. The process includes consideration of the revenues projected to be generated through the capital investment, the time required to recoup both the initial investment and the ongoing operating costs, and how these results compare with alternative uses of the capital asset. Cost-benefit analysis typically includes cost savings, cost avoidance, or quantified financial benefits in both the numerator and the denominator of ratios. Cost-effectiveness analysis includes nonfinancial benefits in the denominators of ratios. Refer to Chapter 15 for more information on these latter two types of analysis.

The following guidelines and principles are useful for evaluating capital planning and investment for technology and are relevant to EMRs and integrated health-care information systems.

- Evaluate the information system by focusing on its unique purpose and objectives and how the system affects the organization's mission. Isolate the impact of the EMR from other changes. Too often, information technology is enmeshed with other organizational changes, such as re-engineering or work redesign. Although the EMR may complement redesign initiatives, the evaluation of its contribution should be separate so that the evaluator can judge the effectiveness of the EMR on its own merit.
- Agree in advance of the investment how the system will contribute to the mission of the organization, how it will affect organizational finances, how work roles will be augmented or changed, and how it will make a contribution to patient care. With financial goals in particular, determine how return on investment, the cost-benefit ratio, and cost effectiveness will be calculated for all stakeholders prior to system implementation. Benefits should be linked to the strategic and operational plans of the organization. Estimate benefits over the life cycle of the EMR, explicitly showing changes resulting from the implementation. Calculate other quantitative measures, such as improved access to information and knowledge (e.g., results reporting and timely access to clinically relevant

resources), early recognition and warning systems (e.g., pharmacy alerts that detect potential fatal drug interactions), efficiency and support systems (e.g., enhanced laboratory and pharmacy ordering), and prevention effectiveness (e.g., mammography and immunization rates).

- Convert system development and implementation benefits and resources to dollars whenever possible. Estimates of charges for "invisible" or "in-kind" resources should be accounted for in the project management and evaluation model. Resource categories include (but are not limited to) management time, overhead support costs, training and support labor costs, physical space requirements, other asset costs (e.g., project management software), and energy costs.
- Evaluate alternatives. To the extent possible, explicitly evaluate the impact of the EMR in the context of legal, regulatory, and accrediting requirements, business strategy decisions, and the most challenging context—quantified patient benefits. Compare the costs and benefits of the EMR with paper-based recording systems.

Substantial direct and indirect costs are involved in the development and maintenance of EMRs. Benefits may include cost containment or reduction in specific areas, but many benefits may be more readily identifiable using other effectiveness indicators.

ECONOMIC ANALYSIS
EVALUATION OF AN ELECTRONIC MEDICAL RECORD SYSTEM

As a nursing representative to your organization's EMR project, you are asked to consider financial issues associated with EMR implementation in your department. To do this, you must be very clear about how your department wants to use the EMR. Detailed considerations of issues that range from hardware to data acquisition, storage, and retrieval across a range of applications will influence decisions about the nature of the system, the cost of the system, and the benefits to users of the EMR. Although vendors should be expected to provide measurement tools to help estimate costs throughout the planning, development, and implementation phase, purchasers of systems share the obligation of determining how the costs and benefits of the EMR will be evaluated.

PREDICTIONS REGARDING THE FUTURE OF ELECTRONIC MEDICAL RECORDS

The rate of technology development and the globalization of all industries, including health care, demands acceptance of the EMR as an organizational imperative. The nursing profession has a unique opportunity to represent itself during the reframing of organizational systems, of which the EMR is a central component. With the EMR, documentation of nursing's contribution to patient care and to efficient and effective organizational productivity is possible through the use of valid, accurate, and responsibly developed and maintained data sources.

The impact of the EMR in the future will be shaped by several forces. The growing importance of information networks is likely to expand as the power of collective knowledge is recognized, as the quality and utility of data and information gained from these electronic systems are improved, and as software and hardware technology continues to improve. For example, active research in new technology concerning human–computer interfaces (such as the ability of computers to accept and process continuous speech) is likely to fundamentally change the nature of clinical data acquired and stored within EMRs.

The need for standards development organizations is widely recognized, and the importance of these groups is likely to increase. Professional organizations such as the ANA serve their members well through continued support of nursing representation and participation in such standards initiatives.

EMRs and integrated information systems in health care raise new issues regarding what is medically possible in a technological age. Areas of active research, such as the inclusion of genetic databases as part of the EMR and fundamental research on the nature of representing clinical concepts within the EMR, are likely to generate many new discussions about resource allocation and ethics.

The EMR will continue to play a central role in integrated information systems within health care. The Institute of Medicine identified five objectives for future patient record systems (Detmer, Steen, & Dick, 1997):

1. Support patient care and improve quality.
2. Enhance the productivity of health-care professionals and reduce administrative costs associated with health-care delivery and financing.
3. Support clinical and health-services research.
4. Accommodate future developments in health-care technology, policy, management, and finance.
5. Have mechanisms in place to ensure patient data confidentiality at all times.

SUMMARY

The EMR can be a boost or a bane to nursing. With concerted leadership effort, including clear thinking about nursing's role in the context of patient care and organizational system effectiveness, an end-user vision about the amount and types of data needed to support practice, and opportunities for clinician education concerning the data management aspects of their service, there is little doubt that the EMR can capture the long-silent voice of nursing's contribution within the health-care system. In the absence of such leadership, or with poorly constructed or optimized data systems and a lack of clarity, an opportunity will have been missed, perhaps never to be recovered. This chapter presented evaluation strategies and issues to support nursing's role in EMR and information systems development and explored where system development is headed and the types of goals that are worthy of achievement.

DISCUSSION QUESTIONS

1. In the setting where you work, what patient data are electronically stored? What type of stored EMR data is used for evaluation purposes?
2. Analyze the issues related to using standardized vocabularies with pre-coordinated phrases for documenting nursing practice compared with using free text.
3. Compare and contrast the clinician's aggregation of data to provide patient care with the need for aggregating data for other purposes, such as quality assessments.
4. Individually or in a small group, describe key data that represent your practice, and diagram the flow of data from the point of care to ultimate use.
5. Imagine that your organization is planning to implement an EMR. Suggest benefits you might expect the EMR system to provide, and the measures that could be used to describe those benefits.
6. Discuss the impact of medical record privacy issues on patient care and the differences between electronic and paper-based records in maintaining confidentiality.
7. Discuss ways your work as a nurse might be influenced by future EMR developments.

REFERENCES

American Medical Informatics Association. (1997). *A proposal to improve quality, increase efficiency, and expand access in the* U.S. *health care system.* Bethesda, MD: Author.

Anderson, J. G., & Aydin, C. E. (1998). Evaluating medical information systems: Social contexts and ethical challenges. In K. W. Goodman (Ed.), *Ethics, computing, and medicine: Informatics and the transformation of health care* (pp. 57–74). New York: Cambridge University Press.

Clayton, P. D. (1998, June). Message from the president. AMIA *News,* 8, 2.

Davidoff, F. (1997). Databases in the next millennium. *Annals of Internal Medicine,* 127(Suppl. 8), 770–774.

Detmer, D. E., Steen, E. B., & Dick, R. S. (1997). *The computer-based patient record: An essential technology for health care* (Rev. ed.). Washington, DC: National Academy Press.

Goossen, W. T. F., Epping, P. J. M. M., & Dassen, T. (1997). Criteria for nursing information systems. *Computers in Nursing,* 15(6), 307–315.

Hardiker, N. R., & Rector, A. L. (1998). Modeling nursing terminology using the GRAIL representation language. *Journal of the American Medical Informatics Association,* 5(1), 120–128.

Henry, S., Warren, J. J., Lange, L., & Button, P. (1998). A review of major nursing vocabularies and the extent to which they have the characteristics required for implementation in computer-based systems. *Journal of the American Medical Informatics Association,* 5(4), 321–328.

McDonald, C. J. (1997). The barriers to electronic medical record systems and how to overcome them. *Journal of the American Medical Informatics Association,* 4(3), 213–221.

Moehr, J. R. (1998). Informatics in the service of health, a look to the future. *Methods of Information in Medicine,* 37, 165–170.

National Research Council. (1997). *For the record: Protecting electronic health information.* Washington, DC: National Academy Press.

Rossi Morri, A., Consorti, F., & Galeazzi, E. (1998). Standards to support development of terminological systems for healthcare telematics. *Methods of Information in Medicine,* 37(4–5), 551–563.

Zielstorff, R. D., Hudgings, C. I., & Grobe, S. J. (1993). *Next-generation nursing information systems.* Washington, DC: American Nurses Publishing.

SUGGESTED READINGS

Bowles, K. H. (1997). The barriers and benefits of nursing information systems. *Computers in Nursing,* 15(4), 191–196.

Chute, C. G. (1997, April). *Medical records vs patient records: Meeting the research agenda.* Paper presented at the Midwest Nursing Research Society, Minneapolis, MN.

Chute, C. G., Cohn, S. P. for the ANSI Healthcare Informatics Standards Board Vocabulary Working Group and the Computer-Based Patient Records Institute Working Group on Codes and Structures. (1998). A framework for comprehensive health terminology systems in the United States. *Journal of the American Medical Informatics Association,* 5, 503–510.

Henry, S. B., Warren, J. J., Lange, L., & Button, P. (1998). A review of major nursing vocabularies and the extent to which they have the characteristics required for implementation in computer-based systems. *Journal of the American Medical Informatics Association,* 5, 321–328.

Button, P., Androwich, I., Hibben, L., Kern, V., Madden, G., Marek, K., Westra, B., Zingo, C., Mead, C. N. (1998). Challenges and issues related to implementation of nursing vocabularies in computer-based systems. *Journal of the American Medical Informatics Association, 5,* 332–334.

Hunt, D. L., Haynes, R. B., Hanna, S. E., & Smith, K. (1998). Effects of computer-based clinical decision support systems on physician performance and patient outcomes. *Journal of the American Medical Association, 280*(15), 1339–1346.

Moorhead, S., Delaney, C. (1998). Information systems innovations for nursings: New visions and ventures. Thousand Oaks, CA: Sage Publications.

Murphy, G. (1997). Making standards work for you: Content vocabulary for computer-based patient records. *Journal of AHIMA, 68*(3), 34–38.

Simpson, R. L. (1997). Nursing data sets are finally beginning to catch up to technology's promise. *Nursing Administration Quarterly, 21*(2), 84–86.

Simpson, R. L. (1998). Why managed care demands information technology. *Nursing Management, 29*(7), 18–19.

Siewicki, B. J., & Hess, J. (1997). Integration challenges in managed care organizations. *Journal of AHIMA, 68*(3), 28–31.

Warren, J. J., Coenen, A. (1998). International classification for nursing practice (ICNP): Most frequently asked questions. *Journal of the American Medical Informatics Association, 5*(4), 335–336.

Appendix A

Glossary

advanced practice nurses (APNs)
Highly skilled nursing personnel who have earned advanced degrees and received clinical training in a variety of specialties. APNs include nurse practitioners, clinical nurse specialists, certified registered nurse anesthetists, and certified nurse midwives.

advertising Marketing activities concerned with making a product or service known to the customers and creating demand for it.

assessment process A mechanism of validating the knowledge, skills, and other values added as a result of the educational process.

asynchronous learning An education product in which students participate in educational experiences at a location convenient to them at a time of their own choosing.

benchmarking 1. A tool used in evaluating outcomes that compares one facility's selected outcomes with those of another facility that is recognized as a standard. 2. Setting the price level of a particular year as a reference point by which future price levels can be measured when calculating the consumer price index.

capitation A prospective payment system that pays health plans or providers a fixed amount per enrollee per month for a defined set of health services.

cartel A group of sellers behaving like a monopoly to raise prices and profits.

case management A professional practice model for identifying resources and using them efficiently and effectively in the provision of client-centered health care by following a set of logical steps and a process of interaction with service networks.

Certificate of Need (CON) laws Laws that require hospitals to obtain approval from regional or state health planning agencies for capital expenditures in excess of a certain threshold amount.

clinical economics Economic evaluations that assist in health-care decision making by assessing the relative merits of alternative courses of medical actions or interventions.

collaboration The process of cooperation and sharing with other health-care professionals that is essential to new nursing practice roles.

community nursing organization (CNO) A nurse-led managed care facility that provides Medicare benefits to elderly people in community-based settings.

competition Rivalry in business; a market situation in which a number of suppliers fight for potential consumers.

complement A service or product that is used with another service or product.

CON See Certificate of Need laws.

consumer price index (CPI) A cost-of-living index that gauges the overall cost (or the price level) of the goods and services bought by a typical household.

cost The dollar value of inputs used in the provision and delivery of goods or services.

cost-benefit analysis A type of clinical economic analysis that compares the benefits created by a program with the costs of resources used by that program.

cost-effectiveness analysis A type of clinical economic analysis that evaluates competing programs that are designed to achieve the same or similar objective.

cost-identification analysis A type of clinical economic analysis that addresses the question of how much something costs.

cost-push theory of inflation A theory that hypothesizes that inflation results from high and rising costs of doing business.

demand The amount of a service or a product that consumers are willing and able to buy at specified prices.

demand-pull theory of inflation A theory that hypothesizes that inflation results from too much spending and not enough supply of goods and services.

derived demand A demand for an input of production, such as labor, that is derived from the demand for the final product that labor helps to produce.

Diagnosis Related Groups The rate-setting prospective payment system used by Medicare to determine payment rates under 495 diagnosis related groups (DRGs). Each DRG represents a particular case type for which Medicare provides a flat dollar amount of reimbursement.

direct medical costs Costs such as hospital charges and physicians' fees that are directly related to a medical intervention.

direct nonmedical costs Costs that significantly disrupt the lives of patients and caregivers.

discounting A method used to calculate the present value of a stream of future benefits or costs.

distribution Marketing activities concerned with delivering a service or product to customers, making it available and easy to purchase.

DRGs *See* Diagnosis Related Groups.

economics The science that studies how consumers, business firms, government entities, and other organizations make choices to overcome the problem of scarcity.

economic shortage of labor A labor shortage that occurs when employers wish to hire more workers at a particular wage level than there are workers willing to work for that wage.

Economic Stabilization Program (ESP) An economic program initiated by President Richard Nixon in 1971 to combat inflation and stagnant economic growth.

economic system The network of institutions, laws, and rules created by society to cope with fundamental economic challenges.

efficiency The absence of waste by gaining productivity from the delivery of goods and services.

electronic medical record (EMR) Electronically stored clinical data that reflect an individual's health status and the health services received. EMRs support patient care, strategic planning, and operational decision making.

employer insurance Health insurance coverage provided by an employer as an employee benefit.

enrollees The employees or association members who are insured by a health plan under the sponsorship of an employer or association.

entrepreneurs Persons who assume the risks associated with a freestanding business.

equilibrium price The market price at which the quantity demanded and the quantity supplied are equal.

equilibrium wage rate The wage level at which the labor market is in balance between demand and supply.

ESP *See* Economic Stabilization Program.

evidence-based practice The use of the best available knowledge upon which to base nursing practice. Such practice should result in achievement of the best client outcomes.

fee-for-service (FFS) system A reimbursement system under which insurance companies reimburse hospitals and physicians after the needed services are delivered.

FFS *See* fee-for-service system.

financial risk The likelihood of unforeseen monetary loss by a health plan because of lack of revenue, excess costs, or both in delivering obligated services.

fixed costs Costs that do not change with patient volume.

gatekeeper A physician or advanced practice nurse who directs and coordinates the care of a group of enrolled members in a managed care plan.

general price level The average price level of the whole economy.

gross domestic product (GDP) The total market value of all the goods and services produced in a country in a year.

health access The timely use of needed, affordable, convenient, acceptable, and effective personal health services.

health-care providers Health-care deliverers, including but not limited to nurses; physicians; dentists; occupational, physical, and respiratory therapists; and pharmacists.

health-care system The system for providing health care that is made up of institutions and facilities such as hospitals, home-care agencies, extended-care facilities, health maintenance organizations, and third-party payers.

health maintenance organization (HMO) A managed care plan that either administers or arranges for health care to be provided to its members for a capitated monthly fee.

health practitioners (HPs) Nonphysician health-care providers, including physician assistants, nurse practitioners, certified nurse midwives, clinical nurse specialists, and certified registered nurse anesthetists.

Healthy People 2000/2010 A comprehensive national health promotion and disease prevention initiative that began in 1990.

indirect morbidity and mortality costs Costs that are borne by society as a result of the loss of productivity either by disability or premature death of an individual.

inferior goods Goods and services that consumers buy less of as their income rises.

inflation Steady and persistent increases in the general price level in an economy.

information Data processed and made available in ways that provide useful information to users.

information system An integrated set of computer applications designed to accomplish specific tasks.

inputs The manpower, materials, and equipment used in the production of outputs or delivery of services.

intrapreneurs Creative and self-directive people who nurture entrepreneurial activities within the organization for which they work.

law of diminishing returns A phenomenon in production such that adding units of an input (e.g., the service of advanced practice nurses) to fixed amounts of other inputs (e.g., the size of a facility and the number of other types of health-care providers) causes the contribution of the additional input to eventually decline.

managed care A health-care system that combines the financing and delivery of health services into a single entity.

managed care organization (MCO) A health-care entity willing to be held clinically and financially accountable for the health outcomes of a group of individuals called health plan enrollees or members.

market An area of economic activity in which buyers and sellers engage in trade.

market economy An economic system that is based on private ownership of resources and that allocates resources through the interactions of individuals and business firms.

marketing A social and managerial process by which individuals and groups obtain what they need and want through creating, offering, and exchanging products of value with others.

marketing mix A key building block of modern marketing practice based on four marketing elements called the four Ps of marketing: product, price, place, and promotion.

marketing research Marketing activities concerned with obtaining information on available products and services, prices, consumer needs, gaps, and so forth.

Medicaid A federal health-care program in which the states and the federal government partner to provide health services for low-income families and individuals.

Medicare A federal health insurance program that provides insurance coverage for elderly people, people with disabilities, and individuals with end-stage renal disease.

national information infrastructure The electronic networks that are capable of communicating through a variety of media.

normal goods Goods and services that consumers buy more of as their income rises.

nurse labor supply equilibrium The point at which the supply of nurses is equal to the demand for them.

nursing demand trends The historical patterns of the number of nurses hired at different points in time for the country as a whole or for different regions of the country.

nursing language Standardized elements within information systems that represent nursing problems, interventions, and outcomes. Nursing languages often consist of precoordinated phrases that describe phenomena of concern to nurses.

nursing minimum data set A set of standard pieces of information recorded for each episode of care that provides comparable information for the evaluation of nursing care.

nursing workforce The predicted number of working nurses required to meet the needs for nursing services in a state, region, or the country as a whole.

opportunity cost The value of the alternative resource use that was not selected.

outputs The end products of production or the clinical outcomes of a procedure.

personal health care expenditures (PHCEs) All purchased services and products that are associated with individual health care, such as hospital,

physician, dental, and nursing-home care; drugs; and medical supplies.

point-of-service (POS) plan A form of HMO in which participants must choose a primary care provider from a list of participating providers, but may choose a specialist who is not in the plan by paying a higher deductible or copayment.

preferences The selection of specific health-care services and products from the variety available.

preferred provider organization (PPO) A health plan that contracts with networks of hospitals, private practice physicians, and other health-care practitioners to provide comprehensive health services to employers and their employees for a negotiated fee.

price elasticity of demand The responsiveness of demand to a change in the price of a product.

pricing Marketing activities concerned with determining the price of a product or service on the basis of costs as well as market factors such as distribution channels, level of prices of competitors' products or services, and the ability or willingness of customers to pay.

process innovations Technological advances that enable providers to deliver the same amount of output more efficiently and cheaply.

product innovations Technological advances that improve the quality and sophistication of a service or product.

product or service planning Marketing activities concerned with developing a product or service so that it satisfies the customers and enables the enterprise or individual to use productive capacities or competencies fully.

productivity The ratio of input to output for a given unit of service.

professional practice model A system of nursing and health-care governance characterized by autonomy, accountability, and authority.

prospective payment system (PPS) A hospital payment system that sets payment rates before treatment begins.

purchasers Employers, groups of employers, trade unions, professional associations, government agencies, and other legal entities that buy health insurance coverage for their participating members or employees. The purchasers arrange for the necessary legal agreements to contract with managed care organizations for health services.

quality outcome A health outcome that meets or exceeds expectations.

rationing function of price The important role played by price in allocating scarce resources in a market economy.

recession A decline in gross domestic product for at least two consecutive quarters.

salary The money received by an employee for services rendered under a contract between an employer and employee.

sales promotion Marketing activities covering all aids to sales other than advertising. Sales promotion stimulates demand and increases purchases or contracts for services.

scarcity Not having enough resources to satisfy all existing human wants or desires.

SCHIP *See* State Children's Health Insurance Program.

sensitivity analysis An analysis that allows researchers to test the robustness of study results to see if variations in the values of important variables will significantly change the conclusions.

shortage A market situation in which the quantity demanded exceeds the quantity supplied.

State Children's Health Insurance Program (SCHIP) A national insurance program initiated in 1997 to provide $24 billion over 5 years to help states offer affordable health insurance to previously uninsured children, especially those in working families whose income exceeds the Medicaid eligibility level but is not enough to afford private insurance coverage.

substitute A service or product that can be used to take the place of another service or product.

supply The quantity of a service or product that providers are willing to sell at particular prices.

surplus A market situation in which the quantity supplied exceeds the quantity demanded.

telehealth An evolving system for health care that uses telecommunications technologies to provide health-care services at a distance.

third-party payment system A system of health-care financing in which providers deliver services to patients, and a third party or a financial intermediary, usually an insurance company or a government agency, pays the bill.

transcultural care Nursing care delivered with an understanding of the culture of another country or region.

UCR charges The usual, customary, and reasonable charges submitted by providers to third-party payers for reimbursements for services rendered.

underinsurance Health insurance that does not provide coverage for prescriptions and services such as home care and long-term care.

unlicensed assistive personnel (UAP) Health-care workers who have no personal licensure who perform delegated tasks in an assistive role as a substitute for licensed personnel. UAP function under the supervision of a licensed provider.

utilization review A process through which an insurer or health plan reviews the appropriateness of the care delivered by physicians and other providers.

value The relative importance of an entity, such as health, compared with other choices.

variable costs Dollar amounts of costs that vary with the number of patients treated in a health-care facility.

VE *See* Voluntary Effort.

Voluntary Effort (VE) A program proposed by President Jimmy Carter in late 1977 to control hospital inflation.

workforce forecasting The process of predicting the demand for labor and the supply of labor at a particular point in the future.

workforce planning Coordinated efforts by government and professional organizations to study, plan, and make recommendations to bring the labor supply in line with labor demand.

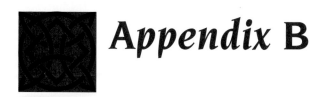

Appendix B

Internet Resources Related to Nursing and Health Care Economics

Disclaimer: This appendix lists a variety of Internet resources of use to nurses and other health care professionals. Since the Internet changes rapidly, not all of these locations may be active at this time. You may use search engines to look for additional sites related to a topic of interest.

Search Engines
These commonly used search engines help the Internet user to find information and sites related to a topic of interest.

Alta Vista	http://www.altavista.com
Dogpile	http://www.dogpile.com
Excite	http://www.excite.com
Hotbot	http://www.hotbot.com
Infoseek	http://infoseek.go.com
Lycos	http://www.lycos.com/mssearch.html
Metafind	http://www.metafind.com
Webcrawler	http://www.webcrawler.com
Yahoo	http://www.yahoo.com or
	http://www.yahoo.com/health

Library and Database Sources
These sites connect you to libraries or other data sources.

Cancerlit	http://cancernet.nci.nih.gov
Cinahl (subscription based)	http://www.cinahl.com
Directory of Library Catalogs	http://library.uask.ca/hytelnet/sites1.html
Electric Library: A database that is searchable using questions	http://www.elibrary.com/id/2525
Embase (subscription based)	http://www.elsevier.com
ERIC: Education database	http://ericir.syr.edu/eric
Michigan Electronic Library	http://mel.lib.mi.us/health
Nursing information	http://mel.lib.mi.us/health/health-nursing.htm.
National Institutes of Health	http://www.nih.gov
National Library of Congress	http://www.loc.gov

473

National Library of Medicine (NLM)	http://www.nlm.nih.gov
NLM Grateful Med	http://igm.nlm.nih.gov
AIDSLINE	http://igm.nlm.nih.gov
Bioethicsline through	http://www.nlm.nih.gov
Grateful Med	http://igm.nlm.nih.gov
PubMed	http://ncbi.nem.nih.gov/PubMed
UMI Document Delivery Services: Dissertations and other documents	http://www.umi.com/
Virginia Henderson International Nursing Library	http://www.stti.iupui.edu/library
Virtual Hospital: Digital library that makes information for client care and distance education available	http://www.vh.org

Sources with Multiple Listings for Nursing and Health Care

CeWEB: Continuing education	http://www.ce-web.com
Hardin MD: An excellent catalog of nursing and health care resources	http://www.lib.uiowa.edu/hardin/md
HealthWeb	http://www.healthweb.org
Healthweb Nursing	http://lib.umich.edu/hw/nursing.html
Idea Nurse	http://www.ideanurse.com
LearnWell RN Online: On-line continuing education	http://www.learnwell.org
Licensed to Care	http://nurseid.com
MedConnect: Information services for the medical community; interactive education job line, educational programs, and search engine	http://www.medconnect.com
Medical Matrix: Guide to Internet clinical medicine resources	http://www.medmatrix.org/index.asp
Medweb	http://www.gen.emory.edu/medweb
National Health Information Center (NHIC)	http://nhic-nt.health.org
Nurseweek/ Healthweek: Links for nursing, health care, and allied health professionals by category	http://www.nurseweek.com
Nursing Index: Annotated reference to nursing sites on the Web	http://www.lib.umich.edu/hw/nursing.html
Nursing Net: Links, chat rooms, and messageboards for communication	http://www.nursingnet.org
Whole Nurse: Provides articles, chats, and book reviews	http://www.wholenurse.com
World Wide Nurse	http://www.allnurses.com

Government Data Sites

Bureau of the Census	http://www.census.gov
Centers for Disease Control	http://www.cdc.gov
Morbidity and Mortality Weekly Report	http://www.cdc.gov/epo/mmwr/mmwr.html
Department of Health and Human Services (DHHS)	http://www.os.dhhs.gov
DHHS, GrantsNet: On-line tool for federal grants	http://www.hhs.gov/proorg/grantsnet
Federal Statistics: Organized site for statistics from 70 federal agencies	http://www.fedstats.gov
Fedworld: Government site with databases	telnet://fedworld.gov
Food and Drug Administration (FDA)	http://www.fda.gov
Healthfinder: Focus on health and nutrition	http://healthfinder.gov
Healthy People 2010	http://web.health/gov/healthypeople
National Institutes of Health	http://www.nih.gov
National Institute of Occupational Safety and Health	http://www.cdc.gov/niosh/homepage.html
National Library of Medicine	http://www.nlm.nih.gov
Occupational Safety and Health Administration (OSHA)	http://osha.gov
Thomas: On-line information on legislation	http://thomas.loc.gov
Unified Medical Language System	http://www.nlm.nih.gov/pubs factsheets/umls.html
U.S. government documents	http://www.access.gpo.gov
The Visible Human Project	http://www.nlm.nih.gov/research/visible/ visible_human.html

Nursing Organizations

This list contains the Web sites of selected professional nursing organizations.

American Academy of Nursing	http://www.nursingworld.org/aan/index.htm
American Assembly of Men in Nursing	http://www.freeyellow.com/members3/aamn
American Association of Colleges of Nursing	http://www.aacn.nche.edu
American Association of Critical Care Nurses	http://www.aacn.org
American Association for the History of Nursing	http://aahn.org
American Association of Managed Care Nurses	http://www.aamcn.org

American Association of Nurse Anesthetists	http://www.aana.com
American Association of Occupational Health Nurses	http://www.aaohn.org
American College of Nurse-Midwives	http://www.acnm.org
American College of Nurse Practitioners	http://www.nurse.org/acnp
American Forensic Nurses	http://www.amrn.com
American Holistic Nurses Association	http://www.ahna.org
American Nurses Association	http://www.ana.org or http://www.nursingworld.org
American Nurses Credentialing Center: Information on criteria for certification	http://www.nursingworld.org/ancc/index.htm
American Medical Informatics Association (AMIA) Nursing Informatics Working Group	http://www.gl.umbs.edu/~abbott/nurseinfo.html
American Nursing Informatics Association	http://www.ania.org
American Organization of Nurse Executives	http://www.aone.com
American Psychiatric Nurses Association	http://www.apna.org
Association of Nurses in AIDS Care	http://www.anacnet.org
Association of Operating Room Nurses	http://www.aorn.org
Association of Rehabilitation Nurses	http://www.rehabnurse.org
Association of Women's Health, Obstetric, and Neonatal Nurses	http://www.awhonn.org
California Nurses Association	http://www.califnurses.org
Canadian Nurses Association	http://www.can-nurses.ca
Emergency Nurses Association	http://www.ena.org
The Florence Project	http://www.florenceproject.org
International Parish Nurse Resource Center	http://www.advocatehealth.com/about/faith/
National Association of Home Care	http://www.nahc.org
MedWeb: Hypertext list of links to conferences, publications, and organizations	http://www.gen.emory.edu/medweb/keyword/nursing.html
Midwest Alliance for Nursing Informatics	http://www.maninet.org

Midwest Nursing Research Society	http://www.mnrs.org
MilitaryRN	http://www.militaryrn.com
National Association of Neonatal Nurses	http://www.nann.org
National Association of Orthopedic Nurses	http://www.inurse.com/naon
National Association of School Nurses	http://wwwnasn.org
National Black Nurses Association	http://www.nbna.org
National Council of State Boards of Nursing	http://www.ncsbn.org
National Institute of Nursing Research	http://www.nih.gov/ninr
National League for Nursing	http://www.nln.org
National Student Nurses Association	http://www.nsna.org
Nurse.org: Site of nurse practioner support services of Kent, Washington; provides information on nursing organizations and state boards.	http://www.nurse.org/index2.html
NurseWire: List of nurse entrepreneurs	http://ideanurse.com/nursewire
Nursing organizations and publications with e-mail	http://www.nursing.ab.umd.edu/students/~snewbol/skorg.htm
Oncology Nursing Society	http://www.ons.org
Sigma Theta Tau International	http://www.nursingsociety.org
Transcultural Nursing Society	http://www.tcns.org
Wound, Ostomy, and Continence Nurses Society	http://www.wocn.org

Related Health Professions Organizations

American Public Health Association	http://www.apha.org
Center for Health Professions	http://furturehealth.ucsf.edu
National Association of Managed Physicians Care	http://www.namcp.com

Managed Health Care
Commercial Providers

AAHP Online: Industry perspective	http://www.aahp.org/menus/index.cfm
Aetna U.S. Healthcare	http://www.aetnaushc.com
American Medical Specialty Organization: Site contains definitions of terms	http://www.amso.com/index.html
FHP Health Care Information Center: Managed health care organization with links to WAIS Search and HCFA	http://www.fhp.com

Group Health Cooperative: Information for consumers and providers	http://www.ghc.org
Integrated Healthcare Association: Managed care industry association information	http://www.iha.org
Kaiser Permanente	http://www.kaiserpermanente.org

Government Resources

Joint Interim Committee on Managed Care	http://www.senate.state.mo.us/mancare/ mc-main.htm
Health Care Finance Administration (HCFA)	http://www.hcfa.gov
Managed Care	http://www.hcfa.gov/medicare/mgdcar.htm

Accrediting or Regulatory Bodies

CARF for Rehabilitation	http://www.carf.org
COLA: Nonprofit accrediting organization promoting excellence in care	http://www.cola.org
Health Care Financing Administration	http://www.hcfa.gov
Joint Commission on Accreditation of Healthcare Organizations	http://www.jcaho.org

Health-Care Informatics

American Medical Informatics Association	http://www.amia.org
British Computer Society Nursing Specialist Group	http://www.man.ac.uk/bcsnsg
Canada's Health Informatics Association	http://www.coachorg.com
CARING—Capital Area Roundtable on Informatics in Nursing	http://nursing.umaryland.edu/students /~snewbol/caring.htm
Healthcare Informatics Standards: Beginning and advanced information on informatics standards	http://www.mcis.duke.edu/standards/ guide.htm
Maryland Society for Healthcare Information Systems	http://www.mshism.org
Medical Education Page	http://www.scomm.net/~greg/med-ed
Medical Informatics at McGill University	http://mystic.biomed.mcgill.ca
Nursing Informatics Working Group	http://www.gl.umbs.edu/~abbott/ nurseinfo.html
Virtually Informatics Nursing	http://milkman.cac.psu.edu/~dxm12/vin.html

Evidence-Based Practice

These sites describe and discuss best practices in health care.

Agency for Health Care Policy and Research now called Agency for Healthcare Quality and Research	http://www.ahqr.gov
American College of Physicians: Information on ACP Journal Club, EBM journal, and clinical guidelines	http://www.acponline.org
Best Practice Network	http://www.best4health.org
Cochrane Collaboration (subscription based): Keeps systematic reviews	http://linux.chpt.es/cochrane/default.html
Evidence-based care homepage	http://hiru.mcmaster.ca/cochrane/default.htm
Health Web—Evidence Based Health	http://www.uic.edu/depts/lib/health/hw/ebhc/
HealthWeb: This is a collaborative project of organizations, providing links to organizations, journals, tools and tutorials, guides to searching the literature, databases, and so forth.	http://healthweb.org
Netting the Evidence: Evidence-based medicine resources on the Internet from the University of Sheffield	http://www.med.unr.edu/medlib/netting.html
Research Methods Knowledge Base: On-line textbook on research methods and theory	http://trochim.human.cornell.edu/kb/index.htm

Selected Journal Resources on Evidence-Based Health Care

ACP Journal Club Bimonthly	http://www.acponline.org
Bandolier	http://www.jr2.ox.ac.uk/bandolier
Evidence-Based Health Policy and Management: Address for subscription orders	orders@edinburgh.rsh.pearson-pro.com
Evidence-Based Medicine	http://www.bmjpg.com
Evidence-Based Mental Health	http://www.bmjpg.com
Evidence-Based Nursing	http://www.bmjpg.com
User Guides to the Medicine Literature	http://ww.shef.ac.uk/~scharr/ir/userg.html

On-line Publications

Academic Journal Directory University of Texas: Directory of 400 journals in nursing and health care, with publication information	http://www.son.utmb.edu/catalog/catalog.htm

Computers in Nursing: Does not duplicate the printed journal	http://www.cini.com
The Gene Letter	http://www.geneletter.org
The Journal of Neonatal Nursing	http://www.bizjet.com/jnn/default.html
Lippincott's Nursing Center: Many on-line publications	http://www.nursingcenter.com or www.ajn.org
Medscape: Articles and on-line education	http://medscape.com
MMWR: Morbidity and Mortality Weekly Report	http://www2.cdc.gov/epo/mmwr
Nurseweek: Promotes nursing	http://www-nurseweek.webnexus.com
Nursing Editors On-line	http://members.aol.comsuzannehj.htm
NursingNet	http://www.nursingnet.org
Nursing Standard	http://www.nursing-standard.co.uk
On-line Journal of Issues in Nursing	http://www.ana.org/ojin/index.htm
On-line Journal of Knowledge Synthesis	http://www.stti.iupui.edu/library/ojksn
On-line Journal of Nursing Informatics	http://ublib.buffalo.edu/libraries/e-resources/ejournals/ records/ojni.html
Research Nurse: Articles for nurses conducting research	http://www.researchnurse.com
Revolution—the Journal of Nurse Empowerment	http://greatnurse.com

American Psychological Association Reference Guide Sites

Publication Manual FAQ: Frequently asked questions	http://www.apa.org/journals/faq.html
Web Extension to APA	http://www.nyct.net~beads/weapas

Foundations and Organizations Related to Health Care

Center for Health Care Strategies: Medicare and Medicaid resources Information on Medicaid managed care	http://www.chcs.org
The Commonwealth Fund	http://www.cmwf.org
Electronic Policy Network: Clearinghouse for health policy research	http://epn.org
Families USA's Home Page: Reports geared to consumers	http://www.epn.org.families.html
National Committee for Quality Assurance: Assessment of quality	http://www.ncqa.org
Robert Wood Johnson Foundation	http://www.rwjf.org

Roles within Health Care
General Information

ANA position statement index	http://www.nursingworld.org/readroom/position/index.htm

Job description of registered nurse	gopher://gopher.umsl.edu:70/00/library/govdocs/ooha/oohb/oohbjobs/oohb0096
Job descriptions by U.S. Labor Department	gopher://gopher.umsl.edu:70/00/library/govdocs/ooha/oohb/oohbjobs
Legislative summary of nursing practice issues	http://www.nursingworld.org/gova/legsumnp.htm
National Health Care Skill Standards	http://www.fwl.org/nhcssp/health.htm
Nurse staffing and quality of care	http://www.ahcpr.gov:80/news/nursagnd.htm
Prescriptive Authority Chart	http://www.nursingworld.org/readroom/rxauth.htm
President's Advisory Commission on Consumer Protection and Quality	http://www.hcqualitycommission.gov
Robert Wood Johnson report on why health care patterns change with the territory	http://www.rwjf.org/library/hlthpuz1.htm
Strengthening nursing and midwifery	http://www.who.ch:80/programmes/nur/wha455en.htm
Title protection for registered nurses	http://www.nursingworld.org/gova/titlepro.htm

Pew Health Professions Commission

ANA Response to Pew Commission	http://www.nursingworld.org.readroom/pew.htm
California Nurses Association: Response to Pew Commission	http://www.igc.apc.org/can/np/pew2.htm
Center Publications	http://futurehealth.ucsf.edu/pubs.html
Center Task Forces	http://futurehealth.ucsf.edu/taskforces.html
Critical Challenges: Executive summary	http://futurehealth.ucsf.edu/summaries/challenges.html
Medical Education and Residency Issues	http://www.aamc.org/meded/edres/workforc/pewrespo.htm
Pew Commission's Third Report	http://futurehealth.ucsf.edu/pdf_files/challenges.pdf
Pew Health Professions Commission	http://futurehealth.ucsf.edu/pewcomm.html
Pew Health Profession Taskforce on Workforce Regulation: Response by Association of Operating Room Nurses	http://aorn.org/nsgtoday/GOVT/pwe.htm
Response to Taskforce on Health by National Council of State Boards	http://www.ncsbn.org/files/pewresponse.htms

Continuing Education

CeWEB	http://www.ce-web.com
Cyber Learners	http://learnwell.org/~edu
EDNET	http://www.ed-net.com

Health Interactive Nursing	http://wwwmceus.com
Lippincott's Nursing Center	http://www.nursingcenter.com
NurseOne	http://www.nurseone.com
NurseTest	http://www.nursetest.com/aboutnurse.htm
Nursing Spectrum	http://www.nursingspectrum.com
Schools of Nursing in the United States	http://www.lib.umich.edu/hw/nursing/nurseschoolus.html
SpringNet	http://www.springnet.com

Career Resources

Advanced Medical Recruiters, Inc.: Recruitment company for health professionals	http://www.medical-search.com
American Mobile Nurses (AMN): Travel agency that offers temporary positions in the United States	http://amn.travelnurse.com/amn/index.html
CareerPath.com: Database of national ads	http://www.careerpath.com
Healthseek: Private company providing health-care information and staffing to businesses	http://www.healthseek.com
Medistaff: Division of Worldwide Staffing	http://ww2.portal.ca/~wwide/nurses.html
MedSearch America: Features a resume entry form and job listings	http://www.medsearch.com
National Nursesearch: Search for experienced nurses	http://www.nursesearch.net
Nurses' Call: Conference and job opportunities	http://www.nurses-call.org
PRN Med Search: Medical employment	http://www.halcyon.com/prnmed

Current Health Care News

CNN Interactive, health main page	http://cnn.com/HEALTH
Journal of the American Medical Association	http://www.ama-assn.org/public/journals/jama/jamahome.htm
New England Journal of Medicine	http://www.nejm.org/current.htm
NewsPage, Healthcare Current Events	http://www.newspage.com/NEWSPAGE/cgi-bin/walk. cgi/NEWSPAGE/info/d15
Reuters Health Information Services	http://www.reutershealth.com
WebMedlit: Medical headlines service	http://www.webmedlit.com

Listservs

Discussion Groups

NRSINGED: Nursing education issues and research	listserv@uLkyvm.LouisviLLe.edu

NRSING-L: Nursing informatics	listserv@nic.umass.edu
NursRes: International forum on nursing research	listserv@kentvm.bitnet
SNURSE-L: Nursing students' group	listserv@ubvm.cc.buffaLo.edu

Education and Informatics

C+HEALTH: Computer use and effects on health	listserv@iubvm.ucs.ind.iana.edu
COMPUMED: Computers in medicine	listserv@sjuvm.stjohns.edu
HESCA: Educational technology and health sciences education	listserv@listserv.dartmouth.edu
HIM-L: Medical records (Health Information Management)	listserv@umsmed.edu
Hmatrix-1: New on-line health resources	listserv@ukanaix.cc.ukans.edu
MEDINF-L: Medical informatics	listserv@vm.gmd.de
MEDNETS: Computer networks and medicine	listserv@vm1.nodak.edu
MEDPICTS: Medical images on the Web	listproc@ucdavis.edu
PANET: Medical education and health information	listserv@yaLevm.ycc.yaLe.edu

Management and Policy

FINAN-HC: Health care financial matters	listserv@wuvmd.wustL.edu
HEALTHRE: Health care reform	listserv@ukcc.uky.edu
NHCTEN: Mental health and health-care reform	listserv@sjuvm.stjohns.edu
NRCH: Hospital information system issues	listserv@usa.net
RHCFRP-L: Residential health-care facilities	listserv@health.state.ny.us

Listserv Subscription Information

This section categorizes listservs and provides subscription information.

Nursing

Clinical alerts (CLINALERT)	Send e-mail message to listproc@list.ab.umd.edu In message body, write: subscribe clinalrt *yourfirstname yourlastname*
Clinical nurse specialist (CNS-L)	Send e-mail to listserv@vm.utcc.utoronto.ca In message body, write: sub cns-l *yourfirstname yourlastname*
Community Health Information Networks	Send e-mail to chins-request@chin.net In message body, write: subscribe chins

Culture and nursing (GLOBALRN)	Send e-mail to listserv@itssrv1@ucsf.edu In message body, write: subscribe globalrn *yourfirstname yourlastname*
Geriatric nursing (GERINET)	Send e-mail to listsesrv@ubvm.cc.buffalo.edu-bit.listserve.GERINET In message body, write: subscribe GERINET *yourfirstname yourlastname*
Geriatric nursing (GERO-NURSE)	Send e-mail to edu.gero-nurse-request@list.uiowa.edu In message body, write: subscribe
Home-care and hospice nursing	Send e-mail to majordomo@po.cwru.edu In message body, write: subscribe hcarenurs *your email address*
International Telenurses Association (ITNA)	Send e-mail to listserv@listserv.bcm.tmc.edu In message body, write: subscribe ITNA *yourfirstname yourlastname*
Nurse managers (RNMGR)	Send e-mail to RNMGR-request@cue.com In message body, write: subscribe
Nurse practitioners (NPCHAT)	Send e-mail to listproc@lists.missouri.edu In message body, write: subscribe *yourfirstname yourlastname*
Nurse practitioners (NPINFO)	Send e-mail to Majordomo@npl.com In message body, write: SUBSCRIBE NPINFO *Your email address*
Nursing Education (NRSINGED)	Send e-mail to LISTSERV@ULKYVM.LOUISVILLE.EDU In message body, write: SUBSCRIBE NRSINGED *yourfirstname yourlastname*
Nursing informatics (NRSING-L)	Send e-mail to LISTPROC@LISTS.UMASS.EDU In message body, write: SUBSCRIBE NRSING-L *yourfirstname yourlastname*
Nursing issues (NURSENET)	Send e-mail to LISTSERV@LISTSERV.UTORONTO.CA In message body, write: SUBSCRIBE NURSENET *yourfirstname yourlastname*
Nursing jobs (NURSEjobs)	Send e-mail to NURSEjobs-request@med-employ.com In message body, write: subscribe
Nursing jobs (RN-JOBS)	Send e-mail to MAJORDOMO@NPL.COM In message body, write: subscribe
Nursing research (NURSERES)	Send e-mail to LISTSERV@LISTSERV.KENT.ED In message body, write: SUBSCRIBE NurseREs *yourfirstname yourlastname*
Psychiatric nurses (PSYNURSE)	Send e-mail to listserv@sjuvm.stjohns.edu In message body, write: subscribe PSYNURSE *yourfirstname yourlastname*

School nurses (SNURSE-L)	Send e-mail to LISTSERV@UBVM.CC.BUFFALO.EDU In message body, write: SUBSCRIBE SCHLRN-L *yourfirstname yourlastname*
Student nurses (SNURSE-L)	Send e-mail to Listserv@ubvm.cc.buffalo.edu In message body, write: Sub SNURSE-L *yourfirstname yourlastname*
Telenursing (ITNA)	Send e-mail to listserv@listserv.bcm.tmc.edu In message body, write: Subscribe itna *yourfirstname yourlastname*

Health Care

Biomedical ethics (BIOMED-L)	Send e-mail to listserv@VMI.NODAK.Edu-bit.listserv.biomed-l In message body, write: subscribe BIOMED-L *yourfirstname yourlastname*
Health economics (HEALTHECON)	Send e-mail to mailbase@mailbase.ac.uk In message body, write: join healthecon-discuss *yourfirstname yourlastname*
Health informatics (MEDNFORM)	Send e-mail to LISTSERV@SJUVM.stjohns.edu In message body, write: subscribe
Health management (HEALTHMGMT)	Send e-mail to listserv@ursus.jun.alaska.edu In message body, write: Subscribe HLTHMGMT *yourfirstname yourlastname*
Health professionals (HEALTH-PRO)	Send e-mail to Listserv@NETCOM.COM In message body, write: Subscribe health-pro *yourfirstname yourlastname*
Health and wellness issues (WELLNESSLIST)	Send e-mail to majordomo@wellness-mart.com In message body, write: subscribe Wellnesslist *yourfirstname yourlastname*
Home health care (HOMEHEALTH)	Send e-mail to listserv@usa.net In message body, write SUBSCRIBE HOMEHEALTH *yourfirstname yourlastname*
Hospice care (HOSPICE)	Send e-mail to majordomo@po.cwru.edu In message body, write: subscribe hospice *yourfirstname yourlastname*
Public health (PUBLIC-HEALTH)	Send e-mail to mailbase@mailbase.ac.uk In message body, write: subscribe PUBLIC-HEALTH *yourfirstname yourlastname*
Quality in health care (QP-Health)	Send e-mail to majordomo@quality.ort In message body, write: Subscribe qp-health *Your e-mail address*

Index